Complications in Endodontic Surgery

Igor Tsesis
Editor

Complications in Endodontic Surgery

Prevention, Identification and Management

Springer

Editor
Igor Tsesis, DMD
Department of Endodontology
Maurice and Gabriela Goldschleger
School of Dental Medicine
Tel Aviv University
Tel Aviv
Israel

ISBN 978-3-642-54217-6 ISBN 978-3-642-54218-3 (eBook)
DOI 10.1007/978-3-642-54218-3
Springer Heidelberg New York Dordrecht London

Library of Congress Control Number: 2014940753

Printed on acid-free paper

Springer is part of Springer Science+Business Media (www.springer.com)

Acknowledgement

Eyal Rosen
Special acknowledgement for his essential contribution to the book preparation and editing.

Illustrations by Asya Aizenstein.

Contents

Contributors

Alexandre Anesi, MD Unit of Cranio-Maxillofacial Surgery, University of Modena and Reggio Emilia, Modena, Italy

Dipartimento di Scienze Mediche e Chirurgiche Materno-Infantili e dell'Adulto, Chirurgia Maxillofacciale, Policlinico di Modena, Modena, Italy

Thomas von Arx, Prof. Dr. Med. Dent. Department of Oral Surgery and Stomatology, School of Dental Medicine, University of Bern, Bern, Switzerland

Alessia Bari, MD Program of Innovative Therapy in Oncology and Hematology, University of Modena and Reggio Emilia, Modena, Italy

Dipartimento di Medicina Diagnostica, Clinica e di Sanità Pubblica, Centro Oncologico Modenese, Policlinico di Modena, Università di Modena e Reggio Emilia, Modena, Italy

Ilan Beitlitum, DMD Department of Periodontology and Dental Implantology, The Maurice and Gabriela Goldschleger School of Dental Medicine, Tel Aviv University, Tel Aviv, Israel

Lars Bjørndal, DDS, PhD, Dr Odont Section of Cariology & Endodontics and Pediatric & Clinical Genetics, Department of Odontology, University of Copenhagen, Copenhagen, Denmark

Luigi Chiarini, MD Unit of Cranio-Maxillofacial Surgery, University of Modena and Reggio Emilia, Modena, Italy

Dipartimento di Scienze Mediche e Chirurgiche Materno-Infantili e dell'Adulto, Chirurgia Maxillofacciale, Policlinico di Modena, Modena, Italy

Ugo Consolo, MD Unit of Dentistry and Oral-Maxillofacial Surgery, University of Modena and Reggio Emilia, Modena, Italy

Dipartimento Chirurgico, Medico, Odontoiatrico e di Scienze Morfologiche con interesse Trapiantologico, Oncologico e di Medicina Rigenerativa, Odontoiatria, Policlinico di Modena, Università di Modena e Reggio Emilia, Modena, Italy

Stefano Corbella, DDS, PhD Department of Biomedical, Surgical and Dental Science, Dental Clinic, IRCCS Istituto Ortopedico Galeazzi, University of Milan, Milan, Italy

Massimo Del Fabbro, BSc, PhD Department of Biomedical, Surgical and Dental Science, Centre for Research in Oral Health, IRCCS Istituto Ortopedico Galeazzi, University of Milan, Milan, Italy

Luigi Generali, MD Unit of Dentistry and Oral-Maxillofacial Surgery, University of Modena and Reggio Emilia, Modena, Italy

Dipartimento Chirurgico, Medico, Odontoiatrico e di Scienze Morfologiche con interesse Trapiantologico, Oncologico e di Medicina Rigenerativa, Odontoiatria, Policlinico di Modena, Università di Modena e Reggio Emilia, Modena, Italy

Peter Jonasson, DDS, PhD Department of Endodontology, Institute of Odontology at The Sahlgrenska Academy, University of Gothenburg, Gothenburg, Sweden

Sahng G. Kim, DDS, MS Division of Endodontics, Columbia University College of Dental Medicine, New York, NY, USA

Thomas Kvist, PhD, DDS Department of Endodontology, The Sahlgrenska Academy, University of Gothenburg, Göteborg, Sweden

Louis M. Lin, BDS, DMD, PhD Department of Endodontics, New York University College of Dentistry, New York, NY, USA

Marilena Vered, DMD Department of Oral Pathology and Oral Medicine, Maurice and Gabriela Goldschleger School of Dental Medicine, Tel Aviv University, Tel Aviv, Israel

Henrik Nielsen, DDS, PhD Department of Oral and Maxillofacial Surgery, Centre of Head and Orthopaedics, Rigshospitalet, Østerbro, Denmark

Tom C. Pagonis, DDS, MS Division of Endodontics, Department of Restorative Dentistry and Biomaterials Sciences, Harvard School of Dental Medicine, Boston, MA, USA

Samantha Pozzi, MD Program of Innovative Therapy in Oncology and Hematology, University of Modena and Reggio Emilia, Modena, Italy

Dipartimento di Medicina Diagnostica, Clinica e di Sanità Pubblica, Centro Oncologico Modenese, Policlinico di Modena, Università di Modena e Reggio Emilia, Modena, Italy

Domenico Ricucci, MD, DDS Private practice, Cetraro, CS, Italy

Eyal Rosen, DMD Department of Endodontology, Maurice and Gabriela Goldschleger School of Dental Medicine, Tel Aviv University, Tel Aviv, Israel

Vibe Rud, DDS Private practice in Surgery and Endodontics, Copenhagen, Denmark

Aviad Tamse, DMD Department of Endodontology, Maurice and Gabriela Goldschleger School of Dental Medicine, Tel Aviv University, Tel Aviv, Israel

Silvio Taschieri, MD, DDS Department of Biomedical, Surgical and Dental Science, Centre for Research in Oral Health, IRCCS Istituto Ortopedico Galeazzi, University of Milan, Milan, Italy

Igor Tsesis, DMD Department of Endodontology, Maurice and Gabriela Goldschleger School of Dental Medicine, Tel Aviv University, Tel Aviv, Israel

Eric Young, DDS Division of Endodontics, Department of Restorative Dentistry and Biomaterials Sciences, Harvard School of Dental Medicine, Boston, MA, USA

Introduction: An Evidence-Based Approach for Prevention and Management of Surgical Complications

1

Igor Tsesis and Eyal Rosen

Abstract

A modern surgical endodontic treatment is a predictable and efficient procedure. Like any treatment modality, surgical endodontics is exposed to risk of complications. Possible complications should be considered in the decision making process, so they could be anticipated, prevented, diagnosed or managed correctly. Both patient and practitioner related matters, that might affect the risk of complications and the ability to manage those complications in case they occur, need to be recognized.

The application of an evidence-based approach for prevention, identification and management of surgical complications should result in a reduction of mistakes in the clinical decision making process.

More than a century ago, Dr. Farrar stated that endodontic surgery is "The most heroic, and the most interesting of all the operations. The time will come when it will not only be considered as highly scientific, but will be indorsed by all progressive operators" [1]. Since then, endodontic surgery has gone through many transformations, conversions, and developments, till its current application [2, 3].

The main goal of a surgical endodontic treatment is to prevent the invasion of bacteria and their by-products from the root canal system into the periradicular tissues [4, 5]. Surgical endodontic treatment may be indicated for teeth with apical periodontitis, when a nonsurgical retreatment is impractical or unlikely to improve the previous results [2, 3, 6].

A need for a biopsy has been commonly mentioned as an additional indication for endodontic surgery [2, 3]. However, if one considers this from a biological point of view this may represent a typical misconception and misinterpretation of the goal and application of the procedure in clinical endodontics [2, 3]. While the discussion whether every pathologic tissues obtained during endodontic surgery procedures should be routinely submitted for histological evaluation is still controversial [7], when a lesion of nonendodontic origin is suspected based on preoperative clinical and radiographic evaluation, the case becomes primarily a surgically oriented case, and it may be better managed by a maxillofacial surgeon.

I. Tsesis, DMD (✉) • E. Rosen, DMD
Department of Endodontology, Maurice and Gabriela Goldschleger School of Dental Medicine, Tel Aviv University, Tel Aviv, Israel
e-mail: dr.tsesis@gmail.com; dr.eyalrosen@gmail.com

I. Tsesis (ed.), *Complications in Endodontic Surgery*,
DOI 10.1007/978-3-642-54218-3_1, © Springer-Verlag Berlin Heidelberg 2014

A traditional surgical endodontic treatment (traditional technique) consistently was performed by root-end resection with a 45° bevel, retrograde preparation of the canal with bur, and root-end filling [8]. A moderate success rate of approximately 60 % was reported with this technique [9, 10]. This relatively unpredictable outcome was mainly related to the difficulties in locating, cleaning, and sealing the apical part of the root canal system [4]. In order to overcome the drawbacks of this technique and the inability to adequately prepare and seal the root canal space, a modification was proposed by Nygaard-Ostby, who suggested to use a cutoff section of h-file for retrograde canal preparation.

The introduction of the dental operative microscope (OM) in the early 1990s [11] led to a new era in surgical endodontics [2, 3]. The modern surgical endodontic treatment (modern technique) uses magnification devices, such as the dental OM to facilitate a more precise procedure with no or minimal bevel of root-end resection, retrograde canal preparation with the aid of an ultrasonic tip to a depth of 3–4 mm, and root-end filling [12]. The advantages of a modern technique include easier identification of root apices, smaller osteotomies, and shallower resection angles that preserve cortical bone and root length [4]. In addition, the resected root surface under high magnification and illumination readily reveals the isthmus, canal fins, micro-fractures, and lateral canals [4]. The modern technique has shown a much higher long-term success rate (>90 %) compared to the traditional technique (<60 %) and is considered a predictable and efficient treatment modality [2, 3, 5].

Like any treatment modality, surgical endodontics is exposed to risk of complications. Routinely a surgical complication (complication) was defined as "any undesirable, unintended and direct result of surgery affecting the patient, which would not have occurred had the surgery gone as well as could reasonably be hoped" [13], thus suggesting that not always a direct action-result relation exists between the surgeon's actions and the ensuing adverse outcomes. On the other hand, a procedural error (error) was defined as "a failed process that is clearly linked to adverse outcome" [14], and some authors stated that "complications occur, whereas errors are committed" [13, 14].

Risk management in endodontics is the active daily process aimed to prevent, identify, assess, prioritize, and manage potential medical and medicolegal risks [15]. Thus, a clinician should always expect the unexpected and be actively prepared to prevent and manage any undesirable results of the surgical procedure.

The classification of "un-undesirable/unintended results" of surgical complications versus errors based on their traditional definitions is too simplistic and incomplete and may not reflect the true clinical scenario.

Procedural errors (error) can be defined as "improper action or inaction of the practitioner prior during or following the surgical procedure." Thus, in some cases errors may have little or no adverse effect, and in other cases they may lead to complications.

The possible complications of surgery may be divided into two categories:

1. Patient-related complications (i.e., undesirable, unintended, and direct result of surgery affecting the patient, which are related to the patient-specific characteristics, rather than to a procedural error).
2. Practitioner-related complications (i.e., errors that directly led to undesirable and unintended results affecting the patient). In some cases the practitioner-related complications may also be a result of a faulty technique, rather than a specific error (e.g., a complication that occurs due to surgical endodontic treatment performed by a traditional technique, even when a procedure was done flawlessly).

"Errare humanum est" (meaning: "to err is human") – errors by clinicians in medical practice will occur and unfortunately may result in harm to patients. However, what matters is the ability to learn from one's errors and to recognize or anticipate these errors in order to avoid or prevent their reoccurrence [16].

Thus, the practitioner's goals are as follows:

1. Minimizing errors by the application of an appropriate surgical technique
2. Correct and timely mannered identification and management of errors in case they

happen, in a way that would prevent ensuing complications
3. Adequate and timely mannered management of complications in case they developed

In addition, patient-related complications should be diagnosed and considered in the decision-making process, so they could be anticipated, prevented, or managed correctly.

From a practical clinical point of view, distinguishing errors from complications is mainly looking on the same coin from two different directions. Also, regardless of the exact definition of the adverse outcome of a surgical procedure, surgeons generally feel personal responsibility for complications/errors that occur [13], and those outcomes may bare medical and sometimes even medicolegal consequences. Thus, this book will discuss complications and errors as an unite clinical matter that would be termed for simplicity – complications.

Since complications are an integral part of any surgical modality, the practitioner is required to adopt a reasonable and effective clinical approach in order to prevent and manage those possible complications. Practitioners tend to institute their approach to complication on personal experience, which in some cases may imply "Making the same mistakes with increasing confidence over an impressive number of years" [17]. On the other hand, evidence-based dentistry is an approach to oral healthcare that integrates the best available clinical evidence to support a practitioner's clinical expertise for each patient's treatment needs and preferences [18–20] and should be adopted by practitioners as a routine.

It is based on the process of systematically finding, apprising, and using research findings as the basis for clinical decision making. Systematic reviews constitute the basis for practicing evidence-based dentistry [15, 17, 18]. The application of an evidence-based approach for prevention, identification, and management of surgical complications should result in a reduction of mistakes in the clinical decision-making process [18–21].

In a clinical scenario, the evidence-based process requires a definition of a specific clinical question (i.e., determine the patient population type, the clinical intervention, the comparison methods, and the clinical outcome of interest), followed by a comprehensive literature search in order to identify as much of the relevant literature as possible [17, 18, 21]. Then, by using explicit methodology, a review and synthesis of the research evidence is performed, aimed to minimize bias and explicitly address the issues of the completeness of the identified evidence and assess the quality of the evidence and the evidence combinability [15–18, 21]. Eventually, based on the quality and combinability of the retrieved evidence, evidence-based conclusions can be made. However, in certain cases, the systematic review of the available literature may lead to a conclusion that there is no available evidence-based data and that further research is indicated to elucidate that particular clinical question. On the other hand, in other cases, when sufficient high-quality and combinable data was retrieved during the systematic review process, a meta-analysis of the results across the studies can be performed and might even lead to new insights regarding that particular clinical question.

Figure 1.1 presents an evidence-based algorithm for prevention, identification, and management of surgical complications.

The ultimate goal of surgical endodontic treatment is to preserve natural teeth. A frequent dilemma is the decision whether to preserve the natural tooth by endodontic treatment or to extract the tooth and replace it with an alternative, such as fixed partial dentures or a dental implant [22, 23]. In case a complication occurred during an endodontic treatment, this dilemma may be even more intense since the prognosis of the tooth and the possible further complications may be unpredictable. On the other hand, it should be recognized that not every complication should necessarily lead to a surgical failure. As long as the surgical main goal (i.e., correct management of the apical part of the root [2, 3]) was achieved in spite of the complication, the treatment outcome may not be compromised. However, if the complication development compromised the main surgical goal, a less predictable outcome should be anticipated [2, 3].

The contemporary dentistry principle is that every reasonable effort should be made in order

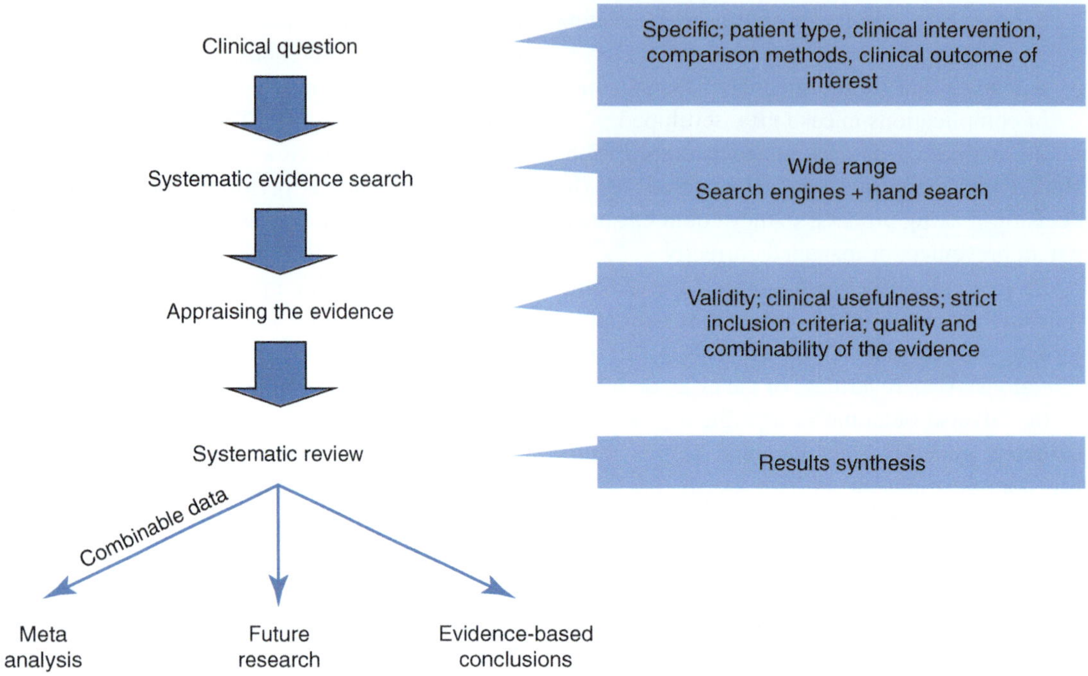

Fig. 1.1 Evidence based algorithm for prevention, identification and management of surgical complications

to preserve natural teeth, since the basic goal of dental implants is to replace missing teeth, and not present teeth [22, 23]. Thus, the long-term prognosis, the capabilities offered by the modern endodontic treatment to address the complication, the alternatives in case of treatment failure, the posttreatment quality of life, and the patient's preferences should all be recognized and incorporated in the practitioner's decision making [22, 23].

Endodontic clinical trials often use "success" as the outcome variable, based on strict clinical and radiographic evaluations. In contrast, implant research often uses "survival," defined as "retention of the tooth or implant, depending on the intervention," as the outcome variable, thus leading to a confusion when attempting to compare these two treatment modalities [22]. Doyle et al. [24] compared the long-term survival of single-tooth implant restorations with matched teeth receiving initial nonsurgical endodontic treatment and restoration and reported a comparable 10-year survival rate of both treatment modalities [24]. Thus, choices between implant and endodontic therapies cannot be solely based on outcomes measurement [25].

The required additional treatments, especially in case of failure, and the patient's quality of life should also be taken under consideration. For example, endodontically treated natural teeth may provide more effective masticatory function compared with implant-supported restorations [26]. In addition, although the success of implant and endodontically treated teeth may be comparable, implants may require more postoperative treatments to maintain them [27]. Thus, natural endodontically treated teeth may grant improved dental function and less required further treatments than implant [24, 26, 27].

As part of the treatment consideration and decision-making process, specific patient- and practitioner-related matters, which might affect the risk of complications and the ability to manage those complications in case they occur, need to be considered. Thus, several questions need to be elucidated:

- Are my patients different from those presented in the literature (i.e., in terms of motivation, socioeconomic status, systemic considerations)?
- Is the treatment feasible in my setting?
- Will the potential benefits of treatment outweigh the potential risks for my patient?

This book is aimed to provide endodontic practitioners with knowledge and practical tools to incorporate an evidence-based approach for prevention, identification, and management of surgical complications, in their daily decision-making process.

References

1. Farrar JN. Radical and heroic treatment of alveolar abscess by amputation of roots of teeth. Dental Cosmos. 1884;26(3):135–9.
2. Tsesis I, Rosen E, Taschieri S, Telishevsky Strauss Y, Ceresoli V, Del Fabbro M. Outcomes of surgical endodontic treatment performed by a modern technique: an updated meta-analysis of the literature. J Endod. 2013;39(3):332–9.
3. Tsesis I, Faivishevsky V, Kfir A, Rosen E. Outcome of surgical endodontic treatment performed by a modern technique: a meta-analysis of literature. J Endod. 2009;35(11):1505–11.
4. Kim S, Kratchman S. Modern endodontic surgery concepts and practice: a review. J Endod. 2006; 32(7):601–23.
5. Tsesis I, Rosen E, Schwartz-Arad D, Fuss Z. Retrospective evaluation of surgical endodontic treatment: traditional versus modern technique. J Endod. 2006;32(5):412–6.
6. Johnson BR, Witherspoon D. Periradicular surgery. In: Cohen S, Hargreaves KM, editors. Pathways of the pulp. 9th ed. St. Louis: Mosby/Elsevier; 2006. p. 724–85.
7. Walton RE. Routine histopathologic examination of endodontic periradicular surgical specimens – is it warranted? Oral Surg Oral Med Oral Pathol Oral Radiol Endod. 1998;86(5):505.
8. Gutmann JL, Harrison JW. Surgical endodontics. Boston: Blackwell Scientific Publications; 1991.
9. Allen RK, Newton CW, Brown Jr CE. A statistical analysis of surgical and nonsurgical endodontic retreatment cases. J Endod. 1989;15(6):261–6.
10. Friedman S. Treatment outcome and prognosis of endodontic therapy. In: Ørstavik D, editor. Essential endodontology: prevention and treatment of apical periodontitis. Oxford: Blackwell Science; 1998. p. 367–401.
11. Carr G. Advanced techniques and visual enhancement for endodontic surgery. Endod Rep. 1992;7(1): 6–9.
12. Rubinstein RA, Kim S. Short-term observation of the results of endodontic surgery with the use of surgical operation microscope and Super-EBA as root end filling material. J Endod. 1999;25:43–8.
13. Angelos P. Complications, errors, and surgical ethics. World J Surg. 2009;33(4):609–11.
14. Hofer TP, Kerr EA, Hayward RA. What is an error? Eff Clin Pract. 2000;3(6):261–9.
15. Givol N, Rosen E, Taicher S, Tsesis I. Risk management in endodontics. J Endod. 2010;36(6):982–4.
16. Wooley CF, Boudoulas H. Clinician. Hellenic J Cardiol. 1993;34:241–3.
17. Isaacs D, Fitzgerald D. Seven alternatives to evidence based medicine. BMJ. 1999;319(7225):1618.
18. Gutmann JL. Evidence-based/guest editorial. J Endod. 2009;35:1093.
19. Mileman PA, van den Hout WB. Evidence-based diagnosis and clinical decision making. Dentomaxillofac Radiol. 2009;38(1):1–10.
20. Rosenberg W, Donald A. Evidence based medicine: an approach to clinical problem-solving. BMJ. 1995;310(6987):1122–6.
21. Sutherland SE, Matthews DC. Conducting systematic reviews and creating clinical practice guidelines in dentistry: lessons learned. J Am Dent Assoc. 2004;135(6):747–53.
22. Iqbal MK, Kim S. A review of factors influencing treatment planning decisions of single-tooth implants versus preserving natural teeth with nonsurgical endodontic therapy. J Endod. 2008;34(5):519–29.
23. Tsesis I, Nemkowsky CE, Tamse E, Rosen E. Preserving the natural tooth versus extraction and implant placement: making a rational clinical decision. Refuat Hapeh Vehashinayim. 2010;27(1):37–46, 75.
24. Doyle SL, Hodges JS, Pesun IJ, Law AS, Bowles WR. Retrospective cross sectional comparison of initial nonsurgical endodontic treatment and single-tooth implants. J Endod. 2006;32(9):822–7.
25. White SN, Miklus VG, Potter KS, Cho J, Ngan AY. Endodontics and implants, a catalog of therapeutic contrasts. J Evid Based Dent Pract. 2006;6(1):101–9.
26. Woodmansey KF, Ayik M, Buschang PH, White CA, He J. Differences in masticatory function in patients with endodontically treated teeth and single-implant-supported prostheses: a pilot study. J Endod. 2009;35(1):10–4.
27. Hannahan JP, Eleazer PD. Comparison of success of implants versus endodontically treated teeth. J Endod. 2008;34(11):1302–5.

Zebra Hunt: Clinical Reasoning and Misdiagnosis

2

Marilena Vered, Aviad Tamse, Igor Tsesis, and Eyal Rosen

Abstract

Diagnosis is the art and science of detecting and distinguishing deviations from health and the cause and nature thereof and should be the foundation for clinical decision making.

Adequate diagnosis is based on sound knowledge and efficient clinical reasoning. Errors during the clinical reasoning process may ultimately lead to misdiagnosis and ensuing complications. This chapter will review misdiagnosis complications in teeth scheduled for endodontic surgery.

Introduction

Diagnosis can be defined as "the art and science of detecting and distinguishing deviations from health and the cause and nature thereof" [1] and should be the foundation for clinical decision making. The ability to effectively diagnose and manage a patient condition is based on sound and updated knowledge base and effective clinical reasoning. The clinical reasoning process is composed of several steps: identification of clinical information that is relevant to the patient's condition, interpretation of its meaning, generation of hypotheses that provides rational explanation of the patient's condition, testing and refining of those hypotheses through further data collection, and eventually establishment of a diagnosis [2]. Errors in one or more of the clinical reasoning steps may ultimately lead to misdiagnosis and ensuing complications.

Errors in diagnosis of a medical condition may be related to the following: manifestation that is not sufficiently noticeable, a condition that is omitted from consideration, excessive consideration is given to some features of the condition, the condition has nonspecific symptoms, and when the condition has a rare clinical presentation [2, 3].

Complications in diagnosis of teeth scheduled for endodontic surgery may occur due to the periodontal condition of the tooth, such as vertical root fracture (VRF), and misdiagnosis of non-endodontic lesions mimicking inflammatory periradicular lesions.

M. Vered, DMD (✉)
Department of Oral Pathology and Oral Medicine,
Maurice and Gabriela Goldschleger
School of Dental Medicine, Tel Aviv University,
Tel Aviv 69978, Israel
e-mail: mvered@post.tau.ac.il

A. Tamse, DMD • I. Tsesis, DMD • E. Rosen, DMD
Department of Endodontology,
Maurice and Gabriela Goldschleger
School of Dental Medicine, Tel Aviv University,
Tel Aviv 69978, Israel
e-mail: tamseaz@post.tau.ac.il; dr.tsesis@gmail.com;
dr.eyalrosen@gmail.com

I. Tsesis (ed.), *Complications in Endodontic Surgery*,
DOI 10.1007/978-3-642-54218-3_2, © Springer-Verlag Berlin Heidelberg 2014

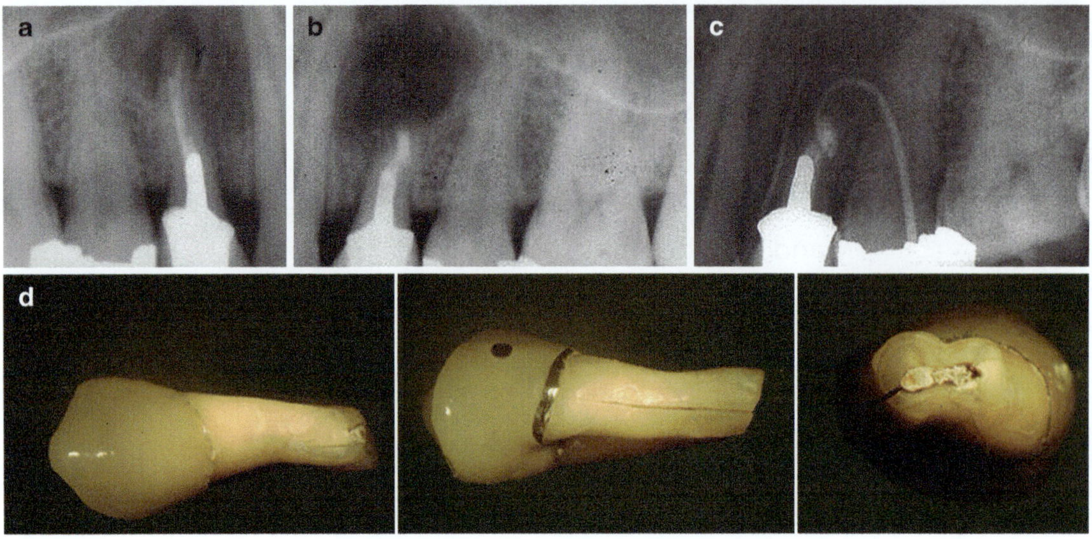

Fig. 2.1 Endodontic surgery on misdiagnosed vertical root fracture on maxillary premolar. (**a**) Presurgical; (**b**) immediately post surgery; (**c**) follow-up (gutta-percha tracing of buccal and palatinal sinus tracts); (**d**) following extraction – a vertical root fracture was diagnosed

Complication of Endodontic Surgery as a Result of Periodontal Condition

The ultimate goal of endodontic surgery is to preserve teeth with apical periodontitis. However, sometimes while it is possible to treat the endodontic pathology, there is still a need to extract the tooth due to uncontrolled periodontal disease [4].

A typical example of misdiagnosis can be a vertical root fracture (VRF). VRFs are longitudinally oriented fractures of the endodontically treated teeth that originate in any location of the root and can propagate coronally or apically [5, 6]. VRF in endodontically treated teeth is a serious complication of root canal therapy which results in the tooth or root extraction [7–10]. The diagnosis of VRF based on clinical and periapical radiographic evaluation may be, at times, complicated for lack of specific signs, symptoms, and/or radiographic features [6] and because several etiologic factors may be involved [5, 6].

The two-dimensional nature of the periapical radiography was suggested as a possible limitation for the radiographic detection of VRF [11]. It was recently suggested that cone beam computed tomography (CBCT) presents superior diagnostic validity over periapical radiography for VRF diagnosis proposes [11–23], and the VRF diagnostic capabilities of CBCT were tested both ex vivo and in vivo, presenting inconsistent and confusing results [11, 12, 14–21, 23–27]. In addition, the long-term health concerns regarding radiation doses associated with CBCT still need to be elucidated [25, 28–34]. Thus, it is therefore an acceptable practice that every effort should be made to minimize the effective radiation dose to the patient in endodontic-specific tasks [28, 35] and that the use of CBCT for VRF diagnosis should be performed based on cost-benefit assessment [28].

The anatomical pattern of the VRF is variable in its direction (vertical to the long axis of the root or sometimes diagonal), and it can be incomplete (on one aspect of the root) or complete (from buccal to palatal/lingual). This variety of clinical presentations might lead to failure to diagnose the VRF during the endodontic surgical procedure [6].

Sometimes the typical deep osseous defect (pocket) is not clinically detectable by probing, since the root fracture is located in the middle part of the root not involving the coronal or apical parts of the root. Thus, the attachment in the coronal part exists and the coronal bone is still intact. This may also lead to failure to diagnose the VRF [6] (Fig. 2.1).

When VRF diagnosis is made, a quick decision to extract the tooth or root is necessary, since that the inflammation in the supporting tissues would otherwise lead to periodontal breakdown followed by the development of a deep osseous defect [7] and resorption of the bone facing the root fracture. Thus, failure to diagnose VRF during the endodontic surgery might lead to treatment failure associated with excessive bone loss that will jeopardize future restoration of the area of the extraction [8].

Non-endodontic Lesions Mimicking Inflammatory Periradicular Lesions in Endodontically Treated Teeth

Pulp sensitivity testing has been frequently suggested for differential diagnosis between apical lesions of endodontic and non-endodontic origin [36]. However, most teeth scheduled for endodontic surgery were previously endodontically treated. Thus, the diagnosis cannot be based on pulp sensitivity testing.

In general, tissue removed from a periradicular area of teeth with apical periodontitis, when submitted to histopathological examination, demonstrates a granuloma or a radicular cyst. However, on rare occasions, histopathological examination of tissues removed from this area will reveal lesions of other entities, which radiologically mimic periradicular inflammatory pathoses. Although radicular cysts and granulomas are very common, we should be aware of the possibility that other noninflammatory lesions may be located in a periradicular location. This is important since these other missed or disregarded diagnoses might result in inappropriate treatment.

Periapical granulomas (PAGs) are formed at the apices of non-vital teeth, most of them being asymptomatic. In general, PAGs represent ~75 % of apical inflammatory lesions and ~50 % of periapical lesions related to lack of response to endodontic treatment [37]. Radiographically, PAGs are radiolucent lesions ranging from small, nearly indistinguishable to lesions of 2 cm in diameter and larger. The involved tooth shows loss of lamina dura (LD) at the apical region. PAGs may be circumscribed or ill defined, with or without a radiopaque rim. Root resorption is quite common. PAGs are biologically dynamic lesions and can transform into periapical cysts (PACs) or periapical abscesses, without necessarily alternating the radiographic features. Although PACs are believed to achieve a larger size than PAGs, distinguishing between these two entities based on the radiographic findings is almost impossible [37].

A cyst associated with a non-vital tooth may develop at the lateral aspect of the root due to spread of the pulpal necrotic material through a lateral root canal and foramen and is termed lateral radicular cyst (LRC). In principle, the radiographic features of LRC are identical to those of PACs/PAGs including the radiolucent nature of the lesion and loss of the LD in the region of the foramen of the root canal [37].

Lesions located at the apices of non-vital teeth that radiographically look like PAGs/PACs, but histologically reveal to be lesions of a large range of entities, have been described in the English language literature, in either single-case reports or limited case series. It is assumed that between 0.65 % and ~6 % of apparently periapical lesions are not of inflammatory origin [38–41]; therefore, comprehensive diagnostic evaluation is needed in order to avoid pitfalls of unnecessary endodontic treatment. The lesions mimicking PAGs/PACs can be classified as follows: anatomical structures and variations, cysts, tumors and diseases, and miscellaneous lesions.

Anatomical Structures and Variations

The incisive canal is located between and apical to the roots of the maxillary central incisors. It is generally accepted that a diameter of 6 mm is the upper limit of the normal size for the incisive canal, so that a radiolucency of 6 mm or smaller in this area is usually considered a normal foramen unless there are clinical signs or symptoms (e.g., swelling, pain, drainage) present [37]. Lesions larger than 6 mm are usually considered as an incisive canal cyst. The incisive canal or the incisive canal cyst usually appears as a symmetrical, well-defined radiolucent lesion between the roots of the upper central incisors, showing a "heart"-like-shaped outline due to its superimposition on the anterior nasal spine. However, occasionally, the canal or its cystic variant is asymmetrical, lying only on one side of the midline, overlapping the apex of the adjacent central incisor, thus mimicking a periapical pathosis. In this case, in particular when the lesion is larger than 6 mm, an occlusal radiograph will aid in determining the spatial relation between the seemingly unilateral "periapical" pathosis and the status of the LD and width of the periodontal ligament of the adjacent tooth [37].

The mental foramen may also have a radiographic appearance of a periapical pathosis in the area of the lower second premolars. If doubts are raised in regard to the true nature of the lesion, then additional periapical x-rays should be taken from different angles in order to analyze changes in the position of the "periapical" finding [37].

The anatomical depression at the angle of the mandible below the inferior alveolar nerve canal, in which part of the submandibular salivary gland or muscle tissue or fibro-fatty tissue resides and has a radiographic appearance of a cyst-like lesion, is known as the mandibular lingual salivary gland depression/Stafne defect/static bone cyst [37]. In a minority of cases, this anatomical mandibular defect has been found more anteriorly, namely, starting from the symphysis area to the premolars. This anterior variation of "Stafne bone defect" is filled by sublingual salivary gland tissue and has the appearance of a periapical pathosis [42].

Anecdotal cases of atypical anatomy of the maxillary sinus with an extension seen on conventional panoramic x-rays as a unilocular, well-defined corticated radiolucency in the second premolar-first molar location were reported [43]. With the aid of adequate CT imaging, when indicated, it could provide valuable information for an exact diagnosis.

Another rare anatomical variation is the canalis sinuosus that carries the anterior superior dental nerve and associated blood vessels [44]. It can rarely take an aberrant route between the medial aspect of the alveolar bone of the maxillary canine and the nasal cavity and as such be interpreted as a periapical pathosis of the canine tooth. Close examination of periapical x-rays will reveal the intact periodontal ligament space of the canine upon which the radiolucency of the canalis sinuosus is superimposed.

Odontogenic Cysts

A true cyst is defined as a pathologic cavity lined by epithelium and filled with fluid or semisolid material [37]. Cysts rarely develop within bones for the simple reason that it is unusual to find epithelium in these locations. The jawbones, however, are a marked exception to this rule, and cysts occur in this region more frequently than in any other bone in the body. The source of epithelium in the jawbones is both odontogenic and non-odontogenic. Corresponding to this epithelium, two major types of bone cysts, odontogenic and non-odontogenic, arise within the jaws. The odontogenic cysts can be further classified as developmental (part originates from the rests of dental lamina and part from reduced enamel epithelium) and as inflammatory (originates from the rests of Malassez) [37]. Cysts of jawbone are well-defined, totally or predominantly radiolucent, sometimes expansile lesions.

The lateral periodontal cyst (LPC) is a rare developmental odontogenic cyst that typically occurs on the lateral surface of a canine or a premolar tooth, predominantly in the lower jaw [37]. Adjacent teeth are vital and as such the LD and periodontal ligament space are expected to be intact. Radiographically, LPC is a well-defined radiolucency on the lateral aspects of the tooth roots with a diameter of ~1 cm. These clinical and radiographic parameters should be enough to distinguish a LPC from a LRC. However, LPC type of lesions can be present in association with a non-vital tooth or with what seems to be lack of healing of an endodontically treated tooth [37]. Upon submitting the lesion to microscopic examination the diagnosis of LPC has to be supported by the typical features of the lining epithelium (that are expected to be preserved, at least in part, even if the cyst is inflamed).

Another rare odontogenic developmental cyst reported at the apex of a non-vital tooth is the orthokeratinized odontogenic cyst [45] that usually has no characteristic clinical or radiographic features to distinguish it from other inflammatory cysts.

Odontogenic Tumors

Odontogenic tumors arise from epithelial and/or mesenchymal components of the developing odontogenic apparatus and are almost always confined to the jaws. These tumors are usually benign but vary widely in their behavior.

Radiographically, they may manifest as totally radiolucent or radiopaque lesions or as mixed radiolucent-radiopaque lesions. The lesions are diagnosed and classified on the basis of their histologic features, usually correlating the clinical and radiographic features.

The keratocystic odontogenic tumor (KCOT), formerly known as odontogenic keratocyst, is a developmental odontogenic lesion, now believed to represent a cystic tumor [37]. KCOT may demonstrate a radiographic picture that, among other possibilities, can mimic that of a PAG/PAC [37]. In fact, when large series of periapical biopsies taken from teeth with clinically necrotic pulps were analyzed, KCOTs were found in a frequency ranging from 0 % [38, 46, 47] to 0.27 % [40], 0.3 % [48], 0.53 % [49], and up to 0.7 % [50]. Comparing KCOT to other periapical noninflammatory types of lesions, it seems that KCOT is the most frequently encountered. In a study of 239 KCOTs, 21 (9 %) were located periradicularly and 12 (57 %) were associated with non-vital teeth or endodontically treated teeth and therefore were considered to be of endodontic origin [51]. Interestingly, in the latter lesions, two-thirds were symptomatic, the mandible-to-maxilla ratio was almost 1:1, 90 % were associated with teeth anterior to the molars, mainly anterior teeth, and the mean age of the patients was 56 years. These features are different than those that characterize the classical nonperiapical, non-vital tooth-related KCOT, in terms of location and age of patients [37]. Periapical lesions that fail to heal after good-quality endodontic treatment require further investigation, in particular if lesions continue to enlarge and/or present aggravating symptomatology during follow-up. A 4-year follow-up period has been suggested in order to assess success or failure [52]. Assuming that the nonhealing periapical lesion could be a KCOT, it is likely that during this follow-up period it would continue to advance and change the radiographic picture, thus demanding a biopsy procedure and a definite microscopic diagnosis. A case of KCOT mimicking a periapical lesion is seen in Fig. 2.2. The treatment of KCOT must take into consideration the tendency for recurrence, and therefore the surgical approach is usually more aggressive than for other developmental cystic lesions nonetheless periapical inflammatory pathoses and usually comprises of removal of the lesion followed by peripheral ostectomy of the bony cavity and/or chemical cauterization. Exceptionally, locally aggressive KCOTs demand local resection and bone grafting [37].

Anecdotal cases of solid ameloblastoma appearing as a periapical, cyst-like radiolucency associated with non-vital teeth have been reported [53, 54]. Similarly, unicystic ameloblastoma adjacent to vital and non-vital teeth was reported [36, 55]. A case of a "periapical" unicystic ameloblastoma considered to be an inflammatory periapical lesion that remained untreated for about 10 years is illustrated in Fig. 2.3. The treatment approach for solid, multicystic ameloblastoma and for unicystic ameloblastoma with mural proliferation is quite aggressive because the tumor infiltrates into the adjacent cancellous bone, beyond the apparent radiographic margins [37]. The most conservative treatment is removal of the tumor after careful study of the CT scans followed by peripheral ostectomy. Escalation of the surgical procedure to marginal resection followed by reconstructive surgery might be mandatory depending on tumor size and pattern of expansion, yet a 15 % recurrence rate still occurs. The other types of unicystic ameloblastoma (i.e., the luminal and intraluminal) are treated as "conventional" cysts by enucleation and close follow-up as recurrence rates of 10–20 % were

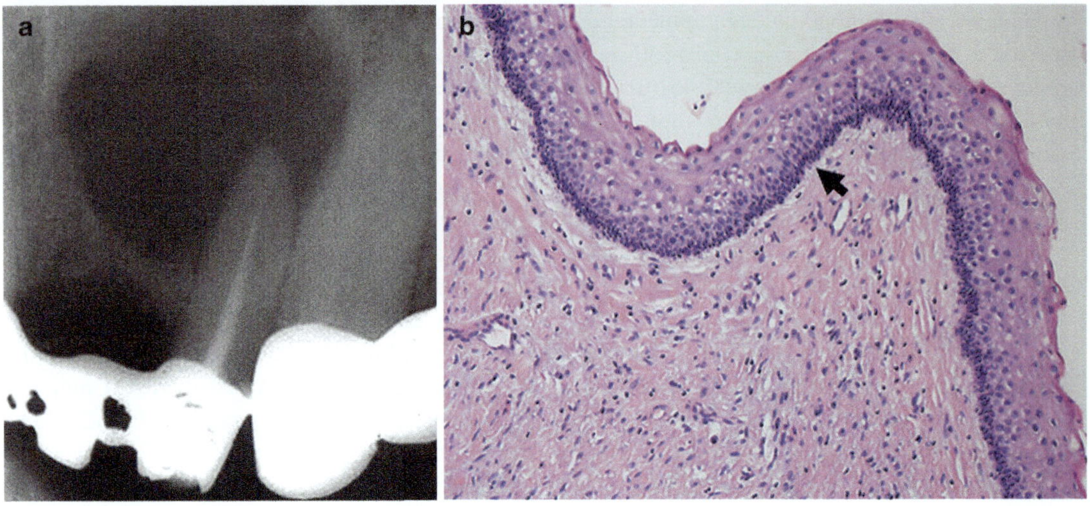

Fig. 2.2 A case of KCOT mimicking a periapical lesion. (**a**) The radiograph shows a radiolucent lesion in the periapical region of the left upper lateral incisor that is noncorticated and defined in the lower portion; however, in the upper portion there is a notion of blurred margins. (**b**) The hematoxylin- and eosin-stained slides showed a cystic lesion lined by stratified squamous epithelium with parakeratin showing a slightly corrugated surface. The epithelium is of regular width and shows a palisading arrangement of the basal nuclei (*arrow*). These histopathological features are consistent with keratocystic odontogenic tumor (KCOT). Original magnification ×200

reported [37]. Additional types of rare odontogenic tumors in a periapical location were published, either as single-case reports or as part of case series on periapical inflammatory lesions, and these include adenomatoid odontogenic tumor, calcifying cystic odontogenic tumor, ameloblastic fibroma, squamous odontogenic tumor, calcifying epithelial odontogenic tumor, and odontogenic myxoma [38, 40, 56, 57]. Part of these reported lesions were not accompanied with photomicrographs of the histopathological findings, so that the accuracy of the diagnoses cannot be always confirmed.

In conclusion, the key to an accurate diagnosis in case of a periapical lesion, even if it looks to be of inflammatory nature, is the collection of all available clinical data and radiographic findings and sufficient follow-up period in those doubtful cases.

Bone Tumors and Diseases

This is a diverse group of lesions of varied etiologies; we will presently focus on two entities that radiologically have features of a radicular cystic lesion, namely, central giant cell granuloma (CGCG) and fibro-osseous lesions.

CGCGs appearing as small periapical lesions constituted 9 % of all examined CGCG cases ($N=75$) in one study [58]. Furthermore, the largest retrospective study on CGCG ($N=79$) found in a periapical location (PA-CGCG) revealed that 20 % of the lesions were associated with teeth with necrotic pulps and that the majority of these necrotic teeth had been endodontically treated [59]. In addition, PA-CGCG was encountered in patients older than 30 years of age, while the non-PA-CGCG is usually diagnosed in younger patients; ~50 % of the PA-CGCGs were in the posterior area of the mandible; in regard to the PA-CGCG found in the maxilla, there was a similar distribution between the anterior and posterior areas. Single cases of PA-CGCG or small case series were also reported [38, 40, 60–62]. All these studies emphasized the need for careful analysis of the radiographic findings in order to decide the lesion-tooth supporting structures relations, both at the initial presentation and during the follow-up period, if teeth were endodontically treated in equivocal cases. Whenever surgical specimens are

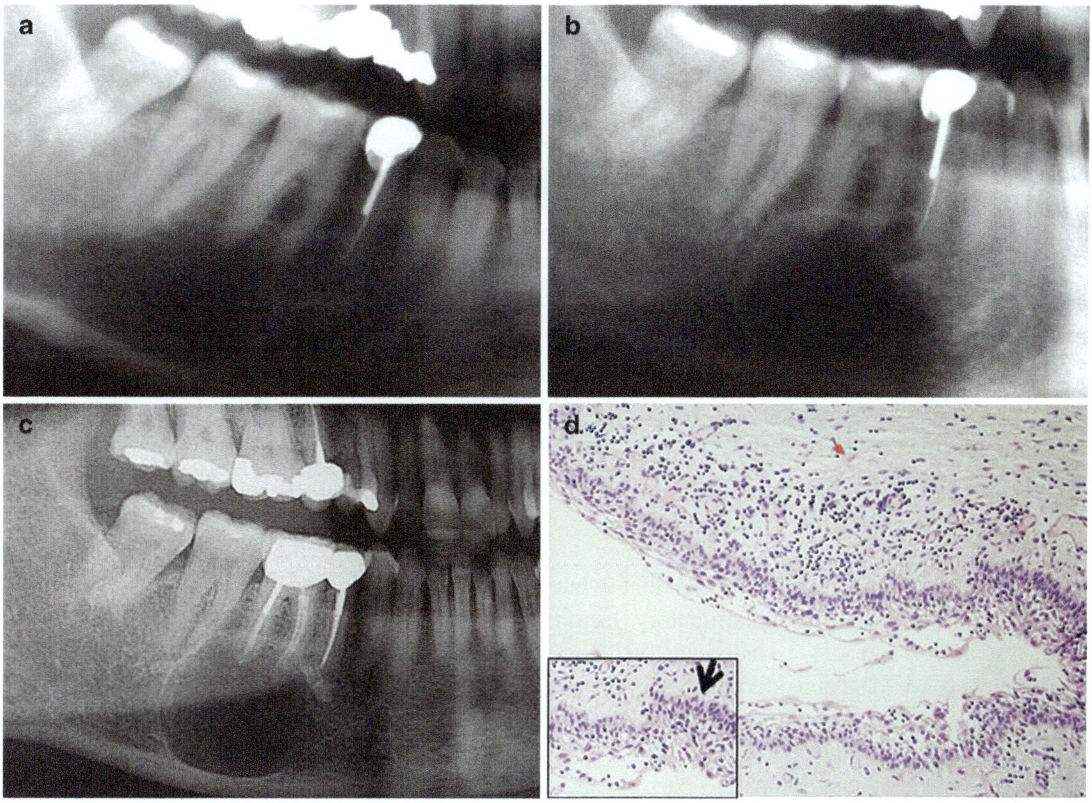

Fig. 2.3 A case of a "periapical" unicystic ameloblastoma (**a**) In 2002, an asymptomatic periapical lesion showing a corticated, round-shaped radiolucency at the apical area of the first right molar. (**b**) In 2005, the lesion continued to grow. (**c**) 2013 – a root canal treatment was performed; however, the lesion continued to grow. (**d**) Histopathologically, a cystic lesion is seen. The lining epithelium shows a basal layer of columnar cells with hyperchromatic nuclei with reverse polarity arranged in a palisading pattern highlighted in the *inset* with an *arrow*. The rest of the epithelial cell layers have an appearance reminiscent of stellate reticulum. There is a mild chronic inflammatory infiltrate. The histopathological features are consistent with a unicystic ameloblastoma, luminal type. Original magnification ×200

taken, submission to microscopic evaluation is mandatory. A case of CGCG mimicking a periapical lesion is seen in Fig. 2.4. CGCGs are usually treated by thorough curettage although recurrence rates of 11 % and up to 50 % were reported, with the higher values being attributed to those lesions that are defined as biologically aggressive and which are characterized by a tendency to recur, especially in young patients [37]. Recurrent CGCGs may be treated by curettage or by a more radical surgical approach, depending on the clinical findings, with optional addition of different pharmacological agents.

Fibro-osseous lesions of the focal or periapical type [focal cemento-osseous dysplasia (FCOD) and periapical cemental dysplasia (PCD)] can be confused with PAGs/PACs in their early, radiolucent stage [63, 64], although, at least PCD, rarely affect only one tooth. Whenever diagnosis based on clinical and radiographic information is doubtful, biopsy of the periapical lesion should be considered before starting a redundant endodontic treatment.

Miscellaneous Rare Lesions That May Mimic Periapical Lesions

This subgroup includes cases of traumatic bone cyst [65, 66], central schwannoma [67, 68], and

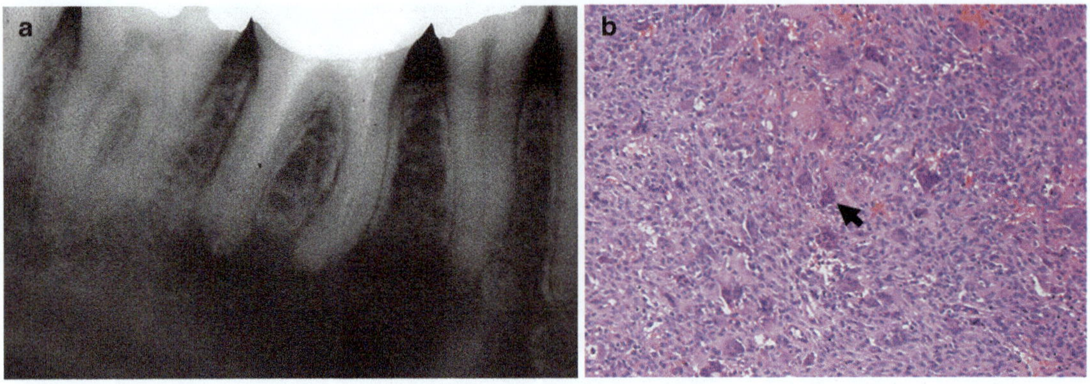

Fig. 2.4 Central giant cell granuloma mimicking a periapical lesion. (**a**) A radiolucent, non-corticated, usually defined lesion is seen at the apical area of the right first mandibular molar. (**b**) Histopathologically, there is a hypercellular mass consisting of multinucleated giant cells (*arrow*) admixed with mononuclear spindle cells in a stroma showing extravasation of red blood cells. Original magnification ×200

lymphangioma [69]. The likelihood that what seems to be a periapical inflammatory lesion could actually represent a malignant lesion is very low but should be considered when it is clinically accompanied by numbness or other sensory disturbances [70].

In conclusion, radiolucent periradicular lesions involving non-vital teeth or endodontically treated teeth usually represent an inflammatory process of a granuloma or a cyst and in some rare cases healing by scar tissue. However, after excluding the possibility of anatomical structures that may resemble a radicular pathosis, lesions of non-endodontic origin should be considered in the differential diagnosis, especially if the clinical signs and symptoms are suggestive of these alternative entities.

When a non-endodontic-related pathology is suspected based on the patient's medical history, anamnesis, and clinical and radiographic evaluation, the practitioner should determine the probability for pathology of non-endodontic origin (Table 2.1). In regard to radiographic findings that are assumed to carry a low-risk for non-endodontic origin, routine endodontic management with a rigorous follow-up is advised. However, radiographic findings suspected of having a high risk for non-endodontic origin, a multi-disciplinary approach including consultation with the primary care dental surgeon and/or oral and maxillo-facial surgeon and/or oral radiologist, is advised.

Table 2.1 Warning signs of conditions mimicking inflammatory periradicular lesions in endodontically treated teeth

Clinical signs	Radiographic signs
Coexistent malignancies or metabolic bone disorders	Multiple teeth involvement
Altered sensation, atypical pain	Large-size lesions
Pathological tooth mobility without evident periodontal disease	Extensive root resorption (especially of the knife-edge type)
Expansion of bone	Tooth displacement
Concomitant mucosal ulcerations	Lesions with undefined, "moth-eaten" border
	Combined radiolucent/ radiopaque
	Multilocular radiolucent lesions

References

1. AAE, editor. Glossary of endodontic terms. Chicago: AAE; 2012. Available at: www.aae.org/glossary.
2. Groves M, O'Rourke P, Alexander H. Clinical reasoning: the relative contribution of identification, interpretation and hypothesis errors to misdiagnosis. Med Teach. 2003;25(6):621–5.
3. Johnson PE, Duran AS, Hassebrock F, Moller J, Prietula M, Feltovich PJ, et al. Expertise and error in diagnostic reasoning. Cognit Sci. 1981;5(3):235–83.
4. Shulman LB, Driskell TD. Dental implants: a historical perspective. In: Block M, Kent J, Guerra L, editors. Implants in dentistry. Philadelphia: W.B. Saunders; 1997.

5. Cracking the cracked tooth code: detection and treatment of various longitudinal tooth fractures. Colleagues for excellence, Summer 2008; Chicago: American Association of Endodontics; 2008. Available at: www.aae.org.
6. Tsesis I, Rosen E, Tamse A, Taschieri S, Kfir A. Diagnosis of vertical root fractures in endodontically treated teeth based on clinical and radiographic indices: a systematic review. J Endod. 2010;36(9):1455–8.
7. Walton RE, Michelich RJ, Smith GN. The histopathogenesis of vertical root fractures. J Endod. 1984;10(2): 48–56.
8. Tamse A. Vertical root fractures in endodontically treated teeth: diagnostic signs and clinical management. Endod Topics. 2006;13(1):84–94.
9. Tamse A, Fuss Z, Lustig J, Kaplavi J. An evaluation of endodontically treated vertically fractured teeth. J Endod. 1999;25(7):506–8.
10. Tamse A. Vertical root fractures of endodontically treated teeth. In: Ingle JI, Bakland LK, Baumgartner JC, editors. Ingle's endodontics. 6th ed. Hamilton: BC Decker Inc.; 2008. p. 676–89.
11. Metska ME, Aartman IH, Wesselink PR, Ozok AR. Detection of vertical root fractures in vivo in endodontically treated teeth by cone-beam computed tomography scans. J Endod. 2012;38(10):1344–7.
12. Ferreira RI, Bahrami G, Isidor F, Wenzel A, Haiter-Neto F, Groppo FC. Detection of vertical root fractures by cone-beam computerized tomography in endodontically treated teeth with fiber-resin and titanium posts: an in vitro study. Oral Surg Oral Med Oral Pathol Oral Radiol. 2013;115(1):e49–57.
13. Fayad MI, Ashkenaz PJ, Johnson BR. Different representations of vertical root fractures detected by cone-beam volumetric tomography: a case series report. J Endod. 2012;38(10):1435–42.
14. da Silveira PF, Vizzotto MB, Liedke GS, da Silveira HL, Montagner F, da Silveira HE. Detection of vertical root fractures by conventional radiographic examination and cone beam computed tomography – an in vitro analysis. Dent Traumatol. 2013;29(1):41–6.
15. Kambungton J, Janhom A, Prapayasatok S, Pongsiriwet S. Assessment of vertical root fractures using three imaging modalities: cone beam CT, intraoral digital radiography and film. Dentomaxillofac Radiol. 2012;41(2):91–5.
16. Wang P, He W, Sun H, Lu Q, Ni L. Detection of vertical root fractures in non-endodontically treated molars using cone-beam computed tomography: a report of four representative cases. Dent Traumatol. 2012;28(4): 329–33.
17. Edlund M, Nair MK, Nair UP. Detection of vertical root fractures by using cone-beam computed tomography: a clinical study. J Endod. 2011;37(6):768–72.
18. Zou X, Liu D, Yue L, Wu M. The ability of cone-beam computerized tomography to detect vertical root fractures in endodontically treated and nonendodontically treated teeth: a report of 3 cases. Oral Surg Oral Med Oral Pathol Oral Radiol Endod. 2011;111(6): 797–801.
19. Varshosaz M, Tavakoli MA, Mostafavi M, Baghban AA. Comparison of conventional radiography with cone beam computed tomography for detection of vertical root fractures: an in vitro study. J Oral Sci. 2010;52(4):593–7.
20. Ozer SY. Detection of vertical root fractures by using cone beam computed tomography with variable voxel sizes in an in vitro model. J Endod. 2011;37(1): 75–9.
21. Ozer SY. Detection of vertical root fractures of different thicknesses in endodontically enlarged teeth by cone beam computed tomography versus digital radiography. J Endod. 2010;36(7):1245–9.
22. Hassan B, Metska ME, Ozok AR, van der Stelt P, Wesselink PR. Comparison of five cone beam computed tomography systems for the detection of vertical root fractures. J Endod. 2010;36(1):126–9.
23. Hassan B, Metska ME, Ozok AR, van der Stelt P, Wesselink PR. Detection of vertical root fractures in endodontically treated teeth by a cone beam computed tomography scan. J Endod. 2009;35(5): 719–22.
24. Bernardes RA, de Moraes IG, Hungaro Duarte MA, Azevedo BC, de Azevedo JR, Bramante CM. Use of cone-beam volumetric tomography in the diagnosis of root fractures. Oral Surg Oral Med Oral Pathol Oral Radiol Endod. 2009;108(2):270–7.
25. Dailey B, Mines P, Anderson A, Sweet M, editors. The use of cone beam computer tomography in endodontics: results of a questionnaire. AAE annual session abstract presentation; 2010. Available at: www.aae.org.
26. de Paula-Silva FW, Wu MK, Leonardo MR, da Silva LA, Wesselink PR. Accuracy of periapical radiography and cone-beam computed tomography scans in diagnosing apical periodontitis using histopathological findings as a gold standard. J Endod. 2009;35(7): 1009–12.
27. Youssefzadeh S, Gahleitner A, Dorffner R, Bernhart T, Kainberger FM. Dental vertical root fractures: value of CT in detection. Radiology. 1999;210(2): 545–9.
28. AAE, AAOMR, editors. AAE and AAOMR joint position statement – use of cone-beam-computed tomography in endodontics. 2010. Available at: www.aaomr.org/news/52024.
29. Berrington de Gonzalez A, Mahesh M, Kim KP, Bhargavan M, Lewis R, Mettler F, et al. Projected cancer risks from computed tomographic scans performed in the United States in 2007. Arch Intern Med. 2009;169(22):2071–7.
30. Brenner D, Elliston C, Hall E, Berdon W. Estimated risks of radiation-induced fatal cancer from pediatric CT. AJR Am J Roentgenol. 2001;176(2):289–96.
31. Brenner DJ, Hall EJ. Computed tomography–an increasing source of radiation exposure. N Engl J Med. 2007;357(22):2277–84.
32. Parker L. Computed tomography scanning in children: radiation risks. Pediatr Hematol Oncol. 2001; 18(5):307–8.

33. Pearce MS, Salotti JA, Little MP, McHugh K, Lee C, Kim KP, et al. Radiation exposure from CT scans in childhood and subsequent risk of leukaemia and brain tumours: a retrospective cohort study. Lancet. 2012; 380(9840):499–505.
34. Rehani MM, Berry M. Radiation doses in computed tomography. The increasing doses of radiation need to be controlled. BMJ. 2000;320(7235):593–4.
35. Patel S. New dimensions in endodontic imaging: Part 2. Cone beam computed tomography. Int Endod J. 2009;42(6):463–75.
36. Gondak RO, Rocha AC, Neves Campos JG, Vargas PA, de Almeida OP, Lopes MA, et al. Unicystic ameloblastoma mimicking apical periodontitis: a case series. J Endod. 2013;39(1):145–8.
37. Neville BW, Damm DD, Allen CM, Bouquot JE. Oral and maxillofacial pathology. 3rd ed. St. Louis: Elsevier.
38. Kuc I, Peters E, Pan J. Comparison of clinical and histologic diagnoses in periapical lesions. Oral Surg Oral Med Oral Pathol Oral Radiol Endod. 2000;89(3):333–7.
39. Nikitakis NG, Brooks JK, Melakopoulos I, Younis RH, Scheper MA, Pitts MA, et al. Lateral periodontal cysts arising in periapical sites: a report of two cases. J Endod. 2010;36(10):1707–11.
40. Ortega A, Farina V, Gallardo A, Espinoza I, Acosta S. Nonendodontic periapical lesions: a retrospective study in Chile. Int Endod J. 2007;40(5):386–90.
41. Spatafore CM, Griffin Jr JA, Keyes GG, Wearden S, Skidmore AE. Periapical biopsy report: an analysis of over a 10-year period. J Endod. 1990;16(5):239–41.
42. Anneroth G, Berglund G, Kahnberg KE. Intraosseous salivary gland tissue of the mandible mimicking a periapical lesion. Int J Oral Maxillofac Surg. 1990;19(2): 74–5.
43. Sekerci AE, Sisman Y, Etoz M, Bulut DG. Aberrant anatomical variation of maxillary sinus mimicking periapical cyst: a report of Two cases and role of CBCT in diagnosis. Case Rep Dent. 2013;2013: 757645.
44. Shelley AM, Rushton VE, Horner K. Canalis sinuosus mimicking a periapical inflammatory lesion. Br Dent J. 1999;186(8):378–9.
45. Hancock MA, Brown Jr CE, Hartman KS. Orthokeratinized odontogenic cyst presenting as a periapical lesion. J Endod. 1986;12(11):539–41.
46. Bhaskar SN. Oral surgery–oral pathology conference No. 17, Walter Reed Army Medical Center. Periapical lesions–types, incidence, and clinical features. Oral Surg Oral Med Oral Pathol. 1966;21(5):657–71.
47. Lalonde ER, Luebke RG. The frequency and distribution of periapical cysts and granulomas. An evaluation of 800 specimens. Oral Surg Oral Med Oral Pathol. 1968;25(6):861–8.
48. Brannon RB. The odontogenic keratocyst. A clinicopathologic study of 312 cases. Part I. Clinical features. Oral Surg Oral Med Oral Pathol. 1976;42(1):54–72.
49. Stockdale CR, Chandler NP. The nature of the periapical lesion–a review of 1108 cases. J Dent. 1988;16(3):123–9.
50. Stajcic Z, Paljm A. Keratinization of radicular cyst epithelial lining or occurrence of odontogenic keratocyst in the periapical region? Int J Oral Maxillofac Surg. 1987;16(5):593–5.
51. Garlock JA, Pringle GA, Hicks ML. The odontogenic keratocyst: a potential endodontic misdiagnosis. Oral Surg Oral Med Oral Pathol Oral Radiol Endod. 1998;85(4):452–6.
52. Nohl FS, Gulabivala K. Odontogenic keratocyst as periradicular radiolucency in the anterior mandible: two case reports. Oral Surg Oral Med Oral Pathol Oral Radiol Endod. 1996;81(1):103–9.
53. Faitaroni LA, Bueno MR, De Carvalhosa AA, Bruehmueller Ale KA, Estrela C. Ameloblastoma suggesting large apical periodontitis. J Endod. 2008; 34(2):216–9.
54. Kashyap B, Reddy PS, Desai RS. Plexiform ameloblastoma mimicking a periapical lesion: a diagnostic dilemma. J Conserv Dent. 2012;15(1):84–6.
55. Cunha EM, Fernandes AV, Versiani MA, Loyola AM. Unicystic ameloblastoma: a possible pitfall in periapical diagnosis. Int Endod J. 2005;38(5):334–40.
56. Curran AE, Miller EJ, Murrah VA. Adenomatoid odontogenic tumor presenting as periapical disease. Oral Surg Oral Med Oral Pathol Oral Radiol Endod. 1997;84(5):557–60.
57. Philipsen HP, Srisuwan T, Reichart PA. Adenomatoid odontogenic tumor mimicking a periapical (radicular) cyst: a case report. Oral Surg Oral Med Oral Pathol Oral Radiol Endod. 2002;94(2):246–8.
58. De Lange J, Van den Akker HP. Clinical and radiological features of central giant-cell lesions of the jaw. Oral Surg Oral Med Oral Pathol Oral Radiol Endod. 2005;99(4):464–70.
59. Dahlkemper P, Wolcott JF, Pringle GA, Hicks ML. Periapical central giant cell granuloma: a potential endodontic misdiagnosis. Oral Surg Oral Med Oral Pathol Oral Radiol Endod. 2000;90(6):739–45.
60. Glickman GN. Central giant cell granuloma associated with a non-vital tooth: a case report. Int Endod J. 1988;21(3):224–30.
61. Lombardi T, Bischof M, Nedir R, Vergain D, Galgano C, Samson J, et al. Periapical central giant cell granuloma misdiagnosed as odontogenic cyst. Int Endod J. 2006;39(6):510–5.
62. Selden HS. Central giant cell granuloma: a troublesome lesion. J Endod. 2000;26(6):371–3.
63. Galgano C, Samson J, Kuffer R, Lombardi T. Focal cemento-osseous dysplasia involving a mandibular lateral incisor. Int Endod J. 2003;36(12):907–11.
64. Drazic R, Minic AJ. Focal cemento-osseous dysplasia in the maxilla mimicking periapical granuloma. Oral Surg Oral Med Oral Pathol Oral Radiol Endod. 1999;88(1):87–9.

65. Rodrigues CD, Estrela C. Traumatic bone cyst suggestive of large apical periodontitis. J Endod. 2008; 34(4):484–9.
66. Abbott PV. Traumatic bone cyst: case report. Endod Dent Traumatol. 1992;8(4):170–5.
67. Martins MD, Taghloubi SA, Bussadori SK, Fernandes KP, Palo RM, Martins MA. Intraosseous schwannoma mimicking a periapical lesion on the adjacent tooth: case report. Int Endod J. 2007;40(1): 72–8.
68. Buric N, Jovanovic G, Pesic Z, Krasic D, Radovanovic Z, Mihailovic D, et al. Mandible schwannoma (neurilemmoma) presenting as periapical lesion. Dentomaxillofac Radiol. 2009;38(3):178–81.
69. Rodrigues CD, Villar-Neto MJ, Sobral AP, Da Silveira MM, Silva LB, Estrela C. Lymphangioma mimicking apical periodontitis. J Endod. 2011;37(1):91–6.
70. Hutchison IL, Hopper C, Coonar HS. Neoplasia masquerading as periapical infection. Br Dent J. 1990; 168(7):288–94.

Case Selection and Treatment Planning

3

Peter Jonasson and Thomas Kvist

Abstract

The first part of this chapter is concerning cases of exploratory surgery. The section about alleviation of symptoms of apical periodontitis focuses on drainage. Indications for endodontic surgery in cases of ongoing root canal treatment are discussed. A method for retrograde root canal treatment in case of difficult orthograde access is presented. The discussion about root-filled teeth without unsatisfactory healing results occupies lion's share of this chapter. Special attention is given to the controversies of "success" and "failure" in endodontics. Factors that generally point to a surgical approach to endodontic retreatment are examined. The meaning of informed consent is in particular focus. This chapter ends up with an examination of the medical considerations, which is the basis for the risk assessment of the individual patient compulsory before any endodontic surgery.

Endodontic Surgery

There is no absolute or generally accepted definition of endodontic surgery. In this chapter, we decided to use the following definition: endodontic surgery is perceived as any method to reach, diagnose and treat the root canal and periradicular region of a tooth by means of surgical access through the oral mucosa and bone surrounding the affected tooth.

There are four main categories of indications for performing such a procedure:

1. To explore the periradicular tissues in order to make a proper diagnosis
2. To drain a periapical abscess in order to relieve symptoms of pain or swelling
3. To get access to and treat a previously untreated root canal
4. To get access to and treat a previously root-filled root canal

P. Jonasson, DDS, PhD • T. Kvist, PhD, DDS (✉)
Department of Endodontology,
Institute of Odontology at The Sahlgrenska Academy,
University of Gothenburg, Box 450,
SE 405 30 Göteborg, Sweden
e-mail: peter.jonasson@odontologi.gu.se;
kvist@odontologi.gu.se

I. Tsesis (ed.), *Complications in Endodontic Surgery*,
DOI 10.1007/978-3-642-54218-3_3, © Springer-Verlag Berlin Heidelberg 2014

In the following, each category will be discussed separately. Medical considerations of endodontic surgery are addressed in the concluding part of this chapter.

Diagnostic and Exploratory Endodontic Surgery

There are a few situations where the clinician decides to enter the periradicular tissues in order to investigate and examine to make a correct diagnosis and at the same time implement an appropriate surgical procedure.

A Root-Filled Tooth That Is Painful to Palpation but Without Other Signs of Apical Periodontitis

As many as 9 % of the teeth have shown to have small window-like openings or defect in the alveolar plate of the bone, frequently exposing a portion of the root, usually located on the facial aspect of the alveolar process [36, 66]. These findings have been confirmed by a recent cone beam computed tomography (CBCT) analysis on patients with periradicular defects of endodontic origin [82].

Pain associated with the presence of apical fenestration may occur after root canal treatment [9, 60]. Even slight instrumentation, irrigation or filling beyond the apical terminus of the root canal may irritate the periosteum and the overlying mucosa. The tooth may be spontaneously sensitive only occasionally, but pain is usually perceived during palpation of the area and masticatory movements. When elevating a flap over a suspicious root tip area, the operator hence could expect to find a root tip without covering cortical bone. The treatment consists of removing all pathological tissue, a root resection, an ultrasonic tip preparation and a root-end filling. Special attention should be done to foreign bodies such as pieces of bone or root and gutta-percha or sealer that sometimes are found embedded in the undersurface of the flap.

A Root-Filled Tooth with a Suspicion of Vertical Fracture or Pathology Other than That of Endodontic Origin

Vertical root fracture may mimic periodontal disease or a persistent apical periodontitis with an endo-perio lesion [84]; these cases often result in referral to a periodontist or endodontist for evaluation.

Newer methods of analysis are currently being studied, such as cone beam computed tomography, in order to help identify longitudinal fractures in a non-destructive fashion [45]. However, when there is doubt about the diagnosis and when the fracture cannot be visualized either on radiographs or clinically despite the use of an operator microscope, there is an indication for an exploratory surgery.

The only predictable treatment is removal of the fractured root or extraction of the tooth. In multirooted teeth, removal of the fractured root may be performed by root amputation (root resection) or hemisection (see Chap. 2).

Caution during endodontic diagnosis is mandatory, because periapical diseases of non-endodontic origin can mimic the more common infections of endodontic origin [19, 20, 22, 42, 67, 69]. If there is a slightest suspicion of disease of nonendodontic origin, a surgery to remove the lesion with subsequent submission for histopathological evaluation is required and compulsory. The records should indicate the size, colour, location and any other characteristics that might be useful for the pathologist (see Chap. 2).

To Drain a Periapical Abscess in Order to Relieve Symptoms of Pain or Swelling

Pulpal and periapical pathology is evolving as a response to microbiological challenges and mainly as a consequence to dental caries. As long as the substantial part of the pulp remains, vital signs of apical periodontitis are usually not evident either clinically or radiographically. Inflammation in the pulp can many times be reversed in its early stages if it is properly treated by withdrawal of the causes of inflammation and protected by proper filling materials. But in many situations, pulpal inflammation will be irreversible and continue and spread throughout the entire pulpal space. This process can be quick or slow and be accompanied by toothache (symptomatic pulpitis) but can also be painless. As the pulp becomes necrotic, the microbiota of the mouth will invade the necrotic pulpal tissue. Outside the root canal system and close and adjacent to the foramina, the host defence will develop an inflammatory reaction, i.e. apical periodontitis. One of the main features of apical periodontitis is the appearance of an osteolytic area due to the increased activity of osteoclasts. In early stages the loss of mineral is not enough to be detected in traditional (i.e. intraoral) radiographs. However, eventually a more or less clearly visible periapical radiolucency will develop. Most inflammatory periapical lesions associated with an infected necrosis of the root canal system prevail without clinical or subjective signs (pain, tenderness, fistulae or swelling). However, symptomatic apical periodontitis may develop spontaneously or in conjunction with a root canal treatment (endodontic flare-up). The symptoms may be associated with or without a soft tissue swelling. The swelling can be categorized into two different types, an abscess or cellulitis.

Apical Abscess

An apical abscess may develop rapidly and be extremely painful. A pressure builds up in the periodontal space or in the bony lesion of the affected tooth by the accumulating pus. As the amount of pus is increasing, the abscess may eventually perforate the cortical bone and mount up under the periosteum. In this stage a distinct clinically visible intra- or extraoral, or both, swelling may well have manifested. On palpation, a subperiosteal abscess often feels hard and very tender. As the process proceeds, the abscess breaks through the periosteum and is amassed in the mucosal tissue. After this event, the pain is usually alleviated but swelling may be substantial. On palpation the lesion fluctuates. The position of the swelling may vary but is usually in direct proximity to the affected tooth. In this situation, there may be an indication for incision for drainage. The objective is to establish a communication between the internally pressurized inflamed and infected tissue and the oral cavity (or sometimes extraoral) in order to alleviate patients' symptoms and prevent spread of infection to anatomical spaces. Spread of an infection may, occasionally, lead to life-threatening conditions that demand immediate hospital care. In particular, abscesses that may spread to the sublingual space and lead to elevation of the tongue followed by occlusion of the airways or towards the eye and ophthalmic vein, which in turn is in contact with the brain through the cavernous sinus, are of concern.

Cellulitis

While the term abscess is used for a localized collection of pus, cellulitis is the term that refers to a disseminated oedematous spreading of inflammation through the connective tissues and fascial planes. The typical clinical feature of cellulitis with endodontic origin is diffuse swelling of facial and cervical tissues. The condition is usually a sequel of an apical abscess and may or may not be accompanied by systemic symptoms such as fever and malaise.

Drainage

Based on the pathophysiological background of apical periodontitis, the traditional "ubi pus, ibi evacua" holds for a rule of thumb. When pus is accumulated in the tissues due to a necrotic or sometimes previously treated and root-filled tooth, drainage is an option that always should be considered. As an alternative to surgical incision of an abscess, drainage through the root canal of the affected tooth may first be taken into account.

Drainage Through the Root Canal

Trying to obtain drainage through the root canal is a potential opportunity in every situation of symptoms from the apical tissue. Even if the patient has not developed any clinically observable swelling, pus may have accumulated in the apical tissues and exert a pressure that can be remedied by leaving the area via the root canal. But even if the patient has developed a clear clinical observable abscess or swelling is more diffuse, a trepanation and instrumentation of the tooth sometimes lead to spontaneous pus drainage from the root canal. After diagnostic procedures, the involved tooth is identified. If the root canal treatment (RCT) is considered suitable as a first choice, it is important to consider any time constraints. If RCT is going to be carried out, the protocol should hold same level of high quality (appropriate access, aseptic technique, working length determination, instrumentation of root canals, rinse with antimicrobial substance and preferably applying an intracanal dressing and temporary restoration) as in any case of RCT. At times drainage occurs immediately when the pulp chamber is exposed. In other cases, drainage starts when root canal instrumentation is initiated or proceeds. Sometimes drainage can be obtained by carefully bypassing the apical foramen using a thin root canal instrument. However, great care should be taken in order to avoid over-instrumentation. Therefore only thin files with apical sizes ISO 06–20 should be used. Otherwise, the procedure may jeopardize the endodontic prognosis in long term. If an abundant amount of pus does drain from the root canal, it may be tempting for the clinician to leave the root canals open for a couple of days. However, many endodontists hesitate to such a procedure because of the severe contamination problem and the potential of endangering the possibilities to healing because of the establishment of a more resistant microbiota. A better approach may be to let the patient sit or lie down for 15–30 min in order to facilitate the apical tissue pressure. Depending on the amount of drainage obtained from the root canal system during the initiated RCT, the clinician can either choose to refrain from further attempts to create drainage or add a surgical incision. If RCT was considered not feasible, surgical incision may also be the only active measure.

Drainage Through Surgical Incision

The indication for a surgical incision is quite clear if the swelling of the soft tissues is well localized and fluctuant, indicating a submucosal abscess. However if the swelling is still localized but feels hard and nonfluctuant on palpation, hence indicating a subperiosteal position of the pus, many clinicians show reluctance to incise since concern exists as to the risk of causing spread of microorganisms and worsening of the condition. In many situations, however, the clinician may have difficulties in distinguishing between a true submucosal or subperiosteal abscess, and incision may be attempted even if an obvious fluctuant abscess is not present. The lack of scientific evidence on this issue leaves the clinician to adhere to his or her clinical experience and judgement [68] (Fig. 3.1).

To Get Access to and Treat a Previously Untreated Root Canal

A Continuously "Weeping" Root Canal

A root canal treatment can usually be completed in one or two visits. However, there are situations in which a root canal treatment is difficult to terminate and close because the root canal system or surrounding tissues continue to give clinical signs of ongoing severe inflammation. Two different situations can easily be recognized.

The first is when the root canal despite proper root canal treatment continues to fill up with serous exudate, pus or blood. The clinician might have postponed the root filling procedure several weeks or even months using an intracanal dressing with calcium hydroxide. Despite these attempts, when opening the tooth, it is still impossible to achieve a dry root canal. Under

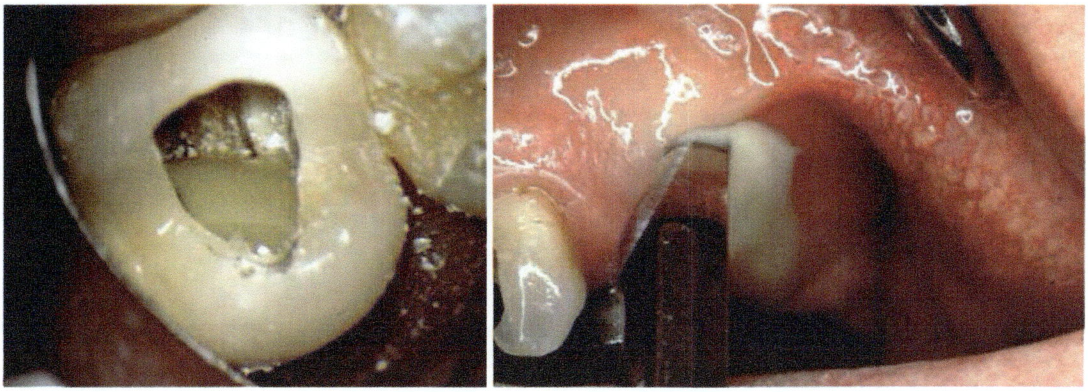

Fig. 3.1 Drainage of pus from a periapical abscess may be obtained through the root canal or by a surgical incision

such circumstances, there is an indication to get surgical access to the periradicular tissues before root canal obturation. Two different strategies may be considered. If the procedure is not foreseen to be too complicated or time-consuming, the surgical access and root canal filling can be accomplished in one treatment session. The first step is to expose the inflamed periapical region by surgical means. The granulation tissue or radicular cyst present in the bony crypt is removed, and before suturing the flap, the root canal is exposed preferably under normal aseptical considerations (rubber dam, sterile instruments). The surgeon covers the wound with the flap without suturing. The root canal is cautiously irrigated with a low concentration of sodium hypochlorite and possibly EDTA. Immediately after finishing the irrigation the canal is dried and root filled with gutta-percha and sealer. Overfill of the canal is of minor concern since any excess of root filling material easily can be removed from the apical area during a final cleaning of the apical area before suturing the flap. As an alternative, the root canal may be filled with gutta-percha with a retrograde root filling technique (see under Situations of unfavourable access through the crown). One other option is that after removal of the periapical pathology, the root end is filled with an MTA plug and the root canal is left with a temporary dressing with calcium hydroxide. The permanent root filling procedure is postponed until a later visit (preferably when the soft tissues have healed and sutures have been removed, usually 1–6 weeks after surgery).

In other situations clinical signs of apical periodontitis, i.e. fistulae, swelling or pain, do not alleviate or cure despite a diligent and proper root canal treatment. The root canal is dry and without signs of remaining infection inside the accessible parts of the root canal. In such a situation, it is considered an option to finalize orthograde root canal treatment and plan for an additional surgical access.

Situations of Unfavourable Access Through the Crown

Orthograde access to the root canal system in abutment teeth or in teeth with significant root canal calcification may pose risks for complications. An extensive drilling to identify and negotiate the canal system through the crown may lead to extensive loss of tooth substance and undermine the abutment and consequently cause prosthodontic failure [44, 47]. The use of the operating microscope obviously makes these procedures more predictable and less daring [37]. But still, a surgical approach as a primary endodontic treatment on specific indications may mean a less invasive procedure and fewer risks of complications [35, 56].

After a conventional method to endodontic surgical intervention, the canal is enlarged and cleaned with Hedstroem files held in a haemostat or with ultrasonic preparation. The root canal is

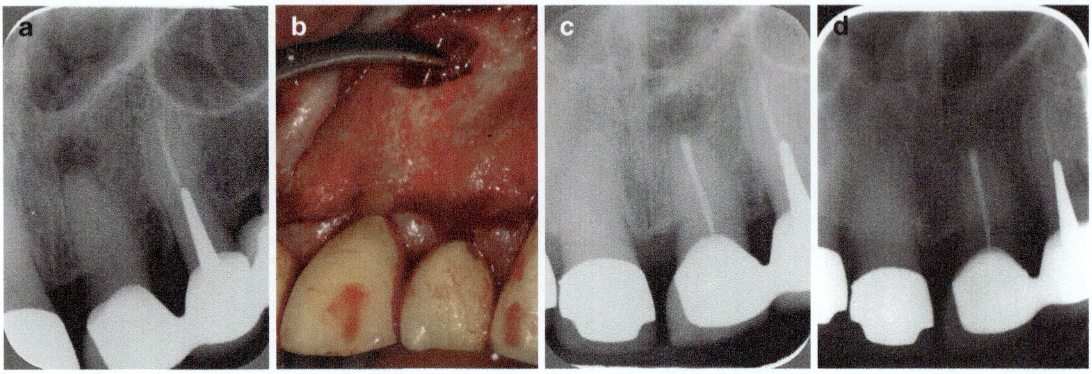

Fig. 3.2 Left central incisor with apical periodontitis and abutment tooth in a bridge. (a) Preoperative radiograph, (b) the root canal was instrumented with hand files in a haemostat, (c) postoperative radiograph with retrograde root canal filling with sealer and warm gutta-percha technique, (d) 1-year postoperative radiograph

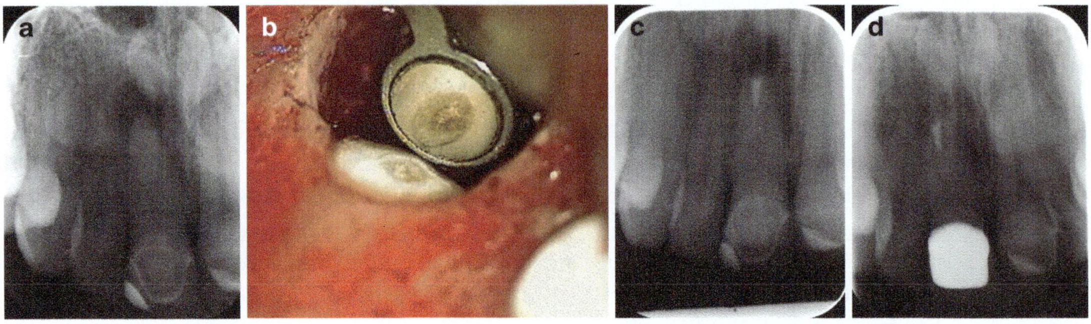

Fig. 3.3 Successful outcome of a surgical root canal treatment of a right central incisor with a root canal obliteration and apical periodontitis after trauma. (a) Preoperative radiograph, (b) the tip of the root-resected central incisor with an extensive root canal calcification, (c) postoperative radiograph with a limited retrograde filling with MTA due to canal obliteration, (d) healing after 1 year

cautiously irrigated during the preparation with a low concentration of sodium hypochlorite and EDTA. Following instrumentation, the canal is dried with paper points and filled with sealer, thermoplasticized gutta-percha and a matched single cone of gutta-percha (Fig. 3.2). In cases where only a limited part of the canal can be explored, alternative materials such as MTA (mineral trioxide aggregate) can be considered for the retrograde filling (Fig. 3.3). Surgical root canal treatment may primarily be considered for incisors and canines and in some two-rooted premolars. However, retrograde access varies between patients and in different parts of the jaws. The feasibility of retrograde root canal treatment should therefore carefully be investigated preoperatively, both clinically and radiographically.

In case reports, it has been shown that surgical root canal therapy has good potential to result in clinically and radiographically healthy periapical tissues [35]. Yet, there are no studies published which systematically compared the outcome of surgical root canal treatment with a conventional treatment protocol. Such studies are now being carried out [34].

To Get Access to and Treat a Previously Root-Filled Root Canal

A root canal treatment can be considered closed as the tooth receives a permanent root filling. Postoperative discomfort sometimes occurs, but after a short period most teeth become asymptomatic. Normally the tooth is restored with a filling or crown as soon as possible.

Successful Root Canal Treatments

For a root canal treatment to be considered completely successful in the long term, it requires not only that the tooth is functional and asymptomatic. When the root-filled tooth is examined clinically and radiographically, it should also be free of clinical signs of inflammation showing normal surrounding bony structures. If radiographic signs of inflammation persist, although presently asymptomatic, it is likely that the root-filled tooth is containing bacteria or other microorganisms. Pain and swelling may thus reoccur. The tooth may also be a source of infectious agents spread both locally and to the body's organs.

Failed Root Canal Treatments

When root-filled teeth cause pain and swelling, it is usually a sign of infection. Similarly, chronic clinical findings at the root-filled tooth in the form of redness, tenderness and fistulas are signs of the presence of microbiota in the root-filled tooth.

In these situations it is usually relatively straightforward to diagnose a persistent, recurrent or arising apical periodontitis. The treatment result is classified as a "failure". There is an obvious indication for a new treatment intervention, retreatment or extraction of the tooth (or sometimes only a root).

However, a common situation is that the root-filled tooth is both subjective and clinically asymptomatic, but an X-ray reveals that bone destruction has emerged or that the original bone destruction remains. In cases where no bony destruction was present when the root canal treatment was completed, and in particular in cases of vital pulp therapy, it can be reasonably assumed that an infection has set in the root canal system. For teeth that exhibited clear bone destruction at treatment start, there must be some time allowed for healing and bone formation to occur. One difficulty is to determine how long is the time required for such a healing process, both in general and in the particular case. The majority of root canal-treated teeth with bone destruction in the initial situation show signs of healing within 1 year [57]. In individual cases, however, the healing process can last for a long time [11, 72]. Molven et al. [46] has reported isolated cases requiring more than 25 years to completely heal. The finding that there are no absolute time limits as to when healing may occur can also be deduced from epidemiological studies [38].

Controversies of "Success" and "Failures" of Root Canal Treatment

Besides the time aspect, there is also a problem of determining what should be considered as a sufficient healing of bone destruction to constitute successful endodontic treatment. And as a consequence also, what establishes a "failure" and hence an indication for retreatment is far from unambiguous. According to the system launched by Strindberg [72], the only satisfactory post-treatment situation, after a predetermined healing period, combines a symptom-free patient with a normal periradicular situation. Only cases fulfilling these criteria were classified as "successes" and all others as "failures". In academic environments and in clinical research, this strict criteria set by Strindberg in 1956 has had a strong position.

However, the diagnosis of periapical tissues based on intra oral radiographs has repeatedly unmasked considerable inter- and intraobserver variation [63].

As an alternative, the periapical index (PAI) scoring system was presented by Orstavik et al. [58]. The PAI provides an ordinal scale of five scores ranging from "healthy" to "severe periodontitis with exacerbating features" and is based on reference radiographs with verified histological diagnoses originally published by Brynolf [10]. In this doctoral dissertation, the radiographic appearance of periapical tissue was compared with biopsies. The results indicated that using radiographs, it was possible to differentiate between normal states and inflammation of varying severity and that the likelihood of a correct diagnosis improved if more than one radiograph were taken. However, the studies were based on a limited patient spectrum, and the biopsy material was restricted to the upper anterior teeth. Among the researchers, the PAI is well established and it has been used in both clinical trials and epidemiological surveys. Researchers often transpose the PAI scoring system to the terms of Strindberg system by dichotomizing score 1 and 2 to "success" and score 3, 4 and 5 into "failure". However, the "cut-off" line is arbitrary and comparisons between the two systems for evaluation are lacking in the literature. The Strindberg system, with its originally dichotomizing structure into "success" and "failure", has achieved status as a normative guide to clinical action. Consequently, when a new or persistent periapical lesion is diagnosed in an endodontically treated tooth, failure is at hand and retreatment (or extraction) is indicated.

However, as early as 1966, Bender et al. [7] suggested that an arrested size of the bone destruction in combination with an asymptomatic patient should be sufficiently conditions for classifying a root canal treatment as endodontic success. More recently, Friedman and Mor [23] as well as Wu et al. [81] have suggested similar less strict classifications of the outcome of root canal treatment.

Uncertainties regarding the validity of the radiographic examination [8, 13, 55] are also of concern. For obvious practical and ethical reasons, only a limited number of studies have compared the histological diagnosis in root-filled teeth with and without radiographic signs of pathology [3, 10, 28]. In these studies, false-positive findings (i.e. radiographic findings indicate apical periodontitis while histological examination does not give evidence for inflammatory lesions) are rare. False-negative findings (i.e. radiographic findings indicate no apical periodontitis while histological examination does give evidence for inflammatory lesions) vary in the different studies. However, it is well known that bone destruction and consequently apical periodontitis may be present without radiographic signs visible in intraoral radiographs (Bender and Seltzer 1961, reprinted in *Journal of Endodontics* [5, 6]).

The advent of cone beam computed tomography (CBCT) has attracted much attention in endodontics in recent years. In vitro studies on skeletal material indicate that the method has higher sensitivity and specificity than intraoral periapical radiography. The higher sensitivity is confirmed in clinical studies. The major disadvantages of CBCT are greater cost and a potentially higher radiation dose, depending on the size of the radiation field being used. However, one benefit of the CBCT method is that it is relatively easy to apply. Moreover it provides a three-dimensional image of the area of interest, an advantage when assessing the condition of multirooted teeth. And the uncertainty of assessing results of endodontic treatment in follow-up using conventional intraoral radiographic technique has been pointed out [80]. Consequently, it has been suggested that CBCT should be used in clinical studies, because of the risk that conventional radiography underestimates the number of unsuccessful endodontic treatments. However, it may be important not to jump into conclusions since long-term studies are required to investigate if healing of periapical bone destruction may take longer than previously assumed. For example, at 1-year postendodontic treatment follow-up, CBCT can show persisting bone destruction, while a conventional intraoral radiograph shows healing [14]. This question is highly relevant and should be addressed in future research.

Prevalence of Failed Root Canal Treatments

The presence of subjective or clinical signs of failed root canal treatment is only occasionally reported in published follow-ups. The results are measured thus exclusively through an analysis of X-rays [52]. In epidemiological cross-sectional studies of periapical disease, the frequency of periapical radiolucencies in root-filled teeth varies between 25 and 50 % [18]. When periapical bone destruction is considered as a treatment failure and an indication for a new intervention, the potential retreatment cases are numerous.

An estimate of the prevalence of endodontic failure cases resulted in 1.7–3.6 million in Sweden, 3.3–7.1 million in Australia and 54–117 million in the USA [21]. The high frequency of root-filled teeth with periapical bone destructions seems to persist despite that the technical quality of root fillings has improved over time [24, 59].

Consequences of Apical Periodontitis in Root-Filled Teeth

Little is known about the frequency of persistent pain in root-filled teeth. From the available data in follow-up studies from university or specialist clinics, in a systematic review, the frequency of persistent pain >6 months after endodontic procedures was estimated to be 5 % [51]. The risks of persistent asymptomatic apical periodontitis in root-filled teeth is not yet very well known. A large majority of lesions remain asymptomatic with only small alteration in radiographically detectable size. It is known that this often silent inflammatory process sometimes turns acute with development of local abscesses that have the potential for life-threatening spreading to other parts of the body. However, the incidence and severity of exacerbation of apical periodontitis at root-filled teeth have met only scarce attention from researchers. Based on epidemiological data Eriksen [18] has estimated the risk of incidence of painful events at 5 % per year. Even lower risk (1–2 %) was reported from a cohort of 1032 root-filled teeth followed over time by Van Nieuwenhuysen et al. [79]. In a report from a university hospital clinic in Singapore, flare-ups in non-healed root-filled teeth occurred only in 5.8 % over a period of 20 years. However, less severe pain was experienced by another 40 % [83]. There have also been studies conducted in order to investigate if inflammatory processes of endodontic origin have an impact on the incidence of cardiovascular disease, but the results are contradictive [12, 15, 25].

Regarding the reason for referrals to specialist clinics, one study showed the main reason to be cases with an already root-filled tooth, followed by inability to control pain or to decide the correct diagnosis [29]. An Australian study found similar results, but with management of pain and technical difficulties outweighing the retreatment cases [1].

Variation in Clinical Decisions Regarding the Failed Root Treatments

The diagnostic difficulties, timing, the question of what should be regarded as healthy and diseased and several other factors partly explain the large variation among dentists regarding retreatment decision-making. This situation has been highlighted in numerous publications in recent years [40, 41, 62, 70]. From the bulk of investigations conducted, it stands clear that the mere diagnosis of apical periodontitis in a root-filled tooth does not consistently result in decisions for retreatment among clinicians. Theoretically four options are available. If retreatment is selected the decision-maker also has to make a choice between a surgical or nonsurgical approach:

- No treatment
- Monitoring
- Extraction
- Retreatment
  - Nonsurgical
  - Surgical

Patient Values

Given equal information and similar diagnostic findings, dentists will not invariably make the same clinical decision of a root-filled tooth with apical periodontitis. Neither will different patients choose the same clinical management despite identical information about apical periodontitis or any other disease by that matter. Both doctors' and patients' values will influence the decision-making process. The concept of value has many aspects, but it is reasonable to suppose that there is a close connection between an individual's values and his or her preferences and value judgements. The concept of personal values in clinical decision-making about apical periodontitis has been explored among both dental students and specialists by Kvist and Reit [39].

Substantial interindividual variation was registered in the evaluation of asymptomatic apical periodontitis in root-filled teeth. From a subjective point of view, some patients will benefit much more from endodontic retreatment than others.

Today patient autonomy is widely regarded as a primary ethical principle, emphasizing the importance of paying attention to the values and preferences of the individual patient.

Informed Consent

In the clinical situation, the requirement of respect for individual autonomy and integrity is managed through the concept of informed consent. The requirement that a medical or dental action should be preceded by informed consent is deemed very important in medical ethics [4].

The informed consent has two components: information and consent. But it is not enough that a patient has received written or oral information and then provided an informed consent. The patient must have accepted and understood the information and not only received it. All the relevant aspects of the situation should be informed about in a relevant way. It is also important that the patient has not misunderstood something he or she thinks is important for the decision. The dentist should not only convey information but also need to ensure that the information is correctly understood. In order to take a position in an independent way in a choice situation, the patient must be informed about the meaning of the alternatives, have understood the information and be free to choose, i.e. not be subjected to compulsion, or in such a position of dependence that the free informed choice becomes an illusion.

In a modern dental surgery, there are many situations that can hamper patient's ability to acquire and rationally process the information given. The environment may seem daunting and lead to both anxiety and worry, which can blur a generally well-functioning sense and judgement. To ascertain that the patient understands the information may thus be difficult. It is therefore important that the dentist is attentive to both verbal and non-verbal expressions.

Since many facts about the consequences of asymptomatic apical periodontitis in root filled are unknown, it is important that patients are free to choose what option they prefer. At the same time, one must have realistic expectations of the patient's ability to understand and evaluate the options – this can vary greatly between individuals. For patients who want to have full control over the decision, doctors should make sure to make this possible, but one must also allow the patient to hand over a part of decision-making if he or she so wishes. A professional reception of each individual patient at the dentist's office creates a seedbed for high confidence that the patient can feel safe with both for the decision-making and the treatment.

The medical ethical debate about informed consent is concerned not only on how information should be handled but also the forms of consent. In everyday clinical practice, an oral consent is normal and also appears naturally. A written agreement could be seen as well formal and might also get the patient to wonder what kind of exceptional measures that require such formalities. However, in many countries and in research contexts, it is quite common or even compulsory with written informed consent documentation.

Information About Treatment

One patient in the dental care can hardly be expected to have knowledge and understanding of all the factors that can and should be taken into consideration before a clinical decision about endodontic surgery. The patient has the right to know what the treatment entails, how risky and painful it is and what impact it is likely to bring with them to undergo treatment and to refrain from it. This implies a corresponding requirement for dental staff to ensure that this information is provided and that it is done in a way that the patient can actually understand. In practice, of course, there is a limit to how detailed the information can and should be. As long as the choice of methods, equipment and materials to carry out an endodontic surgery is considered as the standard, there is no reason to go into small details. If the patient asks many questions about the equipment and methods, this can be an expression of concern or, at worst, distrust rather than a genuine desire for more detailed information. As important as providing answers to all the questions then it is to try to establish or re-establish trust. The patient should be able to rely on dentist's knowledge based on science and proven experience and that they follow both the technological and scientific developments in the field. They should also be confident that the dentist has the best for the patient as their primary goal.

Information About Risks

For completeness of the information something must be said about the risks associated with the suggested treatment and about refraining from treatment. In this particular case, this is complicated significantly due to the fact that evidence is lacking about how the untreated apical periodontitis affects individuals both locally and systemically.

There are two basic aspects of risk: some kind of negative consequence and the probability that it will occur. The negative consequence or injury may be more or less severe. The most serious negative consequences in health care, including dentistry, are life-threatening. Such consequences are also highly unusual in dental practice including surgical procedures.

It is clearly important to inform the patient in the case of relatively high probability of severe consequences (if any treatments at all should be carried out), while it seems unimportant to communicate very unlikely minor damages. In many other cases, it is difficult to know how to do. If there had been only advantages to inform there would have been no reason to hesitate. What complicates the matter is that information in itself can cause injury. First, risk information may cause anxiety, and it can make patients refrain from treatments because of unrest despite that the risks otherwise would be reasonable to accept. This is why there may be reason to wonder, for example, whether to communicate a very small likelihood of great harm. Primarily because it is a concern from dentist's point of view to promote patient's oral health, but also from the autonomy perspective, it is sometimes questionable whether such information should be given. The fear of an unlikely but serious injury may counteract the ability of the patient to rationally reflect on the options and come to an autonomous decision. Exactly what considerations that should be made are debatable. How much and what to inform varies with the situation and who is the patient. Some patients prefer not to know the risks unless it is clearly relevant. The dentist needs to know in advance both those who are keen to get information and those who would prefer to avoid. If the patient visited the practice on a regular basis for several years and is well known, it may be possible for the dentist to give properly balanced information. But as in the case of endodontic surgery, where many patients have been referred to an endodontist or oral surgeon specifically for this treatment, the dentist is lacking this knowledge of the patient. Being in this situation, to ask the patient if he or she wants risk-related information does not work well because the patient will then easily conclude that the caregiver has important risk information because otherwise he or she would not have asked.

Information on Costs

When deciding about a tooth in need of endodontic surgery the economic aspect of the treatment is often one, if not decisive, then at least very important factor. Since surgical endodontics does not require the dismantling of functional prosthodontics constructions, it is often a less expensive alternative for the patient. But the costs of both surgical and nonsurgical treatment of course vary both in different countries between operators and between countries with different systems of reimbursement by insurance. It is important that information about the costs and possible reimbursement by insurance are correct and that it does not change.

Information and Manipulation

When the patient is informed about the facts regarding diagnoses, treatment options, risks and costs, he or she must be allowed to choose what she or he wants to do in the given situation. The individual has a right not to be forced or manipulated to undergo medical or dental treatments. However, it is difficult to imagine that the dentist can completely avoid the influence. The positive approach to good oral and dental health and, in this particular case, the importance of restoring periapical health are likely to affect the patient to some degree. One might think that it is also reasonable, since good periapical health is in the interests of the patient. Here, there is an important balancing act so that patient autonomy is not compromised. The endodontist or oral surgeon must develop sensitivity to patients' varying values and preferences. Particularly important is the responsiveness if the patient's ability to exercise their autonomy is compromised.

Authorized Informed Consent

Many patients lack all or part of the capacity for autonomous decision-making. It may involve children, mentally ill, mentally retarded or demented individuals. It is important to remember that these patients have the right to be treated with care and respect. A fruitful way to address the challenge of information and consent for these patients is to allow them to exercise their autonomy as best they can, and otherwise let them express their willingness or unwillingness to cooperate.

In the absence of the ability to understand, to take a stand and to make decisions, the informed consent can be authorized to a close relative or another person close to the patient.

Summary

Social development has led to the conclusion that we are currently seeing the patient's right to autonomous decision-making as an integral part of both dental care and other health services. Procedures for obtaining informed consent play a key role in safeguarding this right. In the context of endodontic surgery, informed consent means that the patient after having been informed of and understand the relevant aspects of the offered surgical procedure may determine whether to say yes or no to the dentists' suggestion of treatment. The information shall include a description of the course of treatment, the pros and cons of the surgery, and what it costs. Whether to perform a retreatment or not is a complex decision-making situation. Many factors have to be considered. For the dentist who made the diagnosis and who is about to suggest a treatment, both biological considerations and the potential and limitations of different options have to be deliberated. Equally important are the preferences of each individual patient. The subjective meaning of the situation will vary among patients. Only the patient is the expert on how he or she feels about keeping a tooth with or without retreatment or perhaps extracting it, which symptoms are tolerable, which risks are worth taking and what costs are acceptable.

Surgical or Nonsurgical Retreatment

There is insufficient scientific support to determine whether surgical and nonsurgical retreatment of root-filled teeth give systematically different outcomes, both short and long term, with respect to the healing of apical periodontitis or tooth survival [16, 73, 76]. In routine clinical practice, a number of factors influence the choice of treatment. For example, the size of the bone destruction, the technical quality of previous treatment, accessibility to the root canal, future restorative requirements of the tooth and the availability of various types of special equipment are briefly discussed below. Although future comparative studies may provide valuable general information, clinical decisions in every individual case will still have to be made on the basis that the conditions applied to every case are unique.

The Size of the Bone Destruction

Apical periodontitis may develop into cysts [49]. Periapical cysts are classified as "pocket cysts" or "true cysts". In case of a pocket cyst, the cyst cavity is open to the root canal and consequently it is expected to heal after proper conventional root canal treatment. The cavity of a true cyst, on the other hand, is completely enfolded by epithelial lining which may make it nonresponsive to any intracanal treatment efforts. Thus it is supposed that true radicular cysts have to be surgically resected in order to heal [48]. There is no scientific evidence to clinically determine the histological diagnosis of the periapical tissue in general, and in particular there is no method to distinguish between pocket cysts and true cysts [65]. However, cysts are expected to be more predominant among big bone destructions [50].

The Technical Quality of the Previous Treatment

In cases of non-healed apical periodontitis, the quality of the initial root treatment is often poor, which is frequently reflected in the technical quality of the root filling [24, 53]. In molars the reason for treatment failure may be associated with untreated canals [32]. In many cases therefore a nonsurgical retreatment should be considered. In particular this is the case when access is not hindered by a crown and post. Since there is convincing findings that the quality of the restoration also plays a significant role for the periapical status in root-filled teeth, the clinician should always have a critical look at the restoration [26, 61]. If restoration is of poor quality, it may jeopardize the results of an endodontic surgery [2, 86].

The obvious objective for a nonsurgical retreatment is to treat previously untreated parts of root canal system and thus improve the quality of root canal filling. With the help of modern endodontic armament, this is often possible to achieve. Studies have shown that nonsurgical retreatment performed by skilful clinicians results in good chances of achieving periapical healing [27, 54].

Several authors have argued that the result of endodontic surgery is dependent of a good quality of the root filling and consequently argued that any endodontic surgery should be preceded by a nonsurgical retreatment. The benefits of this treatment concept must nevertheless be questioned. No clear evidence exists of the benefit of this approach, and it would moreover, if used orderly, lead to the execution of an insignificant amount of unnecessary surgeries. In many cases the nonsurgical treatment would be sufficient to achieve healing of the periapical tissues.

Accessibility to the Root Canal

Root-filled teeth are often restored with posts and crowns and are frequently used as abutments for bridges and other prosthodontic constructions which have to be removed or passed through in case of a nonsurgical retreatment. In cases where the quality of restorations is adequate, therefore, the more complex the restoration, the more appealing an endodontic surgery approach. Even without hindering restorations, a preoperative analysis of the case may reveal intracanal ledges or fractured instruments that already preoperatively make the accessibility to the site of the residual infection questionable [27].

On the other hand, also access to the site of infection by endodontic surgery can also be judged to imply major difficulties. In particular, surgery involving mandibular molar roots as well as palatal roots of the maxillary teeth sometimes offers significant operator challenges. Preoperative CBCT scans help the surgeon to plan the intervention or sometimes to refrain and choose a nonsurgical approach or even considering extraction and a different treatment plan [64, 78] (Fig. 3.4a–h).

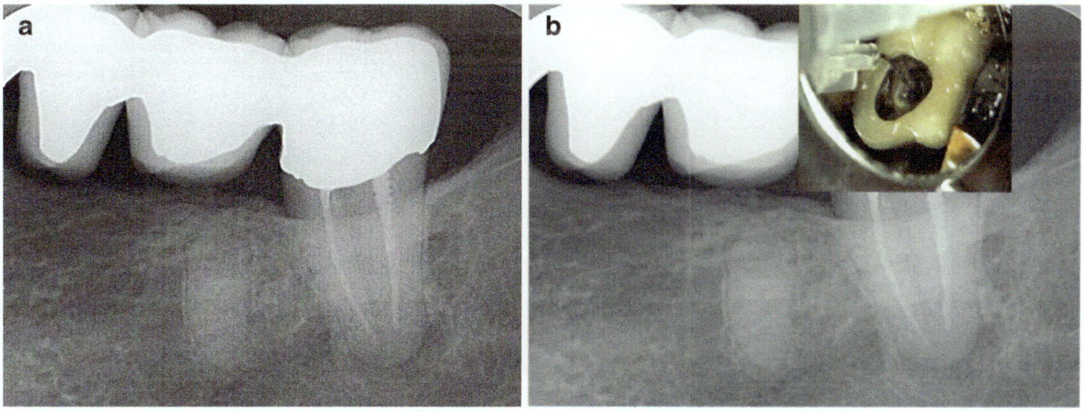

Fig. 3.4 (**a–h**) Persistent apical periodontitis in tooth 37. Abutment in a full arch bridge. Referred for endodontic surgery. CBCT shows difficult surgical access and a possible untreated mesiobuccal canal. Orthograde retreatment performed

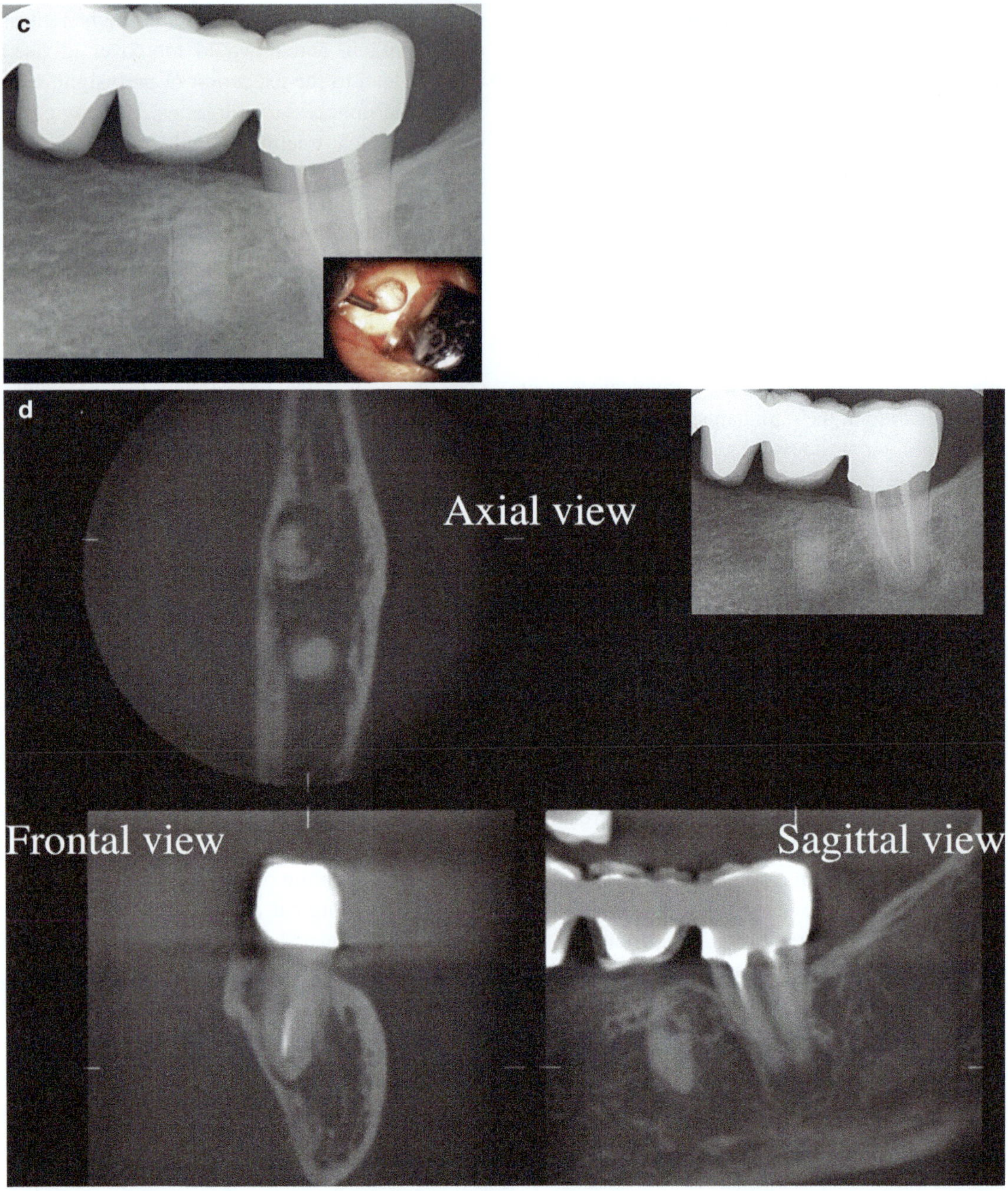

Fig. 3.4 (continued)

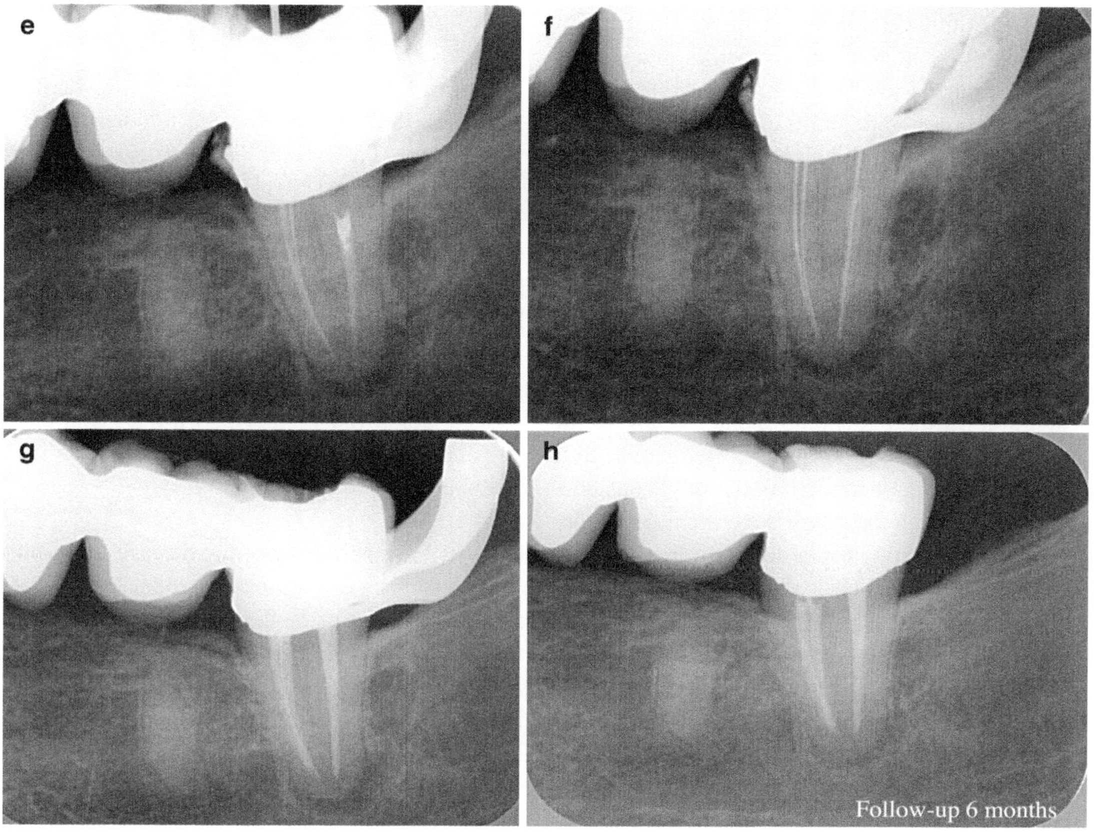

Fig. 3.4 (continued)

Future Restorative Requirements of the Tooth

Before considering retreatment of a previously root-filled tooth, there is a need for a careful deliberation of the overall treatment plan. In many cases, the issue is rather straightforward. It might concern a single tooth, restored with a post and a crown of fully acceptable quality but with an ensured diagnosis of persistent apical periodontitis. The objective is to cure the disease and to "save" the tooth and its restoration in the long term. In other situations, when complete mouth restorations are planned to "build something new", the strategic use of teeth, non-root filled as well as root filled, and dental implants to minimize the risk of failure of the entire restoration must be the first priority [85]. Long-term follow-up studies of teeth that have undergone surgical or nonsurgical retreatment are rare [71].

The Availability of Various Types of Special Equipment

Both endodontic surgery and nonsurgical retreatment techniques are often technically difficult, and the results that can be attained are very much dependent on the professional skills of the operator as well as his or her opportunity to modern equipment. Modern surgical endodontic treatment requires the use of magnification devices, preferably a dental operative microscope. Using the microscope, it has become easier to identify the root tip and to perform resection of the root with minimal bevel. Under the high magnification and illumination of the microscope, the resected root surface can be examined for canal fins, isthmi and lateral canals.

With the aid of an ultrasonic tip, these exits for the microorganisms can be instrumented and cleaned to a depth of at least 3–4 mm and sometimes significantly longer [77]. Finally with high precision, a root-end filling can accurately be placed to seal the root end [14]. Cases considered for endodontic surgery therefore might benefit from being referred to a specialist or an experienced colleague with special interest and training in modern endodontic surgery.

Medical Considerations in Endodontic Surgery

Attention for the patient's life and overall health must always have the highest priority in all health care including dentistry. Consequently, consideration of medical risks is of overarching importance when planning for endodontic surgery. It is a good clinical practice at all times and especially for patients with fragile general health to consider orthograde treatment to an endodontic problem rather than surgery. Conventional endodontics usually involves a minor medical burden on the individual compared to surgery. If endodontic surgery still is the first choice in a patient with serious medical conditions, it may be advantageous to delay the surgical endodontic treatment until other diseases have been medically treated and conditions are stabilized.

A careful medical history is mandatory before all types of dental interventions. If the patient has difficulty accounting for their health status or that it appears there are medical factors that would complicate treatment, a contact should be established with the treating physician. For each treatment, a risk assessment must be performed and it is a crucial part of the treatment planning. An overall estimate of medical risk of a patient can be made due to the physical status classification system adopted by the American Society of Anesthesiologists (ASA) in 1962 with a modification in five categories to the dental treatment situation [43].

ASA I

Patients are considered to be normal and healthy. Patients are able to walk up one flight of stairs or two level city blocks without distress. Little or no anxiety.

Little or no risk for treatment.

ASA II

Patients have mild to moderate systemic disease or are healthy ASA I patients who demonstrate a more extreme anxiety and fear towards dentistry. Patients are able to walk up one flight of stairs or two level city blocks but will have to stop after completion of the exercise because of distress.

Minimal risk during treatment.

Examples: History of well-controlled disease states including non-insulin-dependent diabetes, prehypertension, epilepsy, asthma or thyroid conditions; ASA I with a respiratory condition, pregnancy, and/or active allergies.

May need medical consultation.

ASA III

Patients have severe systemic disease that limits activity, but is not incapacitating. Patients are able to walk up one flight of stairs or two level city blocks, but will have to stop en route because of distress.

If dental care is indicated, stress reduction protocol and other treatment modifications are indicated.

Examples: History of angina pectoris, myocardial infarction, cerebrovascular accident, congestive heart failure over 6 months ago, slight chronic obstructive pulmonary disease and controlled insulin-dependent diabetes or hypertension.

May need medical consultation.

ASA IV

Patients have severe systemic disease that limits activity and is a constant threat to life. Patients are unable to walk up one flight of stairs or two level city blocks. Distress is present even at rest. Patients in this category pose a significant risk. Medical treatment must have priority over planned dental treatment. Whenever possible, elective dental care should be postponed until such time as the patient's medical condition has improved to at least an ASA III classification. Examples: History of unstable angina pectoris, myocardial infarction or cerebrovascular accident within the last 6 months, severe congestive heart failure, moderate to severe chronic obstructive pulmonary disease,

uncontrolled diabetes, hypertension, epilepsy, thyroid condition and extremely elevated hypertension.
Medical consultation is indicated.
ASA V
Patient is moribund and not expected to survive.
Dental treatment is definitely contraindicated.
Examples: End-stage renal, hepatic, infectious disease or terminal cancer.

Conditions and Situations of Special Attention in Endodontic Surgery

Risk of Spread of Infection

In areas with acute infections, surgical interventions should be limited to drainage of abscesses and be carried out to relieve symptoms and reduce the risk for spreading. More invasive surgical treatments might further exacerbate the emergency situation and cause spread of infection to other tissues and organs. Hence, endodontic surgery should only be performed once the infection is under control.

The frequency of bacteraemia is estimated to be between 20 and 100 % after oral surgical procedures [30, 74, 75]. It has been surmised that at least in healthy individuals, the bacteria are scavenged from the bloodstream relatively quickly within minutes up to 1 h by the innate and adaptive defence mechanisms. Due to the potential of microorganisms entering the blood to colonize tissues or artificial surfaces, antibiotics are prescribed to certain risk groups in some countries. However it must be emphasized that bacteraemia with oral microorganisms frequently occurs after daily activities such as tooth brushing and chewing. Even for endocarditis and late prosthetic joint infections, there is no consensus among experts on the need for prophylaxis and little scientific basis for the recommendations. The emerging trend seems to be to avoid the prophylactic use of antibiotics in conjunction with dental treatment unless there is a clear individual risk analysis and indication.

Tumours in Jaws

On suspicion of benignant or malignant jaw tumours adjacent to the area, endodontic surgery will be performed; a diagnosis should first be established by an extended examination with X-ray and biopsy.

Previous high-dose irradiation to the head and neck may have affected the blood vessels of the jaws and as a consequence reduced the blood supply to the actual surgical site in the mandible [33].

An irradiated bone must always be treated with caution, as there is a risk of later developing osteoradionecrosis. Therefore, if possible, dental evaluation and necessary treatment should be a standard of care before irradiation, and questionable teeth should be removed. In case where endodontic surgery is considered after irradiation, more accuracy in considerations must be made based on an increased risk of postoperative infections and poor healing potential.

It may be considering prescribing prophylactic antibiotic, improving oral hygiene prior to surgery, minimizing the invasive interventions, limiting the use of agents for haemostasis control, reducing the time for surgery and more thoroughly cleaning of the surgical site before suturing.

Increased Risk of Bleeding

Patients treated with antiplatelet and anticoagulant agents may have an increased bleeding time and risk of intraoperative and postoperative haemorrhage complications.

Even though several antiplatelet and anticoagulant agents have been developed in recent years, acetylsalicylic acid (ASA) and warfarin are the standard drugs for preventing vascular diseases [17].

Stopping these drugs before a procedure exposes the patient to vascular problems with the potential for significant morbidity. The activity of anticoagulants is expressed using the international normalized ratio (INR). For an individual not taking anticoagulant or antiplatelet drugs, the normal coagulation profile is an INR of 1.0. Patients on medication have an optimal INR of

2.5 (range 2.0–3.0) that minimizes the risk of haemorrhage and thromboembolism [31] during the surgical procedure.

Patients with haemophilia or impaired liver function need special attention and should always be treated in close collaboration with a haematologist and hepatologist.

Immune System Deficiencies

There are several medical conditions and medications that cause a deterioration of the immune system, by the lack of white blood cells or the inability of a patient to produce antibodies. A differential count of white blood cells (leukocytes) gives an indication on whether the body will sustain an infection. Besides the number of cells, also blood cell differentiation and function are important to evaluate before surgery in immunocompromised patients. Those advanced analyses and assessments must be made by the physician who is responsible in treating the patient for his or her underlying disease.

References

1. Abbott PV. Analysis of a referral-based endodontic practice: Part 1. Demographic data and reasons for referral. J Endod. 1994;20(2):93–6.
2. Abramovitz I, Better H, Shacham A, Shlomi B, Metzger Z. Case selection for apical surgery: a retrospective evaluation of associated factors and rational. J Endod. 2002;28:527–30.
3. Barthel CR, Zimmer S, Trope M. Relationship of radiologic and histologic signs of inflammation in human root-filled teeth. J Endod. 2004;30:75–9.
4. Beauchamp TL, Childress JF. Principles of biomedical ethics. 5th ed. New York: Oxford University Press; 2001.
5. Bender IB, Seltzer S. Roentgenographic and direct observation of experimental lesions in bone: II. 1961. J Endod. 2003;29(11):707–12; discussion 701.
6. Bender IB, Seltzer S. Roentgenographic and direct observation of experimental lesions in bone: I. 1961. J Endod. 2003;29(11):702–6.
7. Bender IB, Seltzer S, Soltanoff W. Endodontic success – a reappraisal of criteria. Oral Surg Oral Med Oral Pathol. 1966;22:780–802.
8. Bhaskar SN. Bone lesions of endodontic origin. Dent Clin North Am. 1967;Nov:521–33.
9. Boucher Y, Sobel M, Sauveur G. Persistent pain related to root canal filling and apical fenestration: a case report. J Endod. 2000;26(4):242–4.
10. Brynolf I. Histological and roentgenological study of periapical region of human upper incisors. Odontol Revy. 1967;18 Suppl 11:1–176.
11. Bystrom A, Happonen RP, Sjogren U, Sundqvist G. Healing of periapical lesions of pulpless teeth after endodontic treatment with controlled asepsis. Endod Dent Traumatol. 1987;3:58–63.
12. Caplan DJ, Pankow JS, Cai J, Offenbacher S, Beck JD. The relationship between self-reported history of endodontic therapy and coronary heart disease in the Atherosclerosis Risk in Communities Study. J Am Dent Assoc. 2009;140:1004–12.
13. Carrillo C, Peñarrocha M, Bagán JV, Vera F. Relationship between histological diagnosis and evolution of 70 periapical lesions at 12 months, treated by periapical surgery. J Oral Maxillofac Surg. 2008;66:1606–9.
14. Christiansen R, Kirkevang LL, Gotfredsen E, Wenzel A. Periapical radiography and cone beam computed tomography for assessment of the periapical bone defect 1 week and 12 months after root-end resection. Dentomaxillofac Radiol. 2009;38:531–6.
15. Cotti E, Dessì C, Piras A, Flore G, Deidda M, Madeddu C, Zedda A, Longu G, Mercuro G. Association of endodontic infection with detection of an initial lesion to the cardiovascular system. J Endod. 2011;37:1624–9.
16. Del Fabbro M, Taschieri S, Testori T, Francetti L, Weinstein RL. Surgical versus non-surgical endodontic re-treatment for periradicular lesions (Review). Cochrane Database Syst Rev. 2007;18(3):CD005511
17. Dogné J-M, de Leval X, Benoit P, Delarge J, Masereel B, David JL. Recent advances in antiplatelet agents. Curr Med Chem. 2002;9:577–89.
18. Eriksen HM. Endodontology–epidemiologic considerations. Endod Dent Traumatol. 1991;7:189–95.
19. Estrela C, Decurcio DA, Silva JA, Mendonça EF, Estrela CR. Persistent apical periodontitis associated with a calcifying odontogenic cyst. Int Endod J. 2009;42(6):539–45.
20. Faitaroni LA, Bueno MR, De Carvalhosa AA, Bruehmueller Ale KA, Estrela C. Ameloblastoma suggesting large apical periodontitis. J Endod. 2008;34(2):216–9.
21. Figdor D. Apical periodontitis: a very prevalent problem. Oral Surg Oral Med Oral Pathol Oral Radiol Endod. 2002;94:651–2.
22. Figueiredo MAZ, Figueiredo JAP, Porter S. Root resorption associated with mandibular bone erosion in a patient with scleroderma. J Endod. 2008;34:102–3.
23. Friedman S, Mor C. The success of endodontic therapy-healing and functionality. J Calif Dent Assoc. 2004;32(6):493–503.
24. Frisk F. Epidemiological aspects on apical periodontitis. Studies based on the Prospective Population Study of Women in Göteborg and the Population Study on Oral Health in Jönköping, Sweden. Swed Dent J Suppl. 2007;(189):11–78.
25. Frisk F, Hakeberg M, Ahlqwist M, Bengtsson C. Endodontic variables and coronary heart disease. Acta Odontol Scand. 2003;61:257–62.

26. Gillen BM, Looney SW, Gu LS, Loushine BA, Weller RN, Loushine RJ, Pashley DH, Tay FR. Impact of the quality of coronal restoration versus the quality of root canal fillings on success of root canal treatment: a systematic review and meta-analysis. J Endod. 2011;37:895–902.
27. Gorni FG, Gagliani MM. The outcome of endodontic retreatment: a 2-yr follow-up. J Endod. 2004;30:1–4.
28. Green TL, Walton RE, Taylor JK, Merrell P. Radiographic and histologic periapical findings of root canal treated teeth in cadaver. Oral Surg Oral Med Oral Pathol Oral Radiol Endod. 1997;83:707–11.
29. Harty FJ. A survey of endodontic procedures performed by practitioners in limited practice. Int Endod J. 1992;25:25–8.
30. Heimdahl A, Hall G, Hedberg M, Sandberg H, Söder P-Ö, Tunér K, Nord CE. Detection and quantitation by lysis-filtration of bacteremia after different oral surgical procedures. J Clin Microbiol. 1990;28:2205–9.
31. Hirsh J, Dalen J, Anderson DR, Poller L, Bussey H, Ansell J, Deykin D. Oral anticoagulants: mechanism of action, clinical effectiveness, and optimal therapeutic range. Chest. 2001;119(suppl):8S-21.
32. Huumonen S, Kvist T, Gröndahl K, Molander A. Diagnostic value of computed tomography in retreatment of root fillings in maxillary molars. Int Endod J. 2006;39(10):827–33.
33. Jereczek-Fossa BA, Orecchia R. Radiotherapy-induced mandibular bone complications. Cancer Treat Rev. 2002;28:65–74.
34. Jonasson P, Lennholm C, Kvist T. Surgical versus conventional root canal treatment. A randomized controlled trial. 2014. In manuscript.
35. Jonasson P, Reit C, Kvist T. A preliminary study on the technical feasibility and outcome of retrograde root canal treatment. Int Endod J. 2008;41:807–13.
36. Jorgić-Srdjak K, Plancak D, Bosnjak A, Azinović Z. Incidence and distribution of dehiscences and fenestrations on human skulls. Coll Antropol. 1998;22(Suppl):111–6.
37. Khayat BG. The use of magnification in endodontic therapy: the operating microscope. Pract Periodontics Aesthet Dent. 1998;10:137–44.
38. Kirkevang LL, Vaeth M, Wenzel A. Ten-year follow-up observations of periapical and endodontic status in a Danish population. Int Endod J. 2012; 45(9):829–39.
39. Kvist T, Reit C. The perceived benefit of endodontic retreatment. Int Endod J. 2002;35:359–65.
40. Kvist T, Reit C, Esposito M, Mileman P, Bianchi S, Pettersson K, Andersson C. Prescribing endodontic retreatment: towards a theory of dentist behaviour. Int Endod J. 1994;27(6):285–90.
41. Kvist T, Heden G, Reit C. Endodontic retreatment strategies used by general dental practitioners. Oral Surg Oral Med Oral Pathol Oral Radiol Endod. 2004;97:502–7.
42. Lee JJ, Cheng SJ, Lin SK, Chiang CP, Yu CH, Kok SH. Gingival squamous cell carcinoma mimicking a dentoalveolar abscess: report of a case. J Endod. 2007;33(2):177–80.
43. Malamed SF. Medical emergencies in the dental office. 5th ed. St. Louis: Mosby; 2000. p. 41–4.
44. McMullen 3rd AF, Himel VT, Sarkar NK. An in vitro study of the effect endodontic access preparation has upon the retention of porcelain fused to metal crowns of maxillary central incisors. J Endod. 1989;15: 154–6.
45. Metska ME, Aartman IH, Wesselink PR, Özok AR. Detection of vertical root fractures in vivo in endodontically treated teeth by cone-beam computed tomography scans. J Endod. 2012;38:1344–7.
46. Molven O, Halse A, Fristad I, MacDonald-Jankowski D. Periapical changes following root-canal treatment observed 20–27 years postoperatively. Int Endod J. 2002;35:784–90.
47. Mulvay PG, Abbott PV. The effect of endodontic access cavity preparation and subsequent restorative procedures on molar crown retention. Aust Dent J. 1996;41:134–9.
48. Nair PN. New perspectives on radicular cysts: do they heal? Int Endod J. 1998;31:155–60.
49. Nair PN. Pathogenesis of apical periodontitis and the causes of endodontic failures. Crit Rev Oral Biol Med. 2004;15(6):348–81.
50. Natkin E, Oswald RJ, Carnes LI. The relationship of lesion size to diagnosis, incidence, and treatment of periapical cysts and granulomas. Oral Surg Oral Med Oral Pathol. 1984;57:82–94. Review.
51. Nixdorf DR, Moana-Filho EJ, Law AS, McGuire LA, Hodges JS, John MT. Frequency of persistent tooth pain after root canal therapy: a systematic review and meta-analysis. J Endod. 2010;36:224–30.
52. Ng YL, Mann V, Rahbaran S, Lewsey J, Gulabivala K. Outcome of primary root canal treatment: systematic review of the literature – part 1. Effects of study characteristics on probability of success. Int Endod J. 2007;40:921–39.
53. Ng YL, Mann V, Rahbaran S, Lewsey J, Gulabivala K. Outcome of primary root canal treatment: systematic review of the literature – Part 2. Influence of clinical factors. Int Endod J. 2008;41:6–31.
54. Ng YL, Mann V, Gulabivala K. A prospective study of the factors affecting outcomes of nonsurgical root canal treatment: part 1: Periapical health. Int Endod J. 2011;44:583–609.
55. Nobuhara WK, del Rio CE. Incidence of periradicular pathoses in endodontic treatment failures. J Endod. 1993;19:315–8.
56. Nygaard-Östby B. Introduction to endodontics. Oslo: Universitetsförlaget; 1971.
57. Orstavik D. Time-course and risk analyses of the development and healing of chronic apical periodontitis in man. Int Endod J. 1996;29:150–5.
58. Orstavik D, Kerekes K, Eriksen HM. The periapical index: a scoring system for radiographic assessment of apical periodontitis. Endod Dent Traumatol. 1986;2:20–34.
59. Pak JG, Fayazi S, White SN. Prevalence of periapical radiolucency and root canal treatment: a systematic review of cross-sectional studies. J Endod. 2012;38(9):1170–6.

60. Pasqualini D, Scotti N, Ambrogio P, Alovisi M, Berutti E. Atypical facial pain related to apical fenestration and overfilling. Int Endod J. 2012;45(7):670–7.
61. Ray HA, Trope M. Periapical status of endodontically treated teeth in relation to the technical quality of the root filling and the coronal restoration. Int Endod J. 1995;28:12–8.
62. Reit C, Gröndahl H-G. Management of periapical lesions in endodontically treated teeth. A study on clinical decision making. Swed Dent J. 1984;8:1–7.
63. Reit C, Hollender L. Radiographic evaluation of endodontic therapy and the influence of observer variation. Scand J Dent Res. 1983;91:205–12.
64. Rigolone M, Pasqualini D, Bianchi L, Berutti E, Bianchi SD. Vestibular surgical access to the palatine root of the superior first molar: "low-dose cone-beam" CT analysis of the pathway and its anatomic variations. J Endod. 2003;29(11):773–5.
65. Rosenberg PA, Frisbie J, Lee J, Lee K, Frommer H, Kottal S, Phelan J, Lin L, Fisch G. Evaluation of pathologists (histopathology) and radiologists (cone beam computed tomography) differentiating radicular cysts from granulomas. J Endod. 2010;36:423–8.
66. Rupprecht RD, Horning GM, Nicoll BK, Cohen ME. Prevalence of dehiscences and fenestrations in modern American skulls. J Periodontol. 2001;72(6):722–9.
67. Selden HS, Manhoff DT, Hatges NA, Michel RC. Metastatic carcinoma to the mandible that mimicked pulpal/periodontal disease. J Endod. 1998; 24(4):267–70.
68. Shanti RM, Aziz SR. Should we wait for development of an abscess before we perform incision and drainage? Oral Maxillofac Surg Clin North Am. 2011;23(4):513–8.
69. Slutzky-Goldberg I, Heling I. Healing of a fibrous dysplastic lesion in a permanent molar after endodontic therapy. J Endod. 2007;33(3):314–7.
70. Smith J, Crisp J, Torney D. A survey: controversies in endodontic treatment and re-treatment. J Endod. 1981;7:477–83.
71. Song M, Chung W, Lee SJ, Kim E. Long-term outcome of the cases classified as successes based on short-term follow-up in endodontic microsurgery. J Endod. 2012;38(9):1192–6.
72. Strindberg LZ. The dependence of the results of pulp therapy on certain factors. Acta Odontol Scand. 1956;14(Suppl 21):1–175.
73. Swedish Council on Health Technology Assessment. Rotfyllning – en systematisk litteraturöversikt (In Swedish), Swedish Council on Health Technology Assessment. Report 203, 2010. English translation, Methods of diagnosis and treatment in endodontics, available at http://www.sbu.se as well as on the ESE website.
74. Takai S, Kuriyama T, Yanagisawa M, Nakagawa K, Karasawa T. Incidence and bacteriology of bacteremia associated with various oral and maxillofacial surgical procedures. Oral Surg Oral Med Oral Pathol Oral Radiol Endod. 2005;99(3):292–8.
75. Tomas I, Alvarez M, Limeres J, Potel C, Medina J, Diz P. Prevalence, duration and aetiology of bacteraemia following dental extractions. Oral Dis. 2007;13(1):56–62.
76. Torabinejad M, Corr R, Handysides R, Shabahang S. Outcomes of nonsurgical retreatment and endodontic surgery: a systematic review. J Endod. 2009; 35:930–7.
77. Tsesis I, Rosen E, Taschieri S, Telishevsky Strauss Y, Ceresoli V, Del Fabbro M. Outcomes of surgical endodontic treatment performed by a modern technique: an updated meta-analysis of the literature. J Endod. 2013;39(3):332–9.
78. Tyndall DA, Kohltfarber H. Application of cone beam volumetric tomography in endodontics. Aust Dent J. 2012;57 Suppl 1:72–81.
79. Van Nieuwenhuysen JP, Aouar M, D'Hoore W. Retreatment or radiographic monitoring in endodontics. Int Endod J. 1994;27(2):75–81.
80. Wu MK, Shemesh H, Wesselink PR. Limitations of previously published systematic reviews evaluating the outcome of endodontic treatment. Int Endod J. 2009;42:656–66.
81. Wu MK, Wesselink P, Shemesh H. New terms for categorizing the outcome of root canal treatment. Int Endod J. 2011;44:1079–80.
82. Yoshioka T, Kikuchi I, Adorno CG, Suda H. Periapical bone defects of root filled teeth with persistent lesions evaluated by cone-beam computed tomography. Int Endod J. 2011;44(3):245–52.
83. Yu VS, Messer HH, Yee R, Shen L. Incidence and impact of painful exacerbations in a cohort with post-treatment persistent endodontic lesions. J Endod. 2012;38:41–6.
84. Zehnder M, Gold SI, Hasselgren G. Pathologic interactions in pulpal and periodontal tissues. J Clin Periodontol. 2002;29:663–71.
85. Zitzmann NU, Krastl G, Hecker H, Walter C, Waltimo T, Weiger R. Strategic considerations in treatment planning: deciding when to treat, extract, or replace a questionable tooth. J Prosthet Dent. 2010;104(2):80–91.
86. Zuolo ML, Ferreira MO, Gutmann JL. Prognosis in periradicular surgery: a clinical prospective study. Int Endod J. 2000;33:91–8.

Variations in Outcome of Endodontic Surgery

4

Sahng G. Kim

Abstract

Significant advances in the field of surgical endodontics have resulted in more predictable outcomes. A thorough understanding of the etiology of posttreatment endodontic disease will serve as a basis for better surgical treatment. Technically, EMS allows surgeons to have better opportunities to identify and eliminate the etiologies as compared to TES. In this chapter, the variations in outcomes between EMS and TES observed in the literature were identified by contrasting the differences in surgical techniques. A striking difference in success rates between the two surgical treatment modalities exists, and it is explained by the different techniques employed in achieving disinfection and attaining an adequate apical seal. Finally, the results of various outcome studies should be carefully interpreted with a full understanding of prognostic factors, because the hidden heterogeneity in different studies can alter the outcomes significantly.

Introduction

Surgical endodontic treatment may be indicated for teeth with apical periodontitis, when a nonsurgical re-treatment is impractical or unlikely to improve the previous results. Clinicians have long recognized more variations in outcome of endodontic surgery compared with that of nonsurgical endodontic treatment. For example, the success rate of endodontic surgery ranged from 19.40 % [1] to 96.8 % [2], whereas the success rates of nonsurgical root canal treatment were reported to be 68–85 % [3–5]. For this reason, endodontic surgery has been considered a less predictable and preferred method than nonsurgical endodontic treatment for both clinicians and patients. The variations in outcome of endodontic surgery may be due to be the differences in outcome criteria in each of the studies. However, the variations can still be observed even after the outcomes are reevaluated using an identical outcome criterion.

The greater opportunities available to address the etiology of apical periodontitis, facilitated by recent progress in the technical aspects of endodontic surgery, may explain the striking variations in outcomes of endodontic surgery among individual outcome studies. Indeed, a recent

S.G. Kim, DDS, MS
Division of Endodontics, Columbia University
College of Dental Medicine, 630 West 168
Street – PH7Stem #128, New York, NY 10032, USA
e-mail: sgk2114@columbia.edu

I. Tsesis (ed.), *Complications in Endodontic Surgery*,
DOI 10.1007/978-3-642-54218-3_4,

systematic review with a meta-analysis showed a striking difference in success rates between traditional endodontic surgery (TES) and endodontic microsurgery (EMS) [6]. In TES, root-end preparation was made with burs and root-end filling with amalgam with the aid of low-power magnification (0× to 4× loupes), whereas in EMS, root-end preparation was made with ultrasonics and root-end filling with intermediate restorative material (IRM) or ethoxybenzoic acid (EBA) or mineral trioxide aggregate (MTA) with the use of high-power magnification (10× and higher) [6]. The pooled success rate of EMS was 94 %, whereas that of TES was 59 % in the systematic review [6]. Interestingly, great advances in our armamentarium and techniques for nonsurgical therapy have not been translated into outcome improvements as significantly as surgical endodontic therapy [6–11]. It is perhaps due to already favorable outcomes of nonsurgical endodontic treatment compared to those of TES. It is also likely due to the difficulty in disinfecting the anatomically complex root canal system during the nonsurgical endodontic treatment compared to less complicated anatomical structures that challenge the endodontic surgeon.

In this chapter, the variations in outcomes of endodontic surgery will be discussed by contrasting the differences between TES and EMS in addressing the etiology of posttreatment endodontic diseases and the prognostic factors affecting the various outcomes.

Outcome Assessment

How do we define and evaluate the outcome of endodontic surgery? This question is critical for clinicians because if the outcome of endodontic surgery is not adequately assessed, it will lead to inaccurate postoperative clinical diagnosis and thus may result in an unnecessary treatment or failure to perform an adequate post-intervention treatment. Survival/nonsurvival and success/failure are the most widely used outcomes in the endodontic literature for outcome assessment. Survival is referred to as the presence of a tooth without any clinical symptoms. In contrast, success is defined as the presence of a tooth with no clinical signs and symptoms and the absence [12] or decrease [13, 14] in size of periapical radiolucency. Thus, it is reasonable to assume that survival rates are likely to be higher than success rates when outcome assessment is performed in the same group. Clinicians should base their clinical judgments on studies reporting success rather than survival if the outcome of a treatment is assessed from a perspective of wound healing, although survival/nonsurvival is considered useful when the outcomes of different treatment modalities are compared.

Common mistakes associated with outcome assessment include failure to evaluate clinical symptoms by clinical tests such as percussion and palpation or lack of radiographic interpretation at follow-up appointments. While a complete healing and unsatisfactory healing are easily discernible, clinicians may have difficulties in distinguishing incomplete healing (scar tissue) from uncertain healing. Molven et al. [14] illustrated the four radiographic categories of healing based on the Andreasen and Rud's classification of healing [13]. Incomplete healing (scar tissue), generally considered as success, shows no change or decrease in size of periapical radiolucency without any clinical symptoms (Fig. 4.1). Radiographically, scar tissue has an irregular periphery and asymmetrical radiolucency around the root apex and often exists unassociated with the root. Uncertain healing shows a decrease in size of periapical radiolucency, that is, however, still larger than twice the width of normal periodontal ligament space (Fig. 4.2). It shows a circular or semicircular periphery and symmetrical radiolucency around the root apex. Complete healing demonstrates complete bone repair with intact lamina dura and less than twice the width of normal periodontal ligament space with no clinical symptoms (Fig. 4.3). Unsatisfactory healing shows no change or an increase in size of apical radiolucency (Fig. 4.4). Cases showing unsatisfactory healing are considered as failures and require immediate post-intervention treatments. If untreated, patients may experience continued

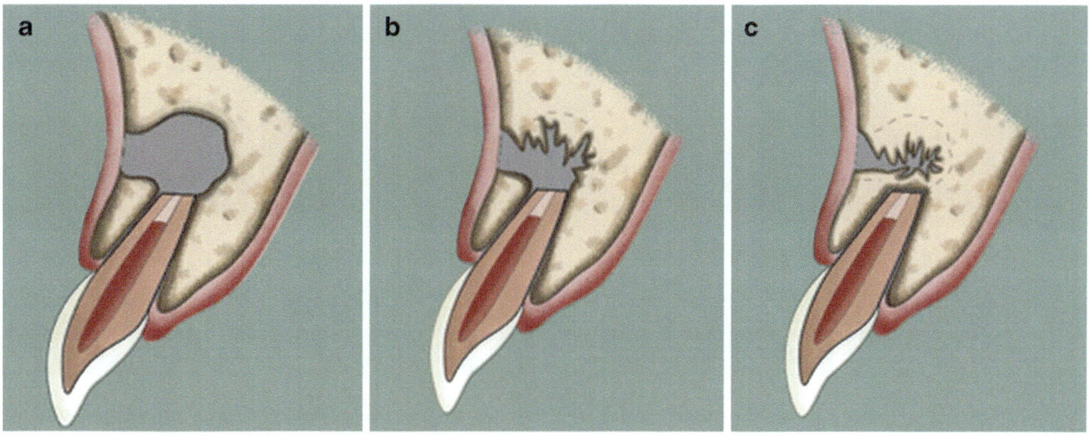

Fig. 4.1 Incomplete healing (scar tissue). (**a**) Surgical bony defect after endodontic surgery. (**b**) Reduction in size of a periapical bony defect by bone formation from periphery. Note the irregular border of the defect. (**c**) Further reduction in size of the periapical bony defect. Note that the residual defect is not associated with the root

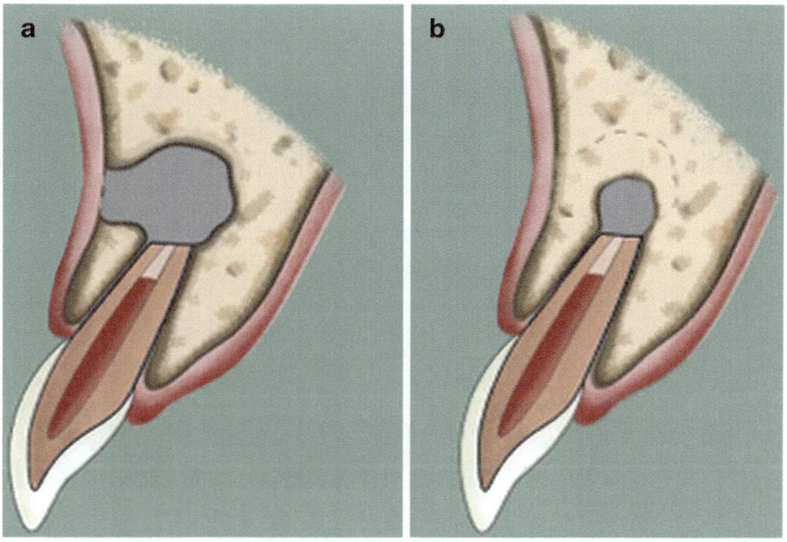

Fig. 4.2 Uncertain healing. (**a**) Surgical bony defect after endodontic surgery. (**b**) Reduction in size of a periapical bony defect by bone formation from periphery. Note that the size of the bony defect is larger than twice the width of normal periodontal ligament space

bone loss as well as other signs and symptoms such as pain, sinus tract, and swelling. The extensive bone loss in these cases may complicate future implant placement, which necessitates guided tissue regeneration or bone grafting after tooth extraction.

Due to the dynamic nature of wound healing, clinicians should be aware that postoperative diagnoses might change in some cases at different follow-up time points. Rud et al. [15] showed that based on the observation of 1,000 endodontic surgery cases, more than half of the cases with incomplete healing and uncertain healing underwent changes into other healing groups while almost all cases with complete healing and unsatisfactory healing remained unchanged. Notably, it was observed that these changes occurred mainly during the first year after the surgery and remained stable after the 4-year follow-up [15]. Therefore, clinicians are advised to have a 1-year follow-up as the first time point for outcome assessment and also

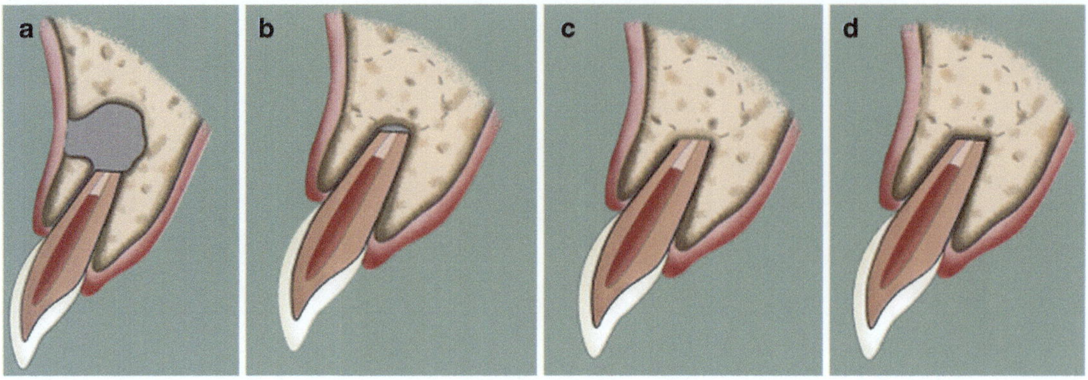

Fig. 4.3 Complete healing. (**a**) Surgical bony defect after endodontic surgery. (**b**) Significant reduction in size of a periapical bony defect by bone formation from periphery. Note that the size of the bony defect is no greater than twice the width of normal periodontal ligament space. (**c**) Complete bone fill without reestablishment of normal periodontal ligament space. (**d**) Complete bone fill with reconstitution of the periodontal ligament and lamina dura

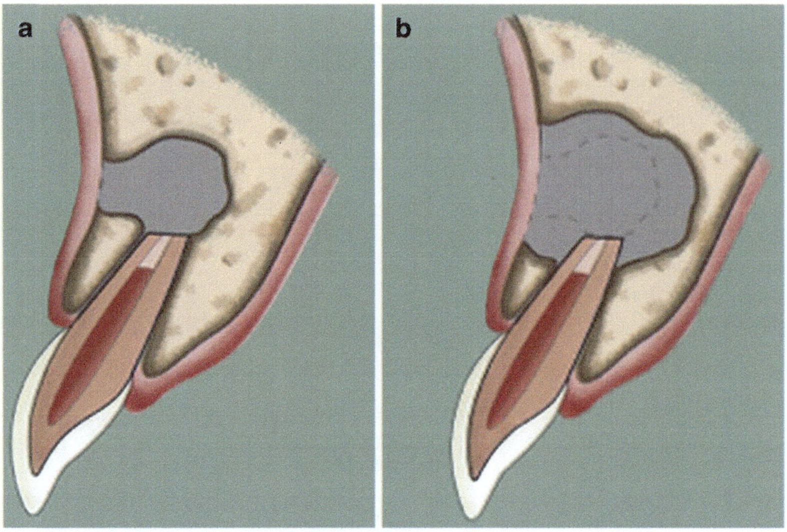

Fig. 4.4 Unsatisfactory healing. (**a**) Surgical bony defect after endodontic surgery. (**b**) Increase in size of a periapical bony defect by bone resorption in periphery

recommended to have follow-ups up to 4 years in cases of uncertain healing before any further treatment is considered.

Etiology of Posttreatment Endodontic Diseases

The key to success of endodontic surgery is to identify and eliminate the origins or causes of apical periodontitis, which could not be addressed by nonsurgical root canal treatment. They include intraradicular infection and extraradicular etiologies.

Can Intraradicular Infection Be Successfully Treated by Root-End Surgery?

Posttreatment endodontic diseases caused by intraradicular infection in most cases can be treated by nonsurgical endodontic re-treatment. Despite technical advances in our disinfection armamentariums, anatomically complex areas in root canals such as isthmuses and fins that potentially harbor pathogenic microorganisms are not easily accessible due to the limitations of our instrumentation techniques during nonsurgical therapy [16–20]. Iatrogenic errors such as canal transportation and separated instruments that impair thorough root canal disinfection may be another significant factor contributing to failure of nonsurgical re-treatment [21, 22].

While endodontic surgery provides less opportunity to disinfect the entire root canal system than nonsurgical root canal treatment, in clinical situations where sufficient intracanal preparation and sealing cannot be obtained, endodontic surgery is a preferred alternative for teeth with apical periodontitis.

Can Extraradicular Etiologies Be Successfully Eliminated by Root-End Surgery?

If the source of infection or the cause of apical periodontitis resides in extraradicular areas [23–29], endodontic surgery is essential for healing. The strategy to cure apical periodontitis in these situations is rather straightforward. The elimination of the origin or cause of the periapical lesion by surgical debridement can lead to the resolution of apical periodontitis.

With the introduction of molecular methods to detect the microorganisms, a growing body of evidence exists to support the view that microorganisms exist in the extraradicular space [30, 31]. The existence of biofilms on the extraradicular surfaces also has been clearly demonstrated in microscopic observational studies [27, 28]. Biofilms can have up to 1,000 times more resistance than their planktonic counterpart [32–34]. Foreign materials beyond the apical foramen may also cause persistent apical periodontitis [35]. Lentil beans [36, 37], cellulose from paper points and cotton wool [38, 39], and small gutta-percha particles [40] may induce chronic inflammatory reaction and foreign body reaction because these materials are not easily degraded by host immune cells [35, 41]. Cholesterols derived from dead host blood and immune cells and plasma lipids [42, 43] are endogenously induced but also cause similar inflammatory reaction and result in persistent apical periodontitis (Fig. 4.1) [44, 45].

The incidence of cysts in periapical pathosis varies greatly between 6 and 54 % [46–50], and it is generally agreed that cystic lesions are less likely to be resolved by nonsurgical endodontic treatment [50–52]. A pocket cyst (bay cyst) where the cyst lumen is continuous with the root canal may resolve with nonsurgical root canal therapy [50, 53, 54]. On the other hand, a true cyst, which is not associated with root canals and is self-sustaining, is less likely to heal by nonsurgical endodontic treatment [50, 53, 54].

Wound Healing After Endodontic Surgery

The knowledge of wound healing processes after endodontic surgery is fundamental to our understanding and evaluation of outcomes, because the outcomes are considered as clinical reflections of wound healing. Harrison and Jurosky [55–57] described soft and hard tissue healing in three basic types of surgical wounds including incisional, dissectional, and excisional osseous wounds based on the histological observations of surgical wound healing in rhesus monkeys. In incisional wounds involving flap tissues, fibrin clot formation was observed at day 1, multilayered epithelial tissue formation at day 2, granulation tissue formation involving collagen synthesis by fibroblasts at days 3–4, and subsequent replacement of granulation tissues with fibrous connective tissues at days 14–28 [55]. Dissectional wounds including mucoperiosteal tissues and cortical bones also showed chronologically similar wound healing processes. The formation of fibrin clots occurred at day 1, granulation tissues were formed at days 3–4, and a new periosteum along the cortical bones and fibrous connective tissues was observed at day 14–28 [56]. In the dissectional wounds, degenerative changes in the cortical bones were closely associated with the absence of periosteal tissues, suggesting a protective effect of the periosteum on cortical bone necrosis [56]. In excisional osseous wounds, the osteotomy site was filled with coagulums at day

1 and replaced by granulation tissues originating from peripheral endosteal tissues at day 4 [57]. At day 14, most of the wound site was occupied with endosteal tissues and newly formed woven bones, which were in contact with dense fibrous connective tissues demarcating between the wound site and the overlying flap tissues [57]. These dense fibrous tissues were thought to participate in the periosteum reformation [57]. At day 28, increased maturation of woven bones and osteoid deposition on the surfaces of both cortical and trabecular bones were observed [57]. Clinicians should note that these healing events are expected to occur in surgical wound sites only if the etiological factors attributing to the posttreatment endodontic diseases are addressed.

Technical Differences and Their Implications for Outcome

The scientific support of outcome variations in endodontic surgery can be found in the different techniques employed in achieving disinfection and attaining an apical seal. Table 4.1 shows the main technical differences between TES and EMS and their implications.

In reviewing these differences, the following definitions will be used, which are generally adopted in the majority of outcome studies [6, 58, 59]. The techniques of TES include root-end preparation with burs and root-end filling with amalgam or zinc oxide eugenol or Cavit™ or gutta-percha without the use of the endoscope or microscope [15, 60–82]. In many instances, TES is also performed without any root-end filling materials [15, 62, 63, 65, 67, 68, 70, 72, 76, 79, 82]. By contrast, EMS techniques include root-end preparation with ultrasonic or sonic tips and root-end filling with IRM or EBA or MTA with the use of the endoscope or microscope [2, 83–91]. Due to insufficient or lack of magnification, TES requires a larger osteotomy than EMS to locate the periapical lesion and resect the root which may influence the progress of healing [83]. In general, both TES and EMS eliminate extraradicular etiologies by similar surgical debridement techniques; however, great technical differences exist between TES and EMS in addressing the intraradicular infection. An adequate apical seal with root-end filling materials is critical to a long-term success of the root-end surgery. The root-end filling materials used in TES such as amalgam or temporary filling materials (zinc oxide eugenol or Cavit™) or burnished gutta-percha are inferior to those in EMS – MTA, EBA, IRM – in their sealing ability and biocompatibility [92–96]. Therefore, it is not surprising to see a gradual deterioration and relapse of apical periodontitis in initially healed cases after TES, leading to remarkable outcome differences between EMS and TES in long-term success.

Table 4.1 Technical differences between TES and EMS and their implications

Surgical procedure	TES	EMS	Implications
Osteotomy	Larger size	Smaller size	Healing time
			Type of wound healing (repair vs. regeneration)
			Periodontal involvement
Root-end resection	Greater bevel (~45°)	Minimal bevel (0–10°)	Removal of etiological factors
	Greater resection (>3 mm)	Minimal (~3 mm) resection	Tooth stability
Retrograde preparation	Deficient inspection of resected root surface	Thorough inspection of resected root surface	Removal of etiological factors
	Altering original root canal morphology	Respecting original root canal morphology	
	Improper canal cleaning	Adequate canal cleaning	
Root-end filling	No or inadequate apical seal	Adequate apical seal	Entombment of microorganisms

Outcome Variations of Endodontic Surgery

The technical advantages conferred by EMS to address the etiological factors have significantly improved the outcome of endodontic surgery. Indeed, outcome studies published about a decade ago have shown significantly higher success rates compared to those published more than two decades earlier [2, 60–68, 70–91]. Interestingly, outcome for nonsurgical root canal treatment has not been changed in this same time period [7–11]. As discussed above, the great technical differences that exist between TES and EMS to address intraradicular infection translate into great outcome differences.

There exists a variation in results of systematic reviews in regard to endodontic surgery. Torabinejad et al. [97] showed that the pooled success rate was 73.8 % with the weighted success rate 75.0 % based on 6,647 teeth from 26 studies. A recent systematic review by Tsesis et al. [59], however, showed that EMS had a pooled success rate of 89 % based on 1,576 teeth from 18 studies. Another systematic review by Tsesis et al. [58] reported that the pooled success rate of EMS was 91.6 % based on 880 teeth from 11 studies. This significant difference in success rates is attributed to the selection criteria of individual systematic reviews. Torabinejad et al. [97] did not distinguish EMS from TES in their criteria. Therefore, the pooled success rate in their systematic review [97] was inevitably lower than those in the systematic reviews of Tsesis et al. [58, 59] that included EMS only.

Naturally, there are fewer EMS outcome studies with long-term follow-ups than TES outcomes studies with long-term follow-ups. Therefore, when long-term success rates of endodontic surgery are reported, TES has more statistical weight on the long-term success rates. Indeed, Torabinejad et al. [97] showed that the pooled success rate was 77.8 % at 2–4-year follow-ups, which dropped to 71.8 % at 4–6-year follow-ups and further deteriorated to 62.9 % at more than 6-year follow-ups. Although limited in number, the EMS outcome studies with long-term follow-ups demonstrated that initial success rates remained high and fairly constant at +90 % over time [2, 83–91]. In contrast, the success rate of TES was initially ~69 % and further declined to ~56 % in long-term follow-ups [60–82]. This noticeable variation was due to the limitations in addressing the intraradicular etiologies in TES. Interestingly, TES still had more than 50 % overall long-term success rates, perhaps due to its ability to eliminate the extraradicular factors.

Prognostic Factors Affecting Outcome Variations

There are overt and hidden heterogeneities between outcome studies in the selection criteria and study designs that potentially affect the outcome. Therefore, one should understand the potential prognostic factors that influence the outcomes and, more importantly, how to assess the individual studies without bias. It is thought that many prognostic factors significantly influence the outcomes. These factors must be reevaluated from the perspective of modern surgical techniques in order to evaluate the outcome variations in current endodontic surgery.

Does Resurgery Have a Poorer Outcome than First-Time Surgery?

Peterson and Gutman [98] reported in their systematic review that only 35.7 % of 350 patients healed successfully after resurgery with 26.3 % uncertain and 38 % failed. This finding is consistent with Gagliani et al. [99] who showed that teeth that underwent resurgery had a poorer outcome compared to that of initial surgery, although this prospective study reported 76 % success rate (59 % complete healing and 17 % incomplete healing). Gagliani et al. [99] used a modern surgical technique including ultrasonic tips, EBA as the root-end filling material, and 4.5× loupes to aid visibility. Another prospective clinical study by Song et al. [100] showed a 92.9 % success rate after endodontic resurgery based on 42 patients with a 77.8 % recall rate. Song et al. [100] used ultrasonic tips and MTA and EBA as root-end filling materials with a surgical operating microscope. The success rate in this study is equivalent to those of first-time EMS and is thought to be due to the ability of EMS to address the causes of posttreatment endodontic disease. Therefore, resurgery may not be considered to affect the outcome negatively if microsurgical techniques are used.

Does High-Power Magnification Affect the Outcome of Endodontic Surgery?

Higher magnification aids in identifying the etiology of persistent apical periodontitis and provide a more precise control of surgical procedures. Surgical operating microscopes and endoscopes are considered to be state-of-the-art magnification tools for endodontic surgery. Any less magnification and illumination is thought to be associated with the lower success rates in TES compared to EMS. However, it should be noted that in order to investigate the effect of magnification on the outcome, magnification should be the only variable to compare, while the other variables such as surgical techniques and materials are controlled. Del Fabbro and Taschieri [101] reported that there was no significant difference in success rates among loupes, endoscopes, and microscopes. Setzer et al. [102] performed a meta-analysis based on 14 outcome studies, which applied the same ultrasonic root-end preparation and root-end filling with biocompatible materials but different magnification tools, and showed that endodontic surgery with the endoscope or the microscope had a statistically greater success rate than those with insufficient magnification. Interestingly, this systematic review showed that no significant difference was observed for anteriors and premolars, but there was a significant difference for molar surgery [102]. This finding is perhaps due to the low statistical power during the subgroup analysis. However, it may be also due to the easier accessibility and less complex root-end intricacies in anteriors and premolars. A recent meta-analysis by Tsesis et al. [59] showed that significantly higher positive outcomes were found when endoscopes or microscopes were used as a magnification tool compared to when loupes were used. This result is consistent with von Arx et al. [103], who reported that teeth that underwent endodontic surgery with the use of an endoscope had a higher success rate than teeth without the use of an endoscope. Therefore, higher magnification using the endoscope and microscope may be considered a prognostic factor that affects the outcome of endodontic surgery positively.

Does the Type of Root-End Filling Materials Matter?

The limited root canal disinfection can be achieved in endodontic surgery by root-end resection and root-end preparation. Therefore, remaining microorganisms in the root canal system may cause a recurrent apical pathosis if the apical seal is incomplete. In order to have an adequate apical seal, proper root-end filling materials should be used. MTA and EBA appear to have a better sealing ability than amalgam and other filling materials such as Cavit and zinc oxide eugenol [92]. In addition, the depth of root-end filling is an important factor for an adequate apical seal and should be at least 3–4 mm when MTA is used as a root-end filling material [104, 105]. MTA was reported to also have better biocompatibility compared to EBA and amalgam [96]. These results from preclinical studies give us considerable insights into selecting root-end filling materials for endodontic surgery, but we do need clinical outcome studies to validate whether superior sealing ability and biocompatibility of MTA can translate into higher success rates compared with other materials. In a systematic review by von Arx et al. [103], a significantly higher estimated healed rate was found in studies using MTA (91.4 %) as compared to amalgam (57.9 %) and glass ionomer cement (51.2 %). Notably, no significant differences in estimated healed rates were found among MTA, EBA (69.8 %), and

IRM (71.6 %) [103]. A meta-analysis by Tsesis et al. [59], however, showed that use of MTA was associated with significantly higher success rates than the use of IRM or EBA, although MTA did not significantly differ from EBA in success rates when studies with low risk of bias were selected and analyzed. A recent retrospective study by Song et al. [106] demonstrated a significant difference between MTA and IRM, but no difference between MTA and EBA. In contrast, two randomized controlled study showed no significant difference between MTA and IRM [85, 107]. Clearly, there is no doubt as to the better clinical outcomes with MTA compared to other materials, although MTA, EBA, and IRM are considered clinically acceptable root-end filling materials. Therefore, the material selection for root-end filling is considered to affect the outcome significantly.

Does Periodontal Involvement Worsen the Outcome?

When the periapical lesion is limited to the apical area, endodontic surgery with microsurgical techniques offers an excellent outcome as evidenced by the previous systematic reviews [6, 58, 59]. However, when the periapical lesion becomes periodontally involved, the outcome of endodontic surgery may be compromised due to the unfavorable healing patterns characterized by the downgrowth of a long junctional epithelium and subsequent hindrance of bone formation and reattachment. Indeed, Kim et al. [87] showed that 95.2 % of cases with isolated endodontic lesions were healed, but only 77.5 % of cases with periodontal involvements were healed. A study of Skoglund and Persson using traditional surgical techniques showed that cases with total loss of buccal bone plates had a 37 % success rate [108]. Similarly, significantly lower survival time was reported in cases with a large marginal bone loss (>4 mm from CEJ) [109]. Therefore, periodontal involvement in endodontic surgery is considered a prognostic factor that adversely influences the outcome.

Summary

Recent progress in the technical aspects of endodontic surgery provides the opportunity to identify and address the etiology of apical periodontitis. The striking variations in outcomes of endodontic surgery among individual outcome studies are primarily due to the different surgical techniques employed during endodontic microsurgery (EMS) and traditional endodontic surgery (TES). The technical difference between EMS and TES is translated into a significant difference in success rates. Notably, the success rate in TES is shown to deteriorate over time, while the consistent success rate in EMS is observed. It should be kept in mind that covert heterogeneities among outcome studies such as the use of magnification, type of root-end filling material, and presence of periodontal involvement may affect the outcome significantly and contribute greatly to outcome variations.

Acknowledgments I wish to express my sincere gratitude to Dr. Charles Solomon for his proofreading. The author declares no conflicts of interest.

References

1. Rahbaran S, Gilthorpe MS, Harrison SD, Gulabivala K. Comparison of clinical outcome of periapical surgery in endodontic and oral surgery units of a teaching dental hospital: a retrospective study. Oral Surg Oral Med Oral Pathol Oral Radiol Endod. 2001;91(6):700–9.
2. Christiansen R, Kirkevang LL, Hørsted-Bindslev P, Wenzel A. Randomized clinical trial of root-end resection followed by root-end filling with mineral trioxide aggregate or smoothing of the orthograde gutta-percha root filling–1-year follow-up. Int Endod J. 2009;42(2):105–14.
3. Ng YL, Mann V, Gulabivala K. Tooth survival following non-surgical root canal treatment: a systematic review of the literature. Int Endod J. 2010;43(3):171–89.
4. Ng YL, Mann V, Rahbaran S, Lewsey J, Gulabivala K. Outcome of primary root canal treatment: systematic review of the literature – part 1. Effects of study characteristics on probability of success. Int Endod J. 2007;40(12):921–39.
5. Ng YL, Mann V, Rahbaran S, Lewsey J, Gulabivala K. Outcome of primary root canal treatment: systematic

review of the literature – part 2. Influence of clinical factors. Int Endod J. 2008;41(1):6–31.
6. Setzer FC, Shah SB, Kohli MR, Karabucak B, Kim S. Outcome of endodontic surgery: a meta-analysis of the literature–part 1: comparison of traditional root-end surgery and endodontic microsurgery. J Endod. 2010;36(11):1757–65.
7. Kerekes K, Tronstad L. Long-term results of endodontic treatment performed with a standardized technique. J Endod. 1979;5(3):83–90.
8. Sjogren U, Hagglund B, Sundqvist G, Wing K. Factors affecting the long-term results of endodontic treatment. J Endod. 1990;16(10):498–504.
9. Peters LB, Wesselink PR. Periapical healing of endodontically treated teeth in one and two visits obturated in the presence or absence of detectable microorganisms. Int Endod J. 2002;35(8):660–7.
10. Ng YL, Mann V, Gulabivala K. A prospective study of the factors affecting outcomes of nonsurgical root canal treatment: part 1: periapical health. Int Endod J. 2011;44(7):583–609.
11. Paredes-Vieyra J, Enriquez FJ. Success rate of single-versus two-visit root canal treatment of teeth with apical periodontitis: a randomized controlled trial. J Endod. 2012;38(9):1164–9.
12. Strindberg LZ. The dependence of the results of pulp therapy on certain factors. Acta Odontol Scand. 1956;14 Suppl 21:1–175.
13. Rud J, Andreasen JO, Jensen JE. Radiographic criteria for the assessment of healing after endodontic surgery. Int J Oral Surg. 1972;1(4):195–214.
14. Molven O, Halse A, Grung B. Observer strategy and the radiographic classification of healing after endodontic surgery. Int J Oral Maxillofac Surg. 1987;16(4):432–9.
15. Rud J, Andreasen JO, Jensen JE. A follow-up study of 1,000 cases treated by endodontic surgery. Int J Oral Surg. 1972;1(4):215–28.
16. Markvart M, Darvann TA, Larsen P, Dalstra M, Kreiborg S, Bjørndal L. Micro-CT analyses of apical enlargement and molar root canal complexity. Int Endod J. 2012;45(3):273–81.
17. Adcock JM, Sidow SJ, Looney SW, Liu Y, McNally K, Lindsey K, Tay FR. Histologic evaluation of canal and isthmus debridement efficacies of two different irrigant delivery techniques in a closed system. J Endod. 2011;37(4):544–8.
18. Endal U, Shen Y, Knut A, Gao Y, Haapasalo M. A high-resolution computed tomographic study of changes in root canal isthmus area by instrumentation and root filling. J Endod. 2011;37(2):223–7.
19. Dietrich MA, Kirkpatrick TC, Yaccino JM. In vitro canal and isthmus debris removal of the self-adjusting file, K3, and WaveOne files in the mesial root of human mandibular molars. J Endod. 2012; 38(8):1140–4.
20. von Arx T. Frequency and type of canal isthmuses in first molars detected by endoscopic inspection during periradicular surgery. Int Endod J. 2005; 38(3):160–8.
21. Gorni FG, Gagliani MM. The outcome of endodontic retreatment: a 2-yr follow-up. J Endod. 2004;30(1):1–4.
22. Spili P, Parashos P, Messer HH. The impact of instrument fracture on outcome of endodontic treatment. J Endod. 2005;31(12):845–50.
23. Sundqvist G, Reuterving CO. Isolation of Actinomyces israelii from periapical lesion. J Endod. 1980;6(6):602–6.
24. Happonen RP. Periapical actinomycosis: a follow-up study of 16 surgically treated cases. Endod Dent Traumatol. 1986;2(5):205–9.
25. Sjögren U, Happonen RP, Kahnberg KE, Sundqvist G. Survival of Arachnia propionica in periapical tissue. Int Endod J. 1988;21(4):277–82.
26. Sunde PT, Olsen I, Debelian GJ, Tronstad L. Microbiota of periapical lesions refractory to endodontic therapy. J Endod. 2002;28(4):304–10.
27. Noiri Y, Ehara A, Kawahara T, Takemura N, Ebisu S. Participation of bacterial biofilms in refractory and chronic periapical periodontitis. J Endod. 2002;28(10): 679–83.
28. Rocha CT, Rossi MA, Leonardo MR, Rocha LB, Nelson-Filho P, Silva LA. Biofilm on the apical region of roots in primary teeth with vital and necrotic pulps with or without radiographically evident apical pathosis. Int Endod J. 2008;41(8):664–9.
29. Ricucci D, Siqueira Jr JF. Apical actinomycosis as a continuum of intraradicular and extraradicular infection: case report and critical review on its involvement with treatment failure. J Endod. 2008;34(9):1124–9.
30. Slots J, Sabeti M, Simon JH. Herpesviruses in periapical pathosis: an etiopathogenic relationship? Oral Surg Oral Med Oral Pathol Oral Radiol Endod. 2003;96(3):327–31.
31. Yildirim S, Yapar M, Kubar A, Slots J. Human cytomegalovirus, Epstein-Barr virus and bone resorption-inducing cytokines in periapical lesions of deciduous teeth. Oral Microbiol Immunol. 2006;21(2):107–11.
32. Chávez de Paz LE, Bergenholtz G, Svensäter G. The effects of antimicrobials on endodontic biofilm bacteria. J Endod. 2010;36(1):70–7.
33. Gilbert P, Das J, Foley I. Biofilm susceptibility to antimicrobials. Adv Dent Res. 1997;11(1):160–7.
34. Johnson SA, Goddard PA, Iliffe C, Timmins B, Rickard AH, Robson G, Handley PS. Comparative susceptibility of resident and transient hand bacteria to para-chloro-meta-xylenol and triclosan. J Appl Microbiol. 2002;93(2):336–44.
35. Nair PN, Sjögren U, Krey G, Sundqvist G. Therapy-resistant foreign body giant cell granuloma at the periapex of a root-filled human tooth. J Endod. 1990;16(12):589–95.
36. Knoblich R. Pulmonary granulomatosis caused by vegetable particles. So-called lentil pulse pneumonia. Am Rev Respir Dis. 1969;99(3):380–9.
37. Simon JH, Chimenti RA, Mintz GA. Clinical significance of the pulse granuloma. J Endod. 1982;8(3):116–9.
38. Koppang HS, Koppang R, Solheim T, Aarnes H, Stølen SO. Cellulose fibers from endodontic paper points

as an etiological factor in postendodontic periapical granulomas and cysts. J Endod. 1989;15(8):369–72.
39. Koppang HS, Koppang R, Solheim T, Aarnes H, Stölen SO. Identification of cellulose fibers in oral biopsies. Scand J Dent Res. 1987;95(2):165–73.
40. Sjögren U, Sundqvist G, Nair PN. Tissue reaction to gutta-percha particles of various sizes when implanted subcutaneously in guinea pigs. Eur J Oral Sci. 1995;103(5):313–21.
41. Ramachandran Nair PN. Light and electron microscopic studies of root canal flora and periapical lesions. J Endod. 1987;13(1):29–39.
42. Browne RM. The origin of cholesterol in odontogenic cysts in man. Arch Oral Biol. 1971;16(1):107–13.
43. Trott JR, Chebib F, Galindo Y. Factors related to cholesterol formation in cysts and granulomas. J Can Dent Assoc (Tor). 1973;39(8):550–5.
44. Nair PN, Sjögren U, Sundqvist G. Cholesterol crystals as an etiological factor in non-resolving chronic inflammation: an experimental study in guinea pigs. Eur J Oral Sci. 1998;106(2 Pt 1):644–50.
45. Nair PN. Cholesterol as an aetiological agent in endodontic failures–a review. Aust Endod J. 1999;25(1):19–26.
46. Nair PN, Sjögren U, Schumacher E, Sundqvist G. Radicular cyst affecting a root-filled human tooth: a long-term post-treatment follow-up. Int Endod J. 1993;26(4):225–33.
47. Priebe WA, Lazansky JP, Wuehrmann AH. The value of the roentgenographic film in the differential diagnosis of periapical lesions. Oral Surg Oral Med Oral Pathol. 1954;7(9):979–83.
48. Lalonde ER, Luebke RG. The frequency and distribution of periapical cysts and granulomas. An evaluation of 800 specimens. Oral Surg Oral Med Oral Pathol. 1968;25(6):861–8.
49. Bhaskar SN. Oral surgery–oral pathology conference No. 17, Walter Reed Army Medical Center. Periapical lesions–types, incidence, and clinical features. Oral Surg Oral Med Oral Pathol. 1966;21(5):657–71.
50. Simon JH. Incidence of periapical cysts in relation to the root canal. J Endod. 1980;6(11):845–8.
51. Nair PN. Apical periodontitis: a dynamic encounter between root canal infection and host response. Periodontol 2000. 1997;13:121–48.
52. Nair PN. New perspectives on radicular cysts: do they heal? Int Endod J. 1998;31(3):155–60.
53. Ramachandran Nair PN, Pajarola G, Schroeder HE. Types and incidence of human periapical lesions obtained with extracted teeth. Oral Surg Oral Med Oral Pathol Oral Radiol Endod. 1996;81(1):93–102.
54. Nair PN. Pathogenesis of apical periodontitis and the causes of endodontic failures. Crit Rev Oral Biol Med. 2004;15(6):348–81.
55. Harrison JW, Jurosky KA. Wound healing in the tissues of the periodontium following periradicular surgery. I. The incisional wound. J Endod. 1991;17(9):425–35.
56. Harrison JW, Jurosky KA. Wound healing in the tissues of the periodontium following periradicular surgery. 2. The dissectional wound. J Endod. 1991;17(11):544–52.
57. Harrison JW, Jurosky KA. Wound healing in the tissues of the periodontium following periradicular surgery. III. The osseous excisional wound. J Endod. 1992;18(2):76–81.
58. Tsesis I, Faivishevsky V, Kfir A, Rosen E. Outcome of surgical endodontic treatment performed by a modern technique: a meta-analysis of literature. J Endod. 2009;35(11):1505–11.
59. Tsesis I, Rosen E, Taschieri S, Telishevsky Strauss Y, Ceresoli V, Del Fabbro M. Outcomes of surgical endodontic treatment performed by a modern technique: an updated meta-analysis of the literature. J Endod. 2013;39(3):332–9.
60. Ericson S, Finne K, Persson G. Results of apicoectomy of maxillary canines, premolars and molars with special reference to oroantral communication as a prognostic factor. Int J Oral Surg. 1974;3(6):386–93.
61. Finne K, Nord PG, Persson G, Lennartsson B. Retrograde root filling with amalgam and Cavit. Oral Surg Oral Med Oral Pathol. 1977;43(4):621–6.
62. Hirsch JM, Ahlström U, Henrikson PA, Heyden G, Peterson LE. Periapical surgery. Int J Oral Surg. 1979;8(3):173–85.
63. Malmström M, Perkki K, Lindquist K. Apicectomy. A retrospective study. Proc Finn Dent Soc. 1982;78(1):26–31.
64. Persson G. Periapical surgery of molars. Int J Oral Surg. 1982;11(2):96–100.
65. Mikkonen M, Kullaa-Mikkonen A, Kotilainen R. Clinical and radiologic re-examination of apicoectomized teeth. Oral Surg Oral Med Oral Pathol. 1983;55(3):302–6.
66. Ioannides C, Borstlap WA. Apicoectomy on molars: a clinical and radiographical study. Int J Oral Surg. 1983;12(2):73–9.
67. Reit C, Hirsch J. Surgical endodontic retreatment. Int Endod J. 1986;19(3):107–12.
68. Forssell H, Tammisalo T, Forssell K. A follow-up study of apicectomized teeth. Proc Finn Dent Soc. 1988;84(2):85–93.
69. Crosher RF, Dinsdale RC, Holmes A. One visit apicectomy technique using calcium hydroxide cement as the canal filling material combined with retrograde amalgam. Int Endod J. 1989;22(6):283–9.
70. Grung B, Molven O, Halse A. Periapical surgery in a Norwegian county hospital: follow-up findings of 477 teeth. J Endod. 1990;16(9):411–7.
71. Dorn SO, Gartner AH. Surgical endodontic and retrograde procedures. Curr Opin Dent. 1991;1(6):750–3.
72. Molven O, Halse A, Grung B. Surgical management of endodontic failures: indications and treatment results. Int Dent J. 1991;41(1):33–42.
73. Rapp EL, Brown Jr CE, Newton CW. An analysis of success and failure of apicoectomies. J Endod. 1991;17(10):508–12.
74. Zetterqvist L, Hall G, Holmlund A. Apicectomy: a comparative clinical study of amalgam and glass

ionomer cement as apical sealants. Oral Surg Oral Med Oral Pathol. 1991;71(4):489–91.
75. Frank AL, Glick DH, Patterson SS, Weine FS. Long-term evaluation of surgically placed amalgam fillings. J Endod. 1992;18(8):391–8.
76. Cheung LK, Lam J. Apicectomy of posterior teeth–a clinical study. Aust Dent J. 1993;38(1):17–21.
77. Pantschev A, Carlsson AP, Andersson L. Retrograde root filling with EBA cement or amalgam. A comparative clinical study. Oral Surg Oral Med Oral Pathol. 1994;78(1):101–4.
78. Jesslén P, Zetterqvist L, Heimdahl A. Long-term results of amalgam versus glass ionomer cement as apical sealant after apicectomy. Oral Surg Oral Med Oral Pathol Oral Radiol Endod. 1995;79(1):101–3.
79. August DS. Long-term, postsurgical results on teeth with periapical radiolucencies. J Endod. 1996;22(7):380–3.
80. Kvist T, Reit C. Results of endodontic retreatment: a randomized clinical study comparing surgical and nonsurgical procedures. J Endod. 1999;25(12):814–7.
81. Schwartz-Arad D, Yarom N, Lustig JP, Kaffe I. A retrospective radiographic study of root-end surgery with amalgam and intermediate restorative material. Oral Surg Oral Med Oral Pathol Oral Radiol Endod. 2003;96(4):472–7.
82. Wesson CM, Gale TM. Molar apicectomy with amalgam root-end filling: results of a prospective study in two district general hospitals. Br Dent J. 2003;195(12):707–14; discussion 698.
83. Rubinstein RA, Kim S. Short-term observation of the results of endodontic surgery with the use of surgical operation microscope and Super-EBA as root end filling material. J Endod. 1999;25(1):43–8.
84. Rubinstein RA, Kim S. Long-term follow-up of cases considered healed one year after apical microsurgery. J Endod. 2002;28(5):378–83.
85. Chong BS, Pitt Ford TR, Hudson MB. A prospective clinical study of Mineral Trioxide Aggregate and IRM when used as root-end filling materials inendodontic surgery. Int Endod J. 2003;36(8):520–6.
86. Taschieri S, Del Fabbro M, Testori T, Francetti L, Weinstein R. Endodontic surgery using 2 different magnification devices: preliminary results of a randomized controlled study. J Oral Maxillofac Surg. 2006;64(2):235–42.
87. Kim E, Song JS, Jung IY, Lee SJ, Kim S. Prospective clinical study evaluating endodontic microsurgery outcomes for cases with lesions of endodontic origin compared with cases with lesions of combined periodontal-endodontic origin. J Endod. 2008;34(5):546–51.
88. Taschieri S, Del Fabbro M, Testori T, Weinstein R. Microscope versus endoscope in root-end management: a randomized controlled study. Int J Oral Maxillofac Surg. 2008;37(11):1022–6.
89. Taschieri S, Del Fabbro M. Endoscopic endodontic microsurgery: 2-year evaluation of healing and functionality. Braz Oral Res. 2009;23(1):23–30.
90. von Arx T, Hänni S, Jensen SS. Clinical results with two different methods of root-end preparation and filling in apical surgery: mineral trioxide aggregate and adhesive resin composite. J Endod. 2010;36(7):1122–9.
91. Song M, Kim E. A prospective randomized controlled study of mineral trioxide aggregate and super ethoxy-benzoic acid as root-end filling materials in endodontic microsurgery. J Endod. 2012;38(7):875–9.
92. Fernández-Yáñez Sánchez A, Leco-Berrocal MI, Martínez-González JM. Metaanalysis of filler materials in periapical surgery. Med Oral Patol Oral Cir Bucal. 2008;13(3):E180–5.
93. Wu MK, Kontakiotis EG, Wesselink PR. Long-term seal provided by some root-end filling materials. J Endod. 1998;24(8):557–60.
94. Yatsushiro JD, Baumgartner JC, Tinkle JS. Longitudinal study of the microleakage of two root-end filling materials using a fluid conductive system. J Endod. 1998;24(11):716–9.
95. Baek SH, Lee WC, Setzer FC, Kim S. Periapical bone regeneration after endodontic microsurgery with three different root-end filling materials: amalgam, SuperEBA, and mineral trioxide aggregate. J Endod. 2010;36(8):1323–5.
96. Baek SH, Plenk Jr H, Kim S. Periapical tissue responses and cementum regeneration with amalgam, SuperEBA, and MTA as root-end filling materials. J Endod. 2005;31(6):444–9.
97. Torabinejad M, Corr R, Handysides R, Shabahang S. Outcomes of nonsurgical retreatment and endodontic surgery: a systematic review. J Endod. 2009;35(7):930–7.
98. Peterson J, Gutmann JL. The outcome of endodontic resurgery: a systematic review. Int Endod J. 2001;34(3):169–75.
99. Gagliani MM, Gorni FG, Strohmenger L. Periapical resurgery versus periapical surgery: a 5-year longitudinal comparison. Int Endod J. 2005;38(5):320–7.
100. Song M, Shin SJ, Kim E. Outcomes of endodontic micro-resurgery: a prospective clinical study. J Endod. 2011;37(3):316–20.
101. Del Fabbro M, Taschieri S. Endodontic therapy using magnification devices: a systematic review. J Dent. 2010;38(4):269–75.
102. Setzer FC, Kohli MR, Shah SB, Karabucak B, Kim S. Outcome of endodontic surgery: a meta-analysis of the literature–part 2: comparison of endodontic microsurgical techniques with and without the use of higher magnification. J Endod. 2012;38(1):1–10.
103. von Arx T, Peñarrocha M, Jensen S. Prognostic factors in apical surgery with root-end filling: a meta-analysis. J Endod. 2010;36(6):957–73.
104. Lamb EL, Loushine RJ, Weller RN, Kimbrough WF, Pashley DH. Effect of root resection on the apical sealing ability of mineral trioxide aggregate. Oral Surg Oral Med Oral Pathol Oral Radiol Endod. 2003;95(6):732–5.

105. Valois CR, Costa Jr ED. Influence of the thickness of mineral trioxide aggregate on sealing ability of root-end fillings in vitro. Oral Surg Oral Med Oral Pathol Oral Radiol Endod. 2004;97(1):108–11.
106. Song M, Jung IY, Lee SJ, Lee CY, Kim E. Prognostic factors for clinical outcomes in endodontic microsurgery: a retrospective study. J Endod. 2011;37(7):927–33.
107. Lindeboom JA, Frenken JW, Kroon FH, van den Akker HP. A comparative prospective randomized clinical study of MTA and IRM as root-end filling materials in single-rooted teeth in endodontic surgery. Oral Surg Oral Med Oral Pathol Oral Radiol Endod. 2005;100(4):495–500.
108. Skoglund A, Persson G. A follow-up study of apicoectomized teeth with total loss of the buccal bone plate. Oral Surg Oral Med Oral Pathol. 1985;59(1):78–81.
109. Wang Q, Cheung GS, Ng RP. Survival of surgical endodontic treatment performed in a dental teaching hospital: a cohort study. Int Endod J. 2004;37(11):764–75.

Surgical Anesthesia: When a Tool Becomes a Weapon

5

Eyal Rosen and Igor Tsesis

Abstract

Anesthesia is the loss of feeling or sensation as a result of an anesthetic agent and is an integral part of any endodontic surgical procedure. In certain cases, local anesthesia (LA) administration may result in complications, ranging from mild discomfort for the patient to catastrophical results and even death.

The complications following LA in endodontic surgery may be regional or systemic and may be related to the local anesthetic itself or to the supplementary vasoconstrictor. Severe systemic complications following LA, such as bronchospasm, seizure, anaphylactic shock, or cardiovascular complications, are rare but may have severe implications on the patient's general health. Regional LA complications, such as insufficient anesthesia, hematoma, and soft-tissue injuries, are more common, may cause severe discomfort for the patient, and may alter the ability to achieve the surgical goals.

The most important steps in managing untoward reactions to LA are the following: adopt a clinical practice aimed to prevent possible complications, diagnose the problem promptly when it does occur, treat it if necessary, and reassure the patient.

Introduction

Anesthesia is defined as "the loss of feeling or sensation as a result of an anesthetic agent to permit diagnostic and treatment procedures" [1]. Dental practitioners use local anesthetic (LA) injections every day with infrequent reports of serious complications. However, local anesthesia administration could result in complications, ranging from mild discomfort for the patient to catastrophical results and even death [2]. In addition, patients that are afraid of dental treatments are likely to show psychogenic reactions to the LA administration [3, 4].

LA agents block the inflow of sodium ions and neuronal depolarization. Modern LA agents are weak bases whose molecules consist of a

E. Rosen, DMD (✉) • I. Tsesis, DMD
Department of Endodontology, Maurice and Gabriela Goldschleger School of Dental Medicine, Tel Aviv University, Tel Aviv, Israel
e-mail: dr.eyalrosen@gmail.com; dr.tsesis@gmail.com

I. Tsesis (ed.), *Complications in Endodontic Surgery*,
DOI 10.1007/978-3-642-54218-3_5,

lipophilic portion (an aromatic ring) and a hydrophilic element (a secondary or tertiary amine) linked by an amide chain. The amine group makes it possible for the molecule, in ionized form, to be soluble in water and to act on specific receptors, and when in non-ionized form, it is soluble in fat and therefore able to cross the membranes within the nerve [3, 4].

Complications following LA in endodontic surgery can be classified into two major groups: systemic complications and regional complications. The systemic complications may be further divided to systemic reactions to the local anesthetic itself and to systemic reactions to the vasoconstrictor.

Systemic Complications

Severe systemic complications following LA are possible bronchospasm, seizure, and anaphylactic shock [2–6]. There are relatively few contraindications for the use of LA when it is used with vasoconstrictors, such as unstable angina, recent myocardial infarction, recent coronary artery bypass arrhythmia, severe uncontrolled hypertension, heart failure, uncontrolled hyperthyroidism, uncontrolled diabetes, thyrotoxicosis, cortico-dependent asthma, and pheochromocytoma [3]. In certain cases patients with any of the abovementioned conditions should be treated only in the general hospital settings (see "ASA classification" in Chap. 3).

Systemic complications may occur because of excessive dosage, rapid absorption, or inadvertent intravascular injection [5].

The anamnesis and thorough medical history assessment is mandatory before considering endodontic surgery. More than 45 % of dental patients will have one or more concomitant diseases in their medical histories and about 20 % of all patients will suffer from cardiovascular diseases or allergies [6], while in the elderly patient the numbers are even higher [7].

Allergic reactions have to be well differentiated from psychogenic reactions, since psychogenic reactions can often mimic allergic reactions with same cardiovascular symptoms such as tachycardia and hypotension as well as concomitant nausea, dizziness, sweating, or hyperventilation [6].

Systemic and Allergic Reactions to the Local Anesthetic Itself

Adverse reactions to LA such as tachycardia, hypotension, and subjective feelings of weakness, heat, or vertigo are common and are mostly due to their pharmacological properties and drug combinations or psychogenic origin [8].

Allergic accidents to LA itself are infrequent [8], and the incidence of true allergy to local anesthetics is rare, other ingredients in LA preparations such as preservatives, or latex contaminants, need to be considered.

Most allergic reactions after the use of LA may be due to substances used as preservatives such as methylparaben, in commercial preparations of ester and amide local anesthetics. Preservatives are structurally similar to aminobenzoic acid, the common metabolite of the ester class and a known potential allergen. Thus, most cases of allergy involve agents from the ester class [9].

Practical management of patients with a history of LA reaction includes a careful allergy history and skin-prick and intradermal tests [10].

Patients with histories of adverse reactions to local anesthesia may be under the impression that they are allergic to local anesthetics. However, the frequency of allergy to local anesthetics is less than 1 %. Local anesthetics are some of the rarest drug allergens; however, allergy tests of local anesthetics should be performed in patients in whom it is uncertain whether they are allergic [11].

Systemic Toxicity of Local Anesthetics

Accidental direct intravascular injection of the anesthetic solution may cause systemic toxicity due to an elevated plasma concentration of the anesthetic drug. Absorption of the LA from the site of injection leading to excess plasma concentration is more rare [9].

The extent of systemic absorption depends on the following: the LA dose, the vascularity of the injection site, the presence of vasoconstrictor (the vasoconstrictor decreases the systemic absorption of the LA), and the chemical properties of the drug. The central nervous system (CNS) and the cardiovascular system are involved owing to the systemic toxicity of the LA [9].

All LA can cause *central nervous system (CNS) toxicity* (manifested as anxiety, restlessness, tremor, and death that may occur due to respiratory failure) or *cardiovascular toxicity* (due to arteriole vasodilation and hypotension), if their plasma concentrations are increased by accidental intravenous injection or an absolute overdose [5].

The best clinical approach to toxicity due to LA is prevention and simple means, such as aspiration via the needle before injection, and addition of epinephrine that can increase the safety of the LA [9].

Systemic Reactions to Vasoconstrictor

The use of vasoconstrictor has been widely recommended for endodontic surgery to achieve prolong depth and duration of anesthesia, and to control bleeding [3, 4]. Increases in blood pressure (BP) are common during endodontic surgery and is influenced by anxiety, and painful stimuli. However, a controversy exists regarding the influence of vasoconstrictors on blood pressure and heart rate (HR) [12–15].

Matsumura et al. [12] found that dental surgery using local anesthesia caused significant increases in systolic BP and pulse rate, and the increase in systolic BP was greater in middle-aged and older patients. Zarei et al. [13] compared the anesthetic efficacy of and HR changes after periodontal ligament or intraosseous X-Tip injection in mandibular molars and found that epinephrine-containing local anesthetics result in dose-dependent increased circulating epinephrine levels that are associated with cardiovascular changes [13]. Knoll-Kohler et al. [14] reported that the increase in HR depends on the amount of vasoconstrictor in the anesthetic solution. On the other hand, other clinical trials reported that the rise in BP and HR following injection of lidocaine with epinephrine was not clinically considerable [15, 16].

Regional Complications

LA administration may lead to a variety of regional localized complications, such as needle breakage, pain or burning on injection, nerve injury, trismus, hematoma, infection, soft-tissue injury, self-inflicted soft-tissue trauma, vascular injury, intraglandular or intramuscular injection, as well as sloughing of tissues and postanesthetic intraoral lesions [17].

Trismus Following LA Injection

Trismus is a spasm of the muscles of mastication resulting in difficulty in opening the mouth [1] and oral injections such as inferior alveolar nerve blocks and posterior maxillary infiltration injections may lead to trismus development. The etiology of trismus is trauma by the injection needle to muscles or blood vessels with subsequent hematoma development [17, 18].

Trismus has an acute phase, when pain leads to muscle spasm and limitation of the jaw motion. The acute phase may proceed with an ensuing chronic phase of hypomobility, develops as a result of fibrosis and scar tissue development. Infection increasing the pain levels may cause more tissue scarring [18].

Trismus is prevented by using minimal depth injections, and by avoiding multiple mandibular block injections. When acute trismus develops, its progression to chronic hypomobility is prevented by an early treatment protocol, that includes heat application, analgesics, muscle relaxants, physiotherapy, and by reassuring the patient. Antibiotics should be prescribed considered since infection may developed. In certain cases when chronic hypomobility develops, surgical intervention may be indicated [17, 18].

LA Complications Related to Misjudged Anatomy

One of the main reasons for LA-related complications is misjudged anatomy, such as middle-ear problems following oral LA [19] and unexpected ophthalmic manifestations that can occur both after maxillary and after mandibular local anesthesia [20]. Maxillary LA, given the close proximity to the orbit, may lead to intra-orbital diffusion of the injected solution. During mandibular LA of the anesthetic may follow the maxillary artery to the orbital branch of the medial meningeal artery, reaching the lacrimal artery that serves the lateral rectal muscle. Ischemia of that muscle structure may explain the blurred vision. Intravenous injection of LA and paralysis of the eye muscles may also occur [20]. Mandibular anesthesia may lead to ophthalmic symptoms when cranial nerves are affected. In addition, in case when a needle injures the wall of an alveolar artery, it may activate sympathetic fibers, creating a vasospastic impulse that passes the internal carotid plexus, reaching the orbit via the ophthalmic artery [20].

About 70 % of the reports of adverse ophthalmic complications following LA concerned female subjects. Moreover, these female cases more often reported diplopia compared with male cases, suggesting the possibility of different anatomic features between genders [20] (or it may be explained by the fact that women seeking more dental treatment [21]). Diplopia, the most extensively documented ocular symptom, is a disturbing experience that is often directly noticed by the patient [20].

Nerve Injury Following LA Administration

The exact mechanism of local anesthesia-related nerve injury is not fully elucidated, but it is hypothesized that it may be one or a combination of several factors: direct traumatic injury to the nerve by the needle, hemorrhage following the injection into the nerve sheath, hydrostatic pressure from the injection, or neurotoxicity from the local anesthetic material itself [22, 23].

Neurotoxicity appears to be dependent on the local anesthetic formulation. The use of either prilocaine or articaine may be associated with an increased risk of developing neurotoxicity-related nerve injury. However, it is yet unclear whether those drugs have a relatively higher level of toxicity compared to other anesthetic solutions or that their relative high manufactured concentration is the nerve injury harmful factor (articaine and prilocaine are the only dental local anesthetics formulated as 4 % solutions in the United States, with all others being of lower concentration) [22].

It should be noted that the majority of reported adverse reactions associated with local anesthetics are not due to the drugs themselves but to the act of drug administration [5]. Thus, direct trauma to the nerve bundle during the injection, or indirectly by the development of intra-alveolar edema or hematomas by puncture of nerve surrounding blood vessels, that produces a temporary pressure increase in the vicinity of the nerve bundle [24] is still considered as the most probable and frequent cause of nerve injury following local anesthesia administration [23, 25–28].

On the other hand, the mechanical injury alone may be insufficient to result in permanent damage, and it may be speculated that it is not the drug per se, but the higher dose of the drug combined with mechanical insult that predisposes the nerve to permanent damage [6]. In order to prevent nerve injury during LA, it seems beneficial to use infiltration instead of block anesthesia whenever possible, especially in the vicinity of major nerve bundles.

Bleeding and Hematoma Following LA

If a vein is engaged during injection of LA, the bleeding is expected to be negligible. However, if an artery is damaged, it may produce rapid bleeding with significant hematoma formation and rapidly developing extensive intraoral or extraoral swelling [2], most commonly occurs in the tuberosity area, when one of the terminal branches of the maxillary artery is damaged [2]. It was also reported that during a mandibular block, failure to obtain anesthesia may be associated with hematoma formation in the pterygomandibular space and the dilution and inactivation of the LA by blood [29].

Hematoma formation may result in trismus or infection. The patient should be observed for any signs of recurrent bleeding or for signs of secondary infection of the hematoma. At the first indication of infection, antibiotic therapy should be initiated [2].

Failure to Achieve Profound Anesthesia

For endodontic surgery purposes, LA infiltration in most cases should be sufficient. However, in certain cases the anesthesia wears off during the surgery. Continuing the surgery while the patient is in pain is unacceptable and impractical [4, 30, 31, 32]. Both the patient's cooperation and the surgeon's ability to continue the operation are decreased when the patient is not fully anesthetized [4, 30, 31, 32], The infiltration sites for periradicular surgery should be multiple, throughout the entire surgical field [4, 30, 31, 32].

Failure to achieve LA can be due to LA administration technical mistakes, anatomic variations with accessory innervation, and anxiety of the patient [4, 30, 31, 32].

Usually, anatomic variation would have a less significant impact on infiltration-based LA compared to block anesthesia, and while it is possible to achieve a good anesthesia using infiltration of LA in the maxilla, in the mandible the infiltration may not penetrate through the cortical plate, thus, leading to insufficient anesthesia [4, 30, 31, 32] (Fig. 5.1a, b).

Inflammation and LA Failure

Presence of inflammation may have several effects on local tissue physiology, and it was speculated that local anesthetics are generally much less effective when administered to patients with inflamed tissue probably due to the tissue acidosis [30]. The inflammation induces tissue acidosis that may cause "ion trapping" of local anesthetics: the low tissue pH will result in a greater proportion of the local anesthetic being trapped in the charged acid form of the molecule and, therefore, unable to cross cell membranes [4]. In addition, peripheral vasodilation induced by inflammatory mediators would reduce the concentration of local anesthetics by increasing the rate of systemic absorption [31].

Local inflammation may lead to activation and sensitization of peripheral nociceptors and sprouting of nerve terminals. In addition, local inflammation may also lead to neural central sensitization, accelerated even more when the patient suffers from psychological stress. Thus, the local inflammation may bare both local and central neural effects that may compromise the ability to achieve profound long-lasting LA [32].

Needle Breakage

Faura-Solé et al. [33] reported on a series of cases of broken anesthetic injection needles. The needles were located in the pterygomandibular space or near the maxillary tuberosity.

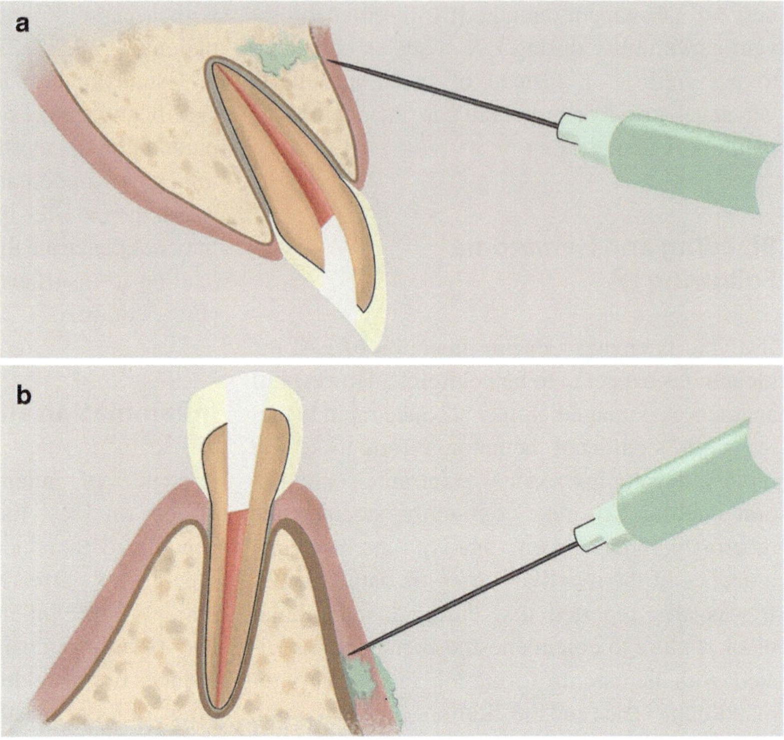

Fig. 5.1 Infiltration of local anesthetic in the maxilla (**a**) and the mandible (**b**). Unlike in the maxilla, in the mandible the LA infiltration may not penetrate the cortical plate, leading to insufficient anesthesia

These complications were the result of an unexpected movement by the patient or an incorrect anesthetic technique. For prevention of needle breakage, it is recommended to routinely inspect dental needles before administering injections and minimize the number of repeated injections using the same needle [34]. The needles should not be bended before use. And short needles are inadequate when performing an inferior alveolar nerve block, since a needle must be of adequate length to ensure that it is never buried to the hub [34].

The management of needle breakage is a clinical dilemma. While there is still controversy as to whether or not to remove a broken dental needle [35], recognition, localization, and documentation are of paramount importance. The removal is warranted not only because of the fear of needle migration toward large blood vessels in the head and neck but also because of the medicolegal considerations [21, 33–38].

Ethunandan et al. [36] recommended in the event that needle breakage does occur, every effort should be made to retrieve the needle immediately, if the tip is visible, using fine hemostats. However, if the broken tip is not visible, an immediate referral is advised. The remaining portion of the broken needle should also be sent along for further determinations of the size of the broken fragment [36]. In addition, when breakage occurs, the patient must be informed immediately and the event must be documented thoroughly. The patient will need reassurance and referral to an oral and maxillofacial surgeon for treatment. In addition, marking the needle entry point with a permanent marker will help the oral surgeon establish orientation [34, 37]. Today, new technologies and surgical techniques allow for complete removal of a broken needle preventing possible complications [38].

Postoperative Soft-Tissue Injury

It is extremely important to warn patients that the effects of anesthesia can persist for several hours which may cause a patient to bite the mucosa of the lower lip, cheek, or tongue or to scratch or rub the chin region resulting in a self-inflicted injury [39].

In Conclusion

The most important steps in managing untoward reactions to LA are to adopt a clinical practice aimed to prevent LA possible complications, diagnose the problem promptly when it does occur, treat it if necessary, and reassure the patient.

References

1. American Association of Endodontics. Glossary of endodontic terms. 7th ed. Chicago: 2003.
2. Blanton PL, Jeske AH. Avoiding complications in local anesthesia induction: anatomical considerations. J Am Dent Assoc. 2003;134(7):888–93.
3. Pipa-Vallejo A, Garcia-Pola-Vallejo MJ. Local anesthetics in dentistry. Med Oral Patol Oral Cir Bucal. 2004;9(5):440–3, 438–40.
4. Hargreaves KM, Keiser K. Local anesthetic failure in endodontics: mechanisms and management. Endod Top. 2002;1:26–39.
5. Naguib M, Magboul MM, Samarkandi AH, Attia M. Adverse effects and drug interactions associated with local and regional anaesthesia. Drug Saf. 1998;18(4):221–50.
6. Daublander M, Muller R, Lipp MD. The incidence of complications associated with local anesthesia in dentistry. Anesth Prog. 1997;44(4):132–41.
7. Umino M, Nagao M. Systemic diseases in elderly dental patients. Int Dent J. 1993;43(3):213–8.
8. Batinac T, Sotosek Tokmadzic V, Peharda V, Brajac I. Adverse reactions and alleged allergy to local anesthetics: analysis of 331 patients. J Dermatol. 2013;40(7):522–7.
9. Cox B, Durieux ME, Marcus MA. Toxicity of local anaesthetics. Best Pract Res Clin Anaesthesiol. 2003;17(1):111–36.
10. Ring J, Franz R, Brockow K. Anaphylactic reactions to local anesthetics. Chem Immunol Allergy. 2010;95: 190–200.
11. Tomoyasu Y, Mukae K, Suda M, Hayashi T, Ishii M, Sakaguchi M, et al. Allergic reactions to local anesthetics in dental patients: analysis of intracutaneous and challenge tests. Open Dent J. 2011;5:146–9.
12. Matsumura K, Miura K, Takata Y, Kurokawa H, Kajiyama M, Abe I, et al. Changes in blood pressure and heart rate variability during dental surgery. Am J Hypertens. 1998;11(11 Pt 1):1376–80.
13. Zarei M, Ghoddusi J, Sharifi E, Forghani M, Afkhami F, Marouzi P. Comparison of the anaesthetic efficacy of and heart rate changes after periodontal ligament or intraosseous X-Tip injection in mandibular molars: a randomized controlled clinical trial. Int Endod J. 2012;45(10):921–6.
14. Knoll-Kohler E, Frie A, Becker J, Ohlendorf D. Changes in plasma epinephrine concentration after dental infiltration anesthesia with different doses of epinephrine. J Dent Res. 1989;68(6):1098–101.
15. Ketabi M, Shamami MS, Alaie M. Influence of local anesthetics with or without epinephrine 1/80000 on blood pressure and heart rate: a randomized double-blind experimental clinical trial. Dent Res J (Isfahan). 2012;9(4):437–40.
16. Silvestre FJ, Verdu MJ, Sanchis JM, Grau D, Penarrocha M. Effects of vasoconstrictors in dentistry upon systolic and diastolic arterial pressure. Med Oral. 2001;6(1):57–63.
17. Haas DA. Localized complications from local anesthesia. J Calif Dent Assoc. 1998;26(9):677–82.
18. Stone J, Kaban LB. Trismus after injection of local anesthetic. Oral Surg Oral Med Oral Pathol. 1979; 48(1):29–32.
19. Brodsky CD, Dower Jr JS. Middle ear problems after a Gow-Gates injection. J Am Dent Assoc. 2001;132(10): 1420–4.
20. Steenen SA, Dubois L, Saeed P, de Lange J. Ophthalmologic complications after intraoral local anesthesia: case report and review of literature. Oral Surg Oral Med Oral Pathol Oral Radiol. 2012;113(6):e1–5.
21. Givol N, Rosen E, Taicher S, Tsesis I. Risk management in endodontics. J Endod. 2010;36(6):982–4.
22. Garisto GA, Gaffen AS, Lawrence HP, Tenenbaum HC, Haas DA. Occurrence of paresthesia after dental local anesthetic administration in the United States. J Am Dent Assoc. 2010;141(7):836–44.
23. Givol N, Rosen E, Bjorndal L, Taschieri S, Ofec R, Tsesis I. Medico-legal aspects of altered sensation following endodontic treatment: a retrospective case series. Oral Surg Oral Med Oral Pathol Oral Radiol Endod. 2011;112(1):126–31.
24. Park SH, Wang HL. Implant reversible complications: classification and treatments. Implant Dent. 2005; 14(3):211–20.
25. Annibali S, Ripari M, La Monaca G, Tonoli F, Cristalli MP. Local accidents in dental implant surgery: prevention and treatment. Int J Periodontics Restorative Dent. 2009;29(3):325–31.
26. Gallas-Torreira MM, Reboiras-Lopez MD, Garcia-Garcia A, Gandara-Rey J. Mandibular nerve paresthesia caused by endodontic treatment. Med Oral. 2003; 8(4):299–303.
27. Grotz KA, Al-Nawas B, de Aguiar EG, Schulz A, Wagner W. Treatment of injuries to the inferior alveolar nerve after endodontic procedures. Clin Oral Investig. 1998;2(2):73–6.
28. Juodzbalys G, Wang H, Sabalys G. Injury of the inferior alveolar nerve during implant placement: a literature review. J Oral Maxillofac Res. 2011;2(1):e1.
29. Traeger KA. Hematoma following inferior alveolar injection: a possible cause for anesthesia failure. Anesth Prog. 1979;26(5):122–3.

30. Walton RE, Torabinejad M. Managing local anesthesia problems in the endodontic patient. J Am Dent Assoc. 1992;123(5):97–102.
31. Vandermeulen E. Pain perception, mechanisms of action of local anesthetics and possible causes of failure. Rev Belge Med Dent (1984). 2000;55(1):29–40.
32. Ingle JI. Ingle's endodontics. 6th ed. BC Decker Inc, Hamilton, Ontario 2008
33. Faura-Sole M, Sanchez-Garces MA, Berini-Aytes L, Gay-Escoda C. Broken anesthetic injection needles: report of 5 cases. Quintessence Int. 1999;30(7):461–5.
34. Bedrock RD, Skigen A, Dolwick MF. Retrieval of a broken needle in the pterygomandibular space. J Am Dent Assoc. 1999;130(5):685–7.
35. Brown LJ, Meerkotter VA. An unusual experience with a broken needle. J Dent Assoc S Afr. 1963;18:74.
36. Ethunandan M, Tran AL, Anand R, Bowden J, Seal MT, Brennan PA. Needle breakage following inferior alveolar nerve block: implications and management. Br Dent J. 2007;202(7):395–7.
37. Rifkind JB. Management of a broken needle in the pterygomandibular space following a Vazirani-Akinosi block: case report. J Can Dent Assoc. 2011;77:b64.
38. Thompson M, Wright S, Cheng LH, Starr D. Locating broken dental needles. Int J Oral Maxillofac Surg. 2003;32(6):642–4.
39. Torrente-Castells E, Gargallo-Albiol J, Rodriguez-Baeza A, Berini-Aytes L, Gay-Escoda C. Necrosis of the skin of the chin: a possible complication of inferior alveolar nerve block injection. J Am Dent Assoc. 2008;139(12):1625–30.

Prevention and Management of Soft Tissue Complications in Endodontic Surgery

6

Igor Tsesis, Ilan Beitlitum, and Eyal Rosen

Abstract

Operator-related factors such as preoperative planning of the surgical procedure, correct flap design, and soft tissue management, as well as patient-related factors such as the gingival biotype and the periodontal condition, may influence the risk of soft tissue complications following endodontic surgery. The clinician should be aware of possible anatomical pitfalls during flap procedure, such as adjacent neurovascular bundles. In order to avoid flap dryness and possible tissue necrosis and delayed healing, it is recommended to perform a short-duration surgery with a constant irrigation of the reflected tissues with saline. Different flap designs may be predisposed to different risks of complications. Intra-sulcular flaps are prone to gingival recession, submarginal and semilunar flaps are prone to scar formation, and a controversy exists whether papilla-based incision is prone to gingival recession and if papilla preservation incision may prevent gingival recession.

Introduction

The outcome evaluation of endodontic surgery usually focuses on clinical and radiographic signs of periapical osseous healing [1–3]. However, endodontic surgery involves also intentional soft tissue wounding, during the flap elevation procedure, and the available information concerning the soft tissue healing and related possible complications following endodontic surgery is relatively scarce [4].

A *Flap* is defined as *a loosened section of tissue separated from the surrounding tissues except at its base* [5] and is aimed to facilitate surgical access to the root apex, a fundamental perquisite for the ability to adequately manage the root end and for the achievement of predictable clinical results [1]. However, adequate flap design, especially in the esthetic zone, is crucial in order to achieve sufficient esthetic results, and failing to take into account the soft tissue considerations may negate all other aspects of the treatment outcome, resulting in esthetic failure [6].

I. Tsesis, DMD (✉) • E. Rosen, DMD
Department of Endodontology,
Maurice and Gabriela Goldschleger
School of Dental Medicine, Tel Aviv University,
Tel Aviv, Israel
e-mail: dr.tsesis@gmail.com; dr.eyalrosen@gmail.com

I. Beitlitum, DMD
Department of Periodontology and Dental Implantology,
The Maurice and Gabriela Goldschleger
School of Dental Medicine, Tel Aviv University,
Ramat Aviv, 69978 Tel Aviv, Israel
e-mail: beilan@bezeqint.net

I. Tsesis (ed.), *Complications in Endodontic Surgery*,
DOI 10.1007/978-3-642-54218-3_6,

Flap procedure, like any other surgical procedure, possesses also inherent risks of complications. Flap necrosis and delayed healing, periodontal defect formation, gingival scarring, and many additional possible complications may emerge during or following the surgery. Some of the complications may adversely affect the long-term survival of the tooth, and some may cause esthetic and functional complexities [4, 6–8].

Flap-related complications may be associated with patient-specific factors, such as the periodontal anatomy and periodontal health status and also with the applied surgical approach and soft tissue management technique [1, 4, 6–11].

This chapter will review possible complications concerning flap management during endodontic surgical procedures, their etiology, prevention, and management.

The Anatomical and Periodontal Aspects of Flap-Related Complications

Understanding the anatomical structure of the periodontium and the specific characteristics of the patient's gingival biotype is essential for a successful soft tissue management during endodontic surgery.

The Normal Periodontal Structure

The periodontium serves as the supporting apparatus for the teeth and consists of the alveolar mucosa, gingiva, cementum, periodontal ligament, and alveolar bone [12] (Fig. 6.1).

The *oral mucosa* is the tissue lining the oral cavity [5] and is termed by its specific anatomical location. For example, the *alveolar mucosa* is the loosely attached and movable mucosa covering the basal part of the alveolar process and continuing into the vestibular fornix and the floor of the mouth [5, 12].

The *gingiva* is the fibrous investing tissue that surrounds a tooth and is contiguous with its periodontal ligament and with the mucosal tissues of the mouth [5]. The gingiva is divided into *free gingiva* and *attached gingiva* and is considered as a part of the *masticatory mucosa,* which covers the alveolar process and surrounds the cervical portion of the teeth. It consists of an epithelial layer and an underlying connective tissue layer. The gingiva obtains its final form and texture with the eruption of the teeth [13].

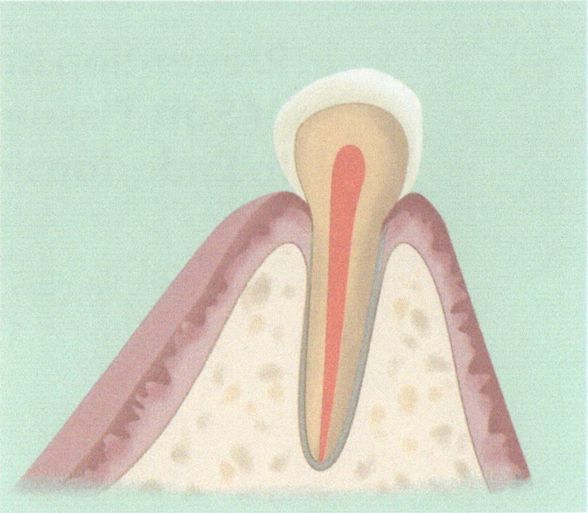

Fig. 6.1 Normal periodontal tissues

The *attached gingiva* is the portion of the gingiva that is firm, dense, stippled, and firmly bound to the underlying periosteum, tooth, and bone [5]. The width of the attached gingiva varies in range from 1 to 9 mm in different parts of the mouth [14]. In the maxilla, the facial attached gingiva is generally widest in incisors and most narrow adjacent to the canine and first premolars. In the mandible, the gingiva on the lingual aspect is particularly narrow in the area of the incisors and canines and widest in the molar region [15]. Facially positioned teeth had narrower zones of attached gingiva compared to well-aligned or lingual positioned teeth [16].

The *free gingiva* is the part of the gingiva that surrounds the tooth and is not directly attached to the tooth surface [5]. The *free gingival margin* is the coronal part of the gingiva and has a scalloped outline. The free gingival margin is situated about 2 mm coronal to the CEJ of the tooth, and the attached gingiva extends from the base of the free gingiva to the mucogingival junction [5, 9, 12].

The gingiva is continuous with the alveolar mucosa that is situated apically. The *mucogingival junction* is the demarcated border between the gingival and the alveolar mucosa and is absent in the palatal aspect of the maxillary teeth where the gingiva is continuous with the palatal mucosa [5, 12]. The mucogingival junction defines the width of the attached gingiva.

The *gingival papilla* is the portion of the gingiva that occupies the interproximal spaces [5]. The shape of the papilla is influenced by the shape of the interproximal contact points, the width of the interproximal area, and the position of the CEJ of the involved teeth, and it may vary from triangular and knife-edge shapes in the anterior regions to a more square shaped in the posterior regions [5, 12].

The *gingival sulcus* is a fissure that is an invagination around a tooth bounded by the free gingival margin [5, 12] and ranges between 0 and 6 mm depth (average depth of 0.7 mm) [12]. The alveolar bone follows a path that parallels the positions of the CEJs of the teeth, and in health the interdental bone is about 1 mm from the CEJ and increases with age to about 3 mm [12].

The *supracrestal connective tissue attachment* is the connective tissue fibers that originate from the osseous crest to the CEJ; the *epithelial attachment (or junctional epithelium)* is the epithelial attachment from the CEJ onto the tooth enamel.

The Etiology and the Possible Risk Factors of Flap-Related Complications

Flap procedures may lead to several complications [4, 6–8, 10, 12, 17], including attachment loss and recession of the gingival margin, flap necrosis, flap tearing, tissue dehiscence, delayed healing, periodontal defect, scarring, hemorrhage, and nerve injury.

Following endodontic surgery, and consistent with the basic biological principles of wound healing, the postsurgical histological wound healing sequel can be *repair* (when the injured tissues are replaced with scar tissue) or *regeneration* (when the injured tissues are reestablished by similar tissue as was originally present) [18].

Clinically, the soft tissue healing can be divided to *healing by first intention*, e.g., primary union of a wound in which the incised tissue edges are approximated and held until union occurs, and to *healing by second intention,* e.g., wound closure wherein the edges remain separated and the wound heals from the base and sides via the formation of granulation tissue [5]. In wounds healing by second intention, continuous local inflammation, infection, wound dehiscence, and foreign bodies are important contributory factors to an ensuing scar formation [19].

Scarring: A scar can be defined as *fibrous tissue replacing normal tissues destroyed by injury or disease* [5]. Macroscopically a scar is a disturbance of the normal structure and function of the tissue architecture, resulting from the end product of the healed wound [10]. Histologically, scars are characterized by their lack of specific organization of cellular and matrix elements when compared with the uninjured tissue [19]. The normal wound healing process includes a combination of biological processes such as hemostasis, inflammation, proliferation, and remodeling. Scar formation may occur as a result of altered regulation of the normal physiological processes in the involved epithelial and submucosal tissues. The scarring may clinically manifest as an elevated or depressed site, with an alteration of the mucosal texture and color and changes in the biomechanical properties of the tissues [4]. From a clinical point of view, scar formation following flap procedure is a significant esthetic problem, especially in the esthetic zone and in patients with a high smile line (i.e., a significant exposure of maxillary anterior gingiva during a full smile) [20] (Fig. 6.2).

Attachment loss refers to the distance between the CEJ and the base of the gingival sulcus and may manifest both as probing pocket depth and\ or gingival recession.

Gingival recession is the location of marginal periodontal tissues apical to the CEJ that may be caused by improper periodontal surgical manipulations [4, 6–8, 10, 12, 17], such as incorrect reposition of the flap, compromised blood circulation of the flap through excessive retraction or poor flap design, and flap contraction

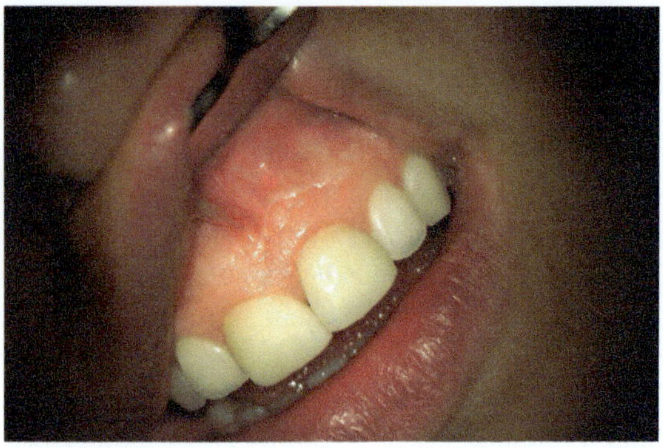

Fig. 6.2 Scar following submarginal incision

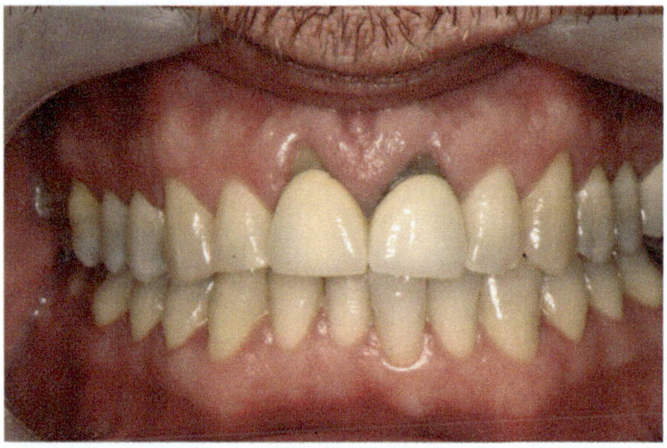

Fig. 6.3 Gingival recession

[4, 7, 8, 10–12, 19, 21] (Fig. 6.3). Thus, it is important to preserve the root-attached tissues and to reposition a tension-free flap.

Flap necrosis may occur because of insufficient blood supply. The prevention of flap necrosis includes vertical releasing incisions that should be parallel or converging to the coronal part of the flap; the base of the flap should be wider than the free margin to allow an adequate blood supply, and it is advised to avoid excessive force or crashing of the tissue with the retractors [1, 7].

Flap tearing may occur as a result of poor flap design with a small and insufficient incision that causes flap tension and may result in tearing (Fig. 6.4). Thus, the flap should be reflected as one unit, with sufficient length of releasing incisions [1, 7]. It should be remembered that the flap incision wound naturally heals from side to side and not end to end. Thus, a long incision does not necessarily heal slower.

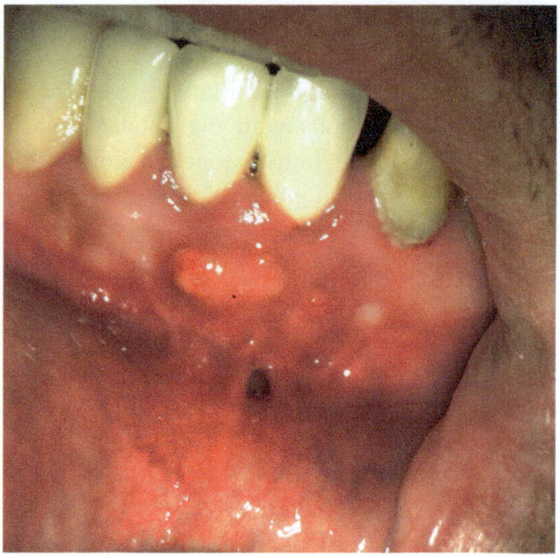

Fig. 6.4 Flap tear following endodontic surgery on the mandibular incisors

Soft tissue dehiscence is usually a result of infection from bacterial contamination of the incisional wound. Partial or total separation of the wound margins may manifest within the first week after surgery. In most instances, the wound dehiscence results from tissue failure rather than improper suturing techniques. The dehisced wound may be closed again or left to heal by secondary intention, depending upon the extent of the disruption and the surgeon's judgment of the clinical situation [22].

Influence of a Periodontal Disease on Soft Tissue Healing Following Endodontic Surgery

Periodontal diseases are infections and are caused by microorganisms that colonize the tooth surface at the gingival margin. Sometimes, a combination of factors (e.g., bacteriological or treatment-related factors) facilitates conditions that may promote either a colonization of newly introduced subset of bacterial species or an overgrowth of existing bacterial species that may eventually lead to a destruction of the periodontium [13].

It has been reported that when performing modern endodontic surgery for teeth with endodontic-periodontal combined lesions, the endodontic success rate is expected to drop to less than 80 %, compared to 95 % for cases with an isolated endodontic lesions [23]. In addition, preoperative factors significant for the prognosis of restored endodontically treated teeth are related to the periodontal status and the attachment loss [24]. Thus, the presence of a significant periodontal disease may adversely affect the success of the endodontic surgery [23], the expected long-term survival of the tooth [24], and the risk and extent of flap-related complications.

The Gingival Biotype Effects on the Surgical Procedure

Recently, it was demonstrated that the gingival biotype could be related to complications following flap procedures [8, 11].

There are two distinctive types of gingival phenotypes: *thick and thin gingival biotypes.*

Thin gingival biotype is more prevalent in women and is characterized by a highly scalloped marginal gingiva with slender teeth, with delicate and almost translucent appearance, and with a minimal narrow zone of attached gingiva [7, 11, 17].

Thick gingival biotype is more prevalent in men and is characterized with a bulky, slightly scalloped marginal gingiva with short and wide teeth, broad zone of attached gingiva, fibrotic and resilient tissue, relatively flat soft tissue, and a relatively large amount of attached gingiva [7, 11, 17].

Several methods were proposed based on the measurement of buccal gingival thickness to assess gingival biotypes, and the simplest method is based on using the transparency of a periodontal probe through the gingival margin. If the outline of the probe could be visually detected through the tissue, it should be categorized as *thin biotype*; if not, it should be categorized as a *thick biotype* [8, 11, 25] (Fig. 6.5). Several periodontal and anatomical parameters were suggested to be associated with a specific gingival biotype, such as the tooth shape and contact point location, papilla height, and the distance from the contact point to the alveolar crest. Additional demographic factors, such as the patient age, may also be associated [11].

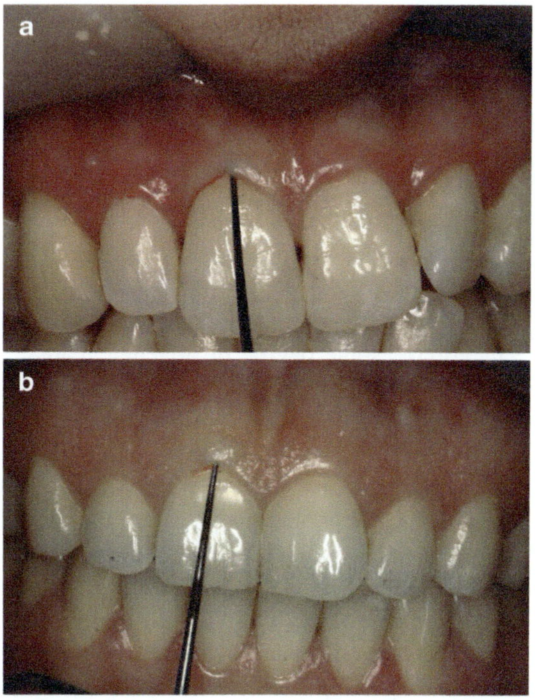

Fig. 6.5 Gingival biotypes assessment. (**a**) thin periodontal biotype, (**b**) thick periodontal biotype

The identification of the gingival biotype is important in planning the type of surgical incision during endodontic surgery, since various gingival biotypes may influence the esthetic outcome of surgery [17]. It may be especially crucial in the esthetic area, since thin gingival biotypes may be a risk factor of postsurgical recession development [8, 11].

Thin gingival biotype is more prone to gingival recession without pocket formation and to a loss of the thin vestibular bone plate [17]. Thus, in surgery of a tooth with a thin biotype, a delicate and unpredictable tissue healing (recession) should be expected [17].

The type of incision is an important predictor for complications following the surgery of a tooth with a thin biotype: higher probability of recession for intra-sulcular incision, more scarring for submarginal incision, more complications during flap elevation such as flap tearing, and dehiscence and difficulties in suturing [4, 6–8, 11, 17].

Thick gingival biotype is more prone to infrabony defect formation and deeper probing pocket depth formation following the surgery. However, thick biotype is less prone to recession formation. Thus, it is less prone to esthetic complications [4, 6–8, 11, 17]. Surgery of a tooth with a thick biotype may also be prone to marginal inflammation, bleeding on probing, and edema [17].

In general, both with thick and with thin gingival biotype, some degree of attachment loss is expected following sulcular flap procedures. However, with thick biotype the attachment loss is a result of increased periodontal probing depth, while with thin biotype it is mainly a result of gingival recession that may cause an esthetic defect in the presence of full coverage crowns [4, 6–8, 11, 17]. It was also reported that teeth with thin gingival biotype led to significantly more recession than thick biotype. In addition, teeth with probing depth less than 2.5 mm had more attachment loss than probing depth more than 2.5 mm [8].

While no differences were reported between the two gingival biotypes with regard to scar formation following apical surgery [4], this conclusion should be perceived with caution since in this study more scar formation was observed, both in the attached and the alveolar mucosa among female patients. Since thin gingival biotype is more common in females, more scar formation following surgery of teeth with a thin gingival biotype is expected [4].

Prevention and Management of Flap-Related Complications

The Surgical Incision and Flap Design

An accurate surgical incision, and adequate flap elevation and repositioning of the reflected soft tissue, will enable sufficient blood supply, root coverage, and proper tissue healing [26]. Thus, several principles should be applied:

1. Avoiding horizontal and severely angled vertical incisions will result in less flap shrinkage and improved flap blood supply.

   When the supplying blood vessels enter the gingiva, they presume a vertical course parallel to the long axis of the teeth, superficial to the periosteum, and are termed *The supra-periosteal vessels* [13, 26–28]. Horizontal and severely angled incisions may serve the gingival blood vessels that scuttle perpendicular to the incision line and may lead to compromised flap blood supply [13, 26].

   In addition, the collagen fibers that attach to the periosteum scuttle in a direction parallel to the long axis of the teeth [13, 26]. Therefore, horizontal and severely angled incisions (such as used in semilunar flaps) may shrink following the surgery as a result of contraction of the severed collagen fibers that run perpendicular to the incision line. As a result, it may be difficult to reposition the flap edges to their original position without applying excessive tension forces on the soft tissues, with increased risk of wound dehiscence and subsequent scar formation from healing by second intention [13, 26].
2. Incisions over radicular eminences should be avoided since they may lead to soft tissue fenestrations.

   Radicular eminences may fenestrate through the cortical bone or be covered by a thin bone layer with relatively poor blood supply. These anatomical defects may lead to soft tissue fenestrations if incisions are made over the eminence. Thus, the vertical-releasing incisions should be parallel to the long axis of the teeth, over solid interdental bone [13, 26].
3. Incisions should be performed in a way that facilitates flap repositioning over a solid bone.

   Areas of bone loss have insufficient blood supply, and flap repositioning over such areas may result in necrosis and sloughing of the soft tissue. Thus, the flap design should take into account the extent of osseous bone defect so that the repositioned flap margins will be supported by a solid bone [13, 26].
4. Incisions should avoid major muscle attachments.

   Muscle attachments may jeopardize the repositioning of the flap and result in healing by second intention and scar tissue formation.

Extended lateral extension of the horizontal incision may allow the vertical incision to bypass muscle attachment and include it in the flap [13, 26].
5. The vertical incision extension should facilitate the positioning of the retractor during surgery on a solid bone. Insufficient vertical incisions may cause the retractor to traumatize the mucosal tissue of the flap and may jeopardize the blood supply of the involved tissues [1, 13, 26].
6. The extent of the horizontal incision should enable adequate surgical access, with minimal tension and stretching of the soft tissue. Excessive soft tissue trauma is expected when performing too short rather than too long incisions [1, 13, 26].

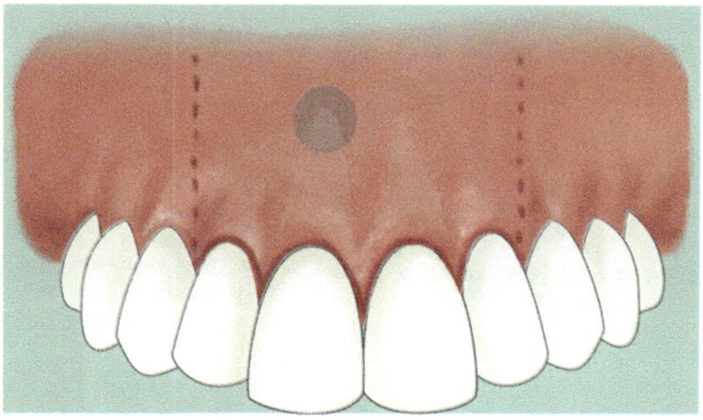

Fig. 6.6 Intra-sulcular incison

The Flap Design

Various preoperative factors should be considered for the flap design in order to achieve predictable results with minimal risks of complications. The gingival biotype, the number of teeth involved, the depth of the vestibulum, presence of high muscle attachment, the width of the attached gingiva, presence of adjacent dental implants (the periodontal anatomy around an implant is more sensitive to additional surgery and more prone to implant recession), adjacent anatomical structures, size and location of the osseous pathology, presence of a periodontal disease, presence of dental crowns, and the patient's smile profile should all be accounted for [7].

In general, the flap should be *full thickness*, thus, include the entire mucoperiosteal tissues (gingiva, alveolar mucosa, and periosteum). Full-thickness flaps maintain the supraperiosteal blood vessels that supply these tissues and result in less trauma and less bleeding [1, 13, 26].

Intra-sulcular Flap

Intra-sulcular flap may be performed with or without releasing incisions, depending on the clinical conditions. A *sulcular flap* (*envelope flap*) is a single continuous incision through the gingival sulcus, without releasing incisions. Advantages: conservative, less scarring, relatively easy and fast procedure, and low morbidity. Disadvantages: limited application for endodontic surgery since it does not permit the visualization of the entire root. The absence of releasing incisions results in flap stretching and tearing and a high risk of gingival recession [1, 7, 21, 22, 29].

Intra-sulcular flap can be also performed with one releasing incision (*triangular flap*) or with two releasing incisions (*rectangular flap*) (Fig. 6.6). Advantages: better visibility and visualization of the entire buccal root surface. Complications: possible dehiscence and pocket formation and recession of the gingival attachment and esthetic complication when crowns are present by exposure of subgingivally placed crown margins at the restoration-tooth interface and damage to the interdental papilla [1, 7, 21, 22, 29].

Submarginal Flap

In this flap, the sulcular incision is replaced with a scalloped submarginal incision. It is made of a horizontal incision along the attached gingival and one or two releasing incisions. The horizontal incision should be confined to the attached gingiva (Fig. 6.7). Advantages: the marginal gingiva is preserved and the risk of dehiscence is minimal. Complications: limited visualization of the coronal part of the root and scarring may occur.

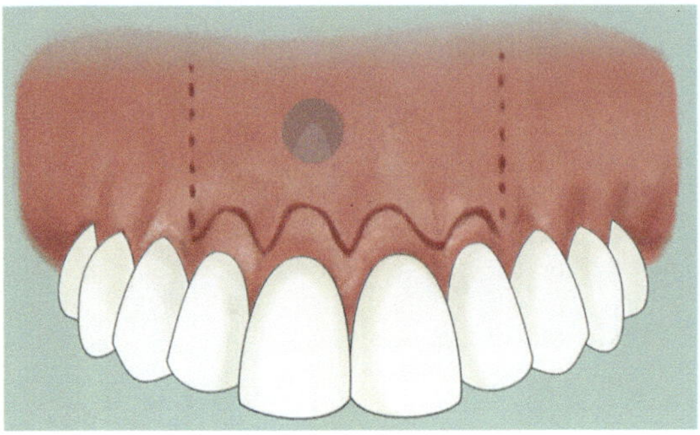

Fig. 6.7 Submarginal incision

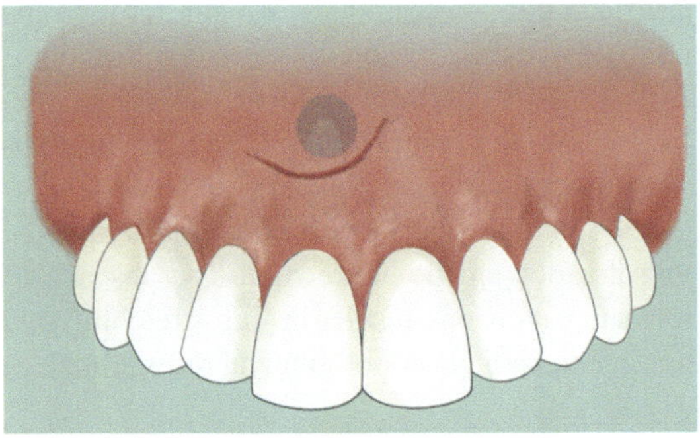

Fig. 6.8 Semilunar incision

Semilunar Flap

A curved horizontal incision in the alveolar mucosa (Fig. 6.8). The semilunar flap is extremely simple to perform. However, it allows limited access and visibility in the surgical area. It may also result in bleeding and in delayed healing. The lack of reference points makes flap repositioning difficult, and scar formation is common. This flap design is not recommended for endodontic surgery.

Papilla Preservation Techniques

Papilla preservation techniques were originally designed for reconstructive procedures, using guided tissue regeneration of intraosseous periodontal defects [7, 13]. The main purposes of this flap design are primary wound closure, maintaining flap integrity, and avoiding early membrane exposure. The procedure could be performed using buccal papilla-based incision (Fig. 6.9)

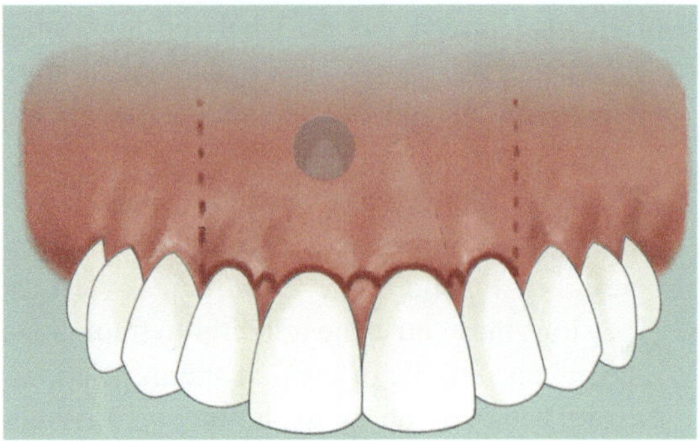

Fig. 6.9 Papilla base incision

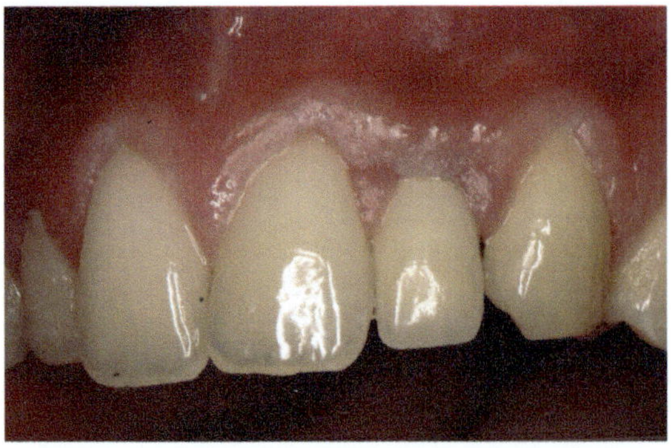

Fig. 6.10 Scar following papilla-based incision

[13, 21]. This technique is complicated and difficult to perform, with a possibility of scar formation in the esthetic area at the base of the papilla (Fig. 6.10). Another alternative is to use a palatal approach to prevent scar formation at the esthetic zone [13] (Fig. 6.11a–e). The advantages of papilla preservation techniques include optimized wound closure leading to primary intention healing and leaving an intact interdental papilla with enhanced gingival esthetics [7, 13].

Flap Elevation General Precautions

The clinician should be aware of several anatomical and procedural pitfalls during flap elevation, such as bone exostoses, high muscle attachment, and proximity of neurovascular bundles. In order to avoid flap dryness, tissue necrosis, and delayed healing, it is recommended to perform a short-duration surgery with a constant irrigation of the reflected tissues with saline.

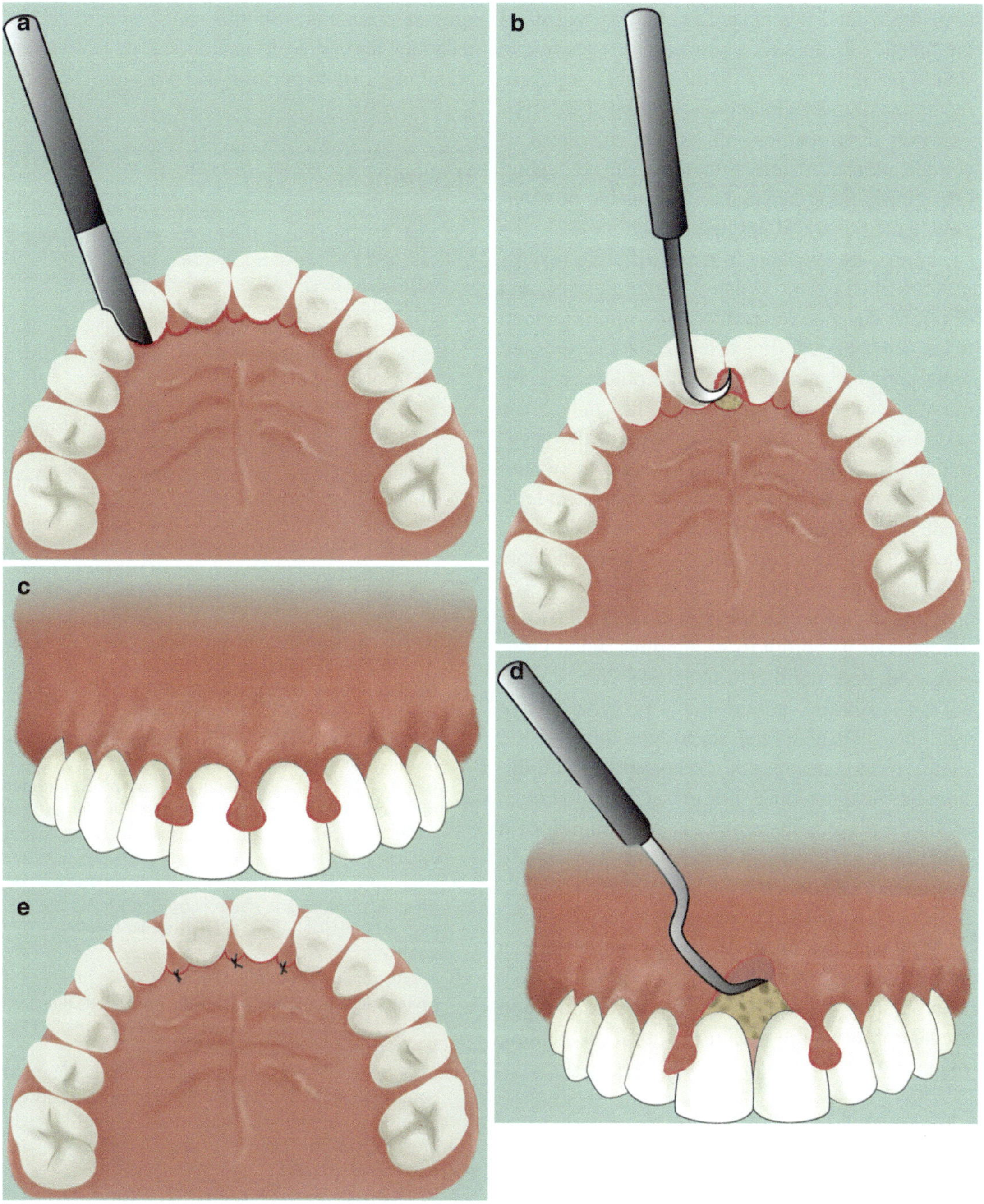

Fig. 6.11 Papilla-preservation flap design. (**a**) Palatal intrasulcular incision, (**b**) Palatal release of the interdental papillae, (**c**) Buccal elevation of the papillae, (**d**) Buccal flap elevation, (**e**) Repositioning of the flap and palatally placed sutures

Flap Repositioning and Suture

While passive repositioning of the flap is imperative, even if a proper tissue approximation is achieved, flap contraction and shrinkage during the early healing phase may result in soft tissue healing complications [7].

Flap suturing is supposed to position and secure the surgical flap in order to promote optimal healing, and it should hold flap edges in apposition until the wound has healed enough to withstand the functional stresses. A proper suture technique should place the tension on the wound margins to facilitate primary intention healing [30, 31]. However, improper use of sutures may lead to complications, inflammation, and delayed healing [26]. In addition, the sutures are capable of strangulating the tissues if applied too tightly [22].

Sutures are available in many different materials (classified by absorbency), different sizes, and different designs (monofilament, multifilament, twisted, or braided). For example, silk sutures are nonabsorbable and easy to manipulate and are made of protein fibers and glue. They may cause severe adverse tissue reactions, due to the accumulation of plaque on the fibers that occurs within a few hours. Gut sutures are absorbable and are made from collagen derived from sheep or bovine intestines. Their absorption rate is unpredictable (may take up to 10 days) [22, 30, 31].

The suturing technique should be evaluated on the basis of its ability to accomplish wound closure and flap stabilization at least for several days. Usually the sutures should provide passive fixation mechanism and avoid stretching of the tissue, tissue tearing, and compromised circulation. Surgical bleeding should be controlled prior to suture placement to prevent a formation of a hematoma under the flap and ensuing culture medium formation for bacterial growth and infection [22, 30, 31].

Synthetic absorbable sutures, when used in a proper suturing technique, may provide easy manipulation, relatively mild tissue reaction, and prevention of suture retention within the healing tissues [30, 31].

Conclusions and Key Learning Point

The design of a surgical flap should be case-specific. The flap extension in endodontic surgery is primarily dictated by the demands for proper root end management.

The flap should permit a proper view of the operative field, should allow adequate blood supply to the flap tissues, should facilitate optimal gingival healing, should not jeopardize the esthetics and adjacent anatomical structures, and should be easy to perform and reposition [4, 6–8].

References

1. Kim S, Kratchman S. Modern endodontic surgery concepts and practice: a review. J Endod. 2006;32(7): 601–23.
2. Tsesis I, Faivishevsky V, Kfir A, Rosen E. Outcome of surgical endodontic treatment performed by a modern technique: a meta-analysis of literature. J Endod. 2009;35(11):1505–11.
3. Tsesis I, Rosen E, Taschieri S, Telishevsky Strauss Y, Ceresoli V, Del Fabbro M. Outcomes of surgical endodontic treatment performed by a modern technique: an updated meta-analysis of the literature. J Endod. 2013;39(3):332–9.
4. von Arx T, Salvi GE, Janner S, Jensen SS. Scarring of gingiva and alveolar mucosa following apical surgery: visual assessment after one year. Oral Surg. 2008;1: 178–89.
5. The American Academy of Periodontology. Glossary of periodontal terms. 4th ed. Chicago: The American Academy of Periodontology; 2001.
6. Ahmad I. Anterior dental aesthetics: gingival perspective. Br Dent J. 2005;199(4):195–202.
7. Trombelli L, Roberto F. Flap designs for periodontal healing. Endod Topics. 2012;25:4–15.
8. von Arx T, Salvi GE, Janner S, Jensen SS. Gingival recession following apical surgery in the esthetic zone: a clinical study with 70 cases. Eur J Esthet Dent. 2009;4(1):28–45.
9. Ainamo J, Loe H. Anatomical characteristics of gingiva. A clinical and microscopic study of the free and attached gingiva. J Periodontol. 1966;37(1): 5–13.
10. Ferguson MW, Whitby DJ, Shah M, Armstrong J, Siebert JW, Longaker MT. Scar formation: the spectral nature of fetal and adult wound repair. Plast Reconstr Surg. 1996;97(4):854–60.
11. Fischer KR, Grill E, Jockel-Schneider Y, Bechtold M, Schlagenhauf U, Fickl S. On the relationship between gingival biotypes and supracrestal gingival height, crown form and papilla height. Clin Oral Implants Res. 2013. doi:10.1111/clr.12196.
12. Palumbo A. The anatomy and physiology of the healthy periodontium. In F. S. Panagakos & R. M. Davies (Eds.), Gingival diseases: Their aetiology, prevention and treatment (pp. 139–154). Rijeka, Croatia: InTech.
13. Lindhe J, Lang NP, Karring T. Clinical periodontology and implant dentistry. 5th ed. Oxford: Blackwell Publishing Ltd; 2008.
14. Bowers GM. A study of the width of attached gingiva. J Periodontol. 1963;34:201–9.

15. Voigt JP, Goran ML, Flesher RM. The width of lingual mandibular attached gingiva. J Periodontol. 1978;49(2):77–80.
16. Andlin-Sobocki A, Bodin L. Dimensional alterations of the gingiva related to changes of facial/lingual tooth position in permanent anterior teeth of children. A 2-year longitudinal study. J Clin Periodontol. 1993; 20(3):219–24.
17. De Rouck T, Eghbali R, Collys K, De Bruyn H, Cosyn J. The gingival biotype revisited: transparency of the periodontal probe through the gingival margin as a method to discriminate thin from thick gingiva. J Clin Periodontol. 2009;36(5):428–33.
18. Tsesis I, Rosen E, Tamse A, Taschieri S, Del Fabbro M. Effect of guided tissue regeneration on the outcome of surgical endodontic treatment: a systematic review and meta-analysis. J Endod. 2011;37(8):1039–45.
19. Enoch S, Moseley R, Stephens P, Thomas DW. The oral mucosa: a model of wound healing with reduced scarring. Oral Surg. 2008;1(1):11–21.
20. Peck S, Peck L, Kataja M. The gingival smile line. Angle Orthod. 1992;62(2):91–100; discussion 1–2.
21. Velvart P, Ebner-Zimmermann U, Ebner JP. Comparison of papilla healing following sulcular full-thickness flap and papilla base flap in endodontic surgery. Int Endod J. 2003;36(10):653–9.
22. Miloro M, Peterson LJ. Peterson's principles of oral and maxillofacial surgery. 3rd ed. Shelton: People's Medical Pub. House-USA; 2012.
23. Kim E, Song JS, Jung IY, Lee SJ, Kim S. Prospective clinical study evaluating endodontic microsurgery outcomes for cases with lesions of endodontic origin compared with cases with lesions of combined periodontal-endodontic origin. J Endod. 2008;34(5): 546–51.
24. Setzer FC, Boyer KR, Jeppson JR, Karabucak B, Kim S. Long-term prognosis of endodontically treated teeth: a retrospective analysis of preoperative factors in molars. J Endod. 2011;37(1):21–5.
25. Kan JY, Rungcharassaeng K, Umezu K, Kois JC. Dimensions of peri-implant mucosa: an evaluation of maxillary anterior single implants in humans. J Periodontol. 2003;74(4):557–62.
26. Morrow SG, Rubinstein RA. Endodontic surgery. In: Ingle JI, Bakland LK, editors. Endodontics. 5th ed. Hamilton: Decker Inc; 2002.
27. Cutright DE, Hunsuck EE. Microcirculation of the perioral regions in the Macaca rhesus. II. Oral Surg Oral Med Oral Pathol. 1970;29(6):926–34.
28. Cutright DE, Hunsuck EE. Microcirculation of the perioral regions in the Macaca rhesus. I. Oral Surg Oral Med Oral Pathol. 1970;29(5):776–85.
29. Grandi C, Pacifici L. The ratio in choosing access flap for surgical endodontics: a review. Oral Implantol (Rome). 2009;2(1):37–52.
30. Selvig KA, Biagiotti GR, Leknes KN, Wikesjo UM. Oral tissue reactions to suture materials. Int J Periodontics Restorative Dent. 1998;18(5): 474–87.
31. Silverstein LH, Kurtzman GM, Shatz PC. Suturing for optimal soft-tissue management. J Oral Implantol. 2009;35(2):82–90.

Esthetic Complications in Endodontic Surgery

7

Tom C. Pagonis and Eric Young

Abstract

The leading measure of successful outcomes in endodontic surgery relies heavily on the ability of the endodontic surgeon to provide conditions that promote resolution of persisting periradicular pathosis. Prevailing criteria for success depend on the preservation and continued function of teeth and radiographic parameters to assess healing (Orstavik, Scand J Dent Res 96:108–11, 1988). However, in an era of high patient expectations, the esthetic consequences of surgical treatment are of paramount concern. Esthetic outcomes are comprised of the natural or idealized shape, color, position, and juxtaposition of teeth to gingival tissues. Esthetic complications of endodontic surgery are best addressed before treatment by careful endodontic diagnosis and periodontal evaluation. This should be followed by adherence to the principle and practice of endodontic microsurgery both at the treatment planning stage and during the surgical procedure. In addition, appropriate surgical management of soft tissues and underlying bony structures is important as persistent endodontic infections are a risk factor for continued marginal attachment loss following endodontic surgery (Jansson et al., Oral Surg Oral Med Oral Pathol Oral Radiol Endod 83:596–601, 1997). While classical measures of success may suggest the positive outcome of a case, failing to achieve an esthetic outcome results in an unhappy patient.

Periodontal Considerations

Epithelial and connective tissues are the primary constituents of gingival tissues. Connective tissue makes up a majority of the supragingival fibers serving the purposes of attachment to the teeth and providing strength and resilience on chewing [3]. The attached gingiva extends from the coronal margin where the tooth meets the gingiva down to the mucogingival junction where

T.C. Pagonis, DDS, MS (✉) • E. Young, DDS
Division of Endodontics, Department of Restorative Dentistry and Biomaterials Sciences, Harvard School of Dental Medicine, 188 Longwood Avenue, REB 222, Boston, MA 02115, USA
e-mail: tom_pagonis@hsdm.harvard.edu; eric_young@hsdm.harvard.edu

I. Tsesis (ed.), *Complications in Endodontic Surgery*,
DOI 10.1007/978-3-642-54218-3_7,

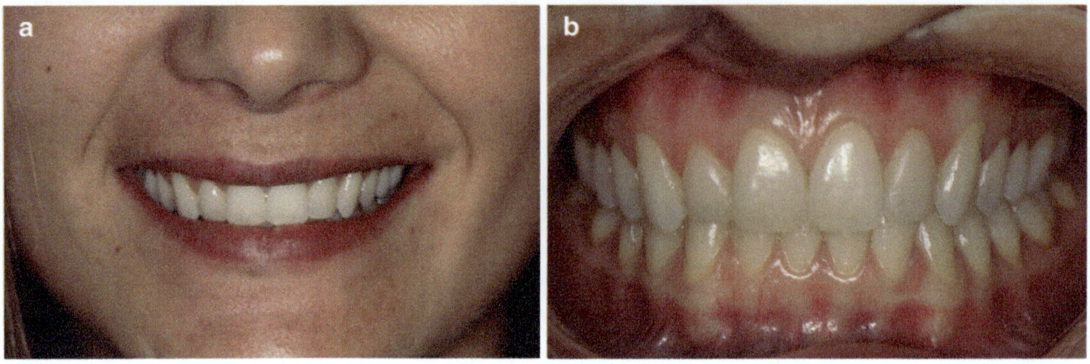

Fig. 7.1 (a, b) Esthetically pleasing smile with papilla that fills the entire embrasure

the firmly bound tissue meets the unattached mucosa. The greatest levels of attached gingiva are found on the facial aspect of the maxillary incisors [4]. The roughly triangular-shaped gingiva filling the embrasure apical to the contact point between two teeth is the papilla. In a lateral view of the papilla, one would observe a facial and lingual peak of the papilla joined by a concave ridge known as the col. Histologically, the col, being derived from junctional epithelium, is composed of nonkeratinized epithelium in the depressed area just apical to the interproximal contact, and more keratinized epithelium occurs laterally as the tissue extends to the gingival epithelial cuff of the papilla [3]. As the papilla is influenced by the embrasure it fills, the col takes on greater concavity where the contact points are the broadest as is the case in posterior teeth [5].

It is both functionally desirable and esthetically pleasing for the papilla to fill the entire embrasure (Fig. 7.1a, b) leaving no "black triangle" (Fig. 7.2). The ability for the gingiva to achieve this is determined by the distance from the contact point to the crest of the bone [4]. It has been shown that when the distance from the crest of bone to the contact point is less than 5 mm, the embrasure was completely filled [6]. At 6 mm, the papilla fills the space in only 56 % of cases, and at 7 mm or more, the papilla successfully filled the space 27 % of the time or less [6]. As the distance from the blood supply at the bone increases, the gingiva is significantly less likely to fill the embrasure. To provide predictable esthetic results, the surgical full thickness flap should avoid apically placed horizontal incisions since the major blood supply originates apically [7, 8].

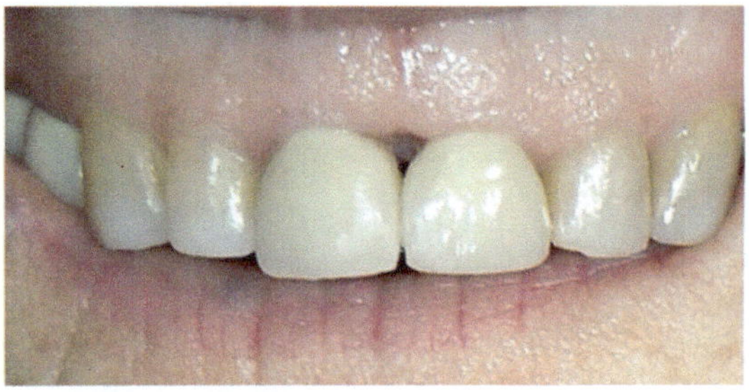

Fig. 7.2 A "black triangle" between maxillary central incisors

Pretreatment periodontal evaluation and accompanying strategic operative planning is essential to avoid postoperative esthetic complications. Specific periodontal parameters should be recorded and include the following:

1. Signs of periodontal inflammation at the surgical site in terms of pocket depths, bleeding upon probing, color, and contour of gingival tissue.
2. Attachment loss.
3. The location and measurement of the mucogingival junction along with measurement of the width of attached gingiva.
4. The position and inclination of the root and thickness of bone over the root.
5. Patient biotype: generally speaking, a thin gingival biotype has greater potential for gingival recession when compared to a thicker gingival biotype.

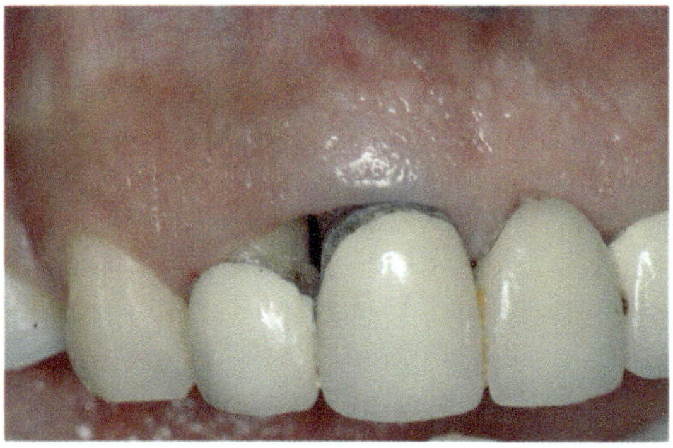

Fig. 7.3 Pretreament presentation of periodontal disease

For the patient that exhibits periodontal disease (Fig. 7.3), treatment of the periodontium should be completed before endodontic surgery [2]. With these periodontal parameters in mind, the endodontic surgeon must consider the patient's esthetic demands along with an evaluation of the quality and type of restoration particularly as it relates to the position of the margin to the gingiva. This represents a critical component of treatment planning especially as it relates to a good esthetic outcome. Finally, these clinical findings must also be considered in the context of location and extent of the existing periradicular pathosis before incision and selection of surgical flap design.

Even with careful consideration of the pretreatment periodontal condition, it has been shown that an ongoing endodontic infection represents a contributing factor for marginal attachment loss after endodontic surgery [2].

Application of Microsurgical Techniques for Prevention of Esthetic Complications

Endodontic microsurgery fundamentally represents the refinement of established and recognized surgical principles by incorporating technology to improve visualization. This is accomplished primarily with the utilization of the operating microscope along with the development and use of microsurgical instrumentation. There are three important principles that are incorporated in endodontic microsurgery [9, 10]:

1. The improvement of motor skills which translates into the enhancement of surgical ability
2. Wound closure by exact primary apposition of the wound edge
3. The adjunctive development and utilization of microsurgical instrumentation

The goal of the endodontic surgeon is to cause minimal tissue damage and provide the environment for primary healing which contemplates gentle handling of both hard and soft tissue with accurate wound closure. Understanding, training, and experience in endodontic microsurgery will allow the surgeon to achieve both excellent treatment outcomes with highly esthetic clinical results.

For the surgeon who practices without an operating microscope, a willingness to adapt this level of magnification is necessary. Surgical magnification will tremendously enhance motor skills which will translate into the enhancement of surgical ability [11]. In addition, greater attention to surgical esthetics, microanatomy, and tissue handling are critical. While tissue handling and microsurgical instrumentation are discussed in other chapters of this text, the incorporation of endodontic microsurgery requires the discussion of some aspects of hand function.

Hand Support and Control

It is well understood that unsupported finger movements in extension or flexion are relatively unstable and not suited for endodontic microsurgery [10, 12]. Therefore, wrist stabilization on a fixed surface with a 20° angulation in dorsiflexion decreases muscle tremor and mitigates unsupported finger flexion and extension thereby providing finely controlled finger movements [10, 12].

Physiologic hand tremor is not unusual and a manifestation of intentional and unintentional actions causing hand and finger movement [13]. The realization of a surgeon's tremor becomes more obvious with visual enhancement of magnification. It typically is associated with tension generated by poor postural control, unsupported hand, and unstable instrument holding position, but several other factors have been associated with hand tremor such as cigarette smoking, alcohol withdrawal, caffeine, hypoglycemia, hyperparathyroidism, pheochromocytoma, and Wilson's disease. Drug-induced hand tremor is a nervous system and muscle response to certain medications which include valproic acid, albuterol, cyclosporine, lithium carbonate, tricyclic antidepressants, antivirals such as acyclovir, and certain blood pressure drugs [14]. To perform endodontic surgery with microsurgical techniques and to minimize hand tremors, the surgeon must be in a relaxed and proper mind-set. To perform highly esthetic results, the endodontic surgeon must consider his/her attitude with mental focus and patience in order to maintain precise motor skills [10, 11].

Hand: Instrument Grips

It is interesting to consider that with the rapid expansion and utilization of technological advances of computers and even text messaging on handheld mobile devices, there is very little emphasis on handwriting or penmanship. In an academic setting or for the contemporary specialist dentist trainee, this lack of emphasis provides little background for good ergonomic habits during training [11, 15].

The three-digit pen or internal precision grip is the most commonly utilized in microsurgery and provides excellent stability particularly when compared to other hand grips [9, 16]. As its name suggests this grip mimics a three-digit pen grip with the thumb, index finger, and middle finger creating an effective tripod [9]. The surgeon's hand should rest on an immovable flat surface with support of the ulnar surface of the wrist and forearm. With this tripod in place, the instrument is supported by the middle finger with the thumb and index finger placed in contact with the instrument. Opening and closing of an instrument requires very fine movements, and any possible tremor is minimized. By utilizing the pen or internal precision grip, the flexor and extensor muscles of the hand remain relaxed facilitating accurate movement. Finally, proper surgical ergonomics not only helps prevent back and neck problems; it provides the functional environment to properly perform endodontic microsurgery and prevent esthetic complications. The patient and chair position should be adjusted to the surgeon and microscope with the surgeon seated in an upright position with thighs approximately at a right angle to the knees [17].

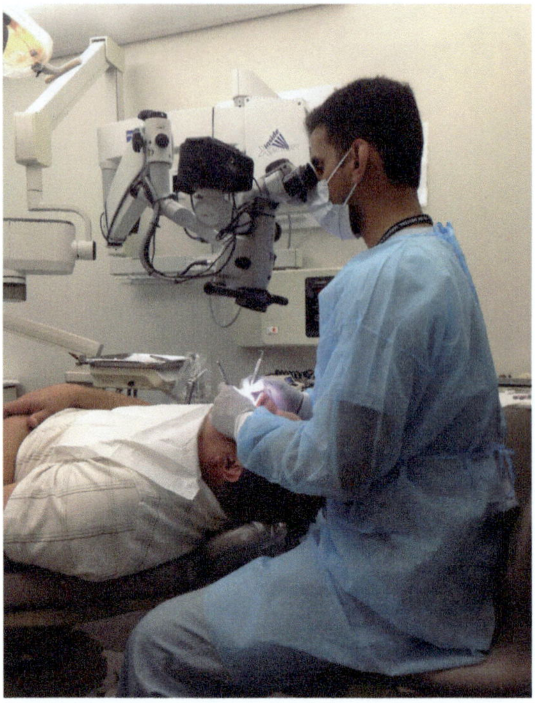

Fig. 7.4 Posture and position of the endodontic surgeon

Microsurgical instrumentation, accurate hand movement with precision hand grip, and correct posture and position of the endodontic surgeon (Fig. 7.4) are critical factors in avoiding esthetic complications.

Tissue Management and Esthetic Considerations

Surgical access has been cited as a major point of concern in endodontic surgery [18]. Appropriate selection of flap design enables proper access reducing the time needed in surgery and thus reducing postoperative morbidity. Poor flap design may lead to failure in treating

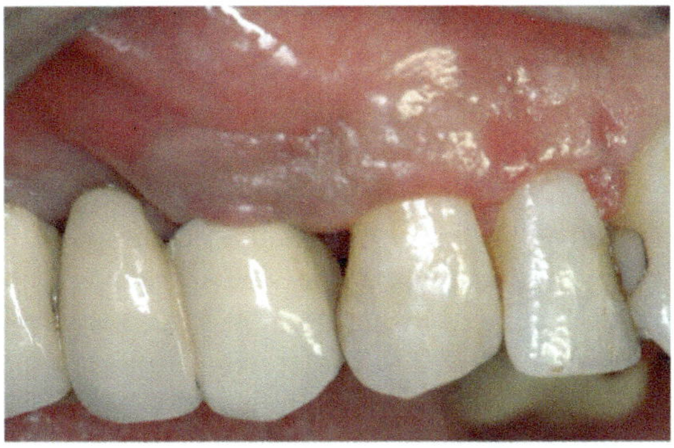

Fig. 7.5 Esthetic consequences of poor flap design and incision

the pathology or to unsightly hard and soft tissue defects leading to unhappy patients (Fig. 7.5). With the introduction of the surgical operating microscope, microsurgical techniques have evolved to improve the handling of soft tissues and reduce the incidence of defects [19].

Incisions should be made in smooth continuous motions pressing the blade to the bone in order to follow the topography of the hard tissue maintaining a full thickness cut. Discontinuous motions lead to jagged irregular edges more likely to leave noticeable scarring [20]. Full thickness flaps are desirable in endodontic surgery as it is essential to have direct access to the bone in order to gain access to the root in question. A full thickness mucoperiosteal flap consists of the marginal, interdental, and attached gingiva, alveolar mucosa, and periosteum [20–22]. This flap reduces the risk of tears and perforations, and upon closure, the periosteum immediately begins to reattach [22]. Furthermore, incisions should be long enough to provide adequate tissue to reflect so that unnecessary tension is not placed on the soft tissue. Tears of the tissue heal more slowly and leave greater scars as approximating the margins becomes more difficult, and associated healing occurs by secondary rather than primary intention [21, 22].

Intrasulcular releasing incisions are full thickness cuts directed toward the crestal bone. This incision is used in full mucoperiosteal flaps such as triangular-, rectangular-, trapezoidal-, and in papilla-base flap designs. The contraindication of this approach is the presence of a dehiscence [23]. A full thickness incision at a point of dehiscence may damage root attachment fibers leading to localized chronic periodontal disease [23]. This is one indication for a split thickness design to preserve gingiva in the compromised location. A split thickness flap will provide a suitable surface for reattachment of the flap, but this is a technically challenging approach. The split thickness flap is contraindicated in areas of normal bone as the incision has a greater likelihood of damaging the supraperiosteal vessels [7]. A simpler alternative is the use of limited mucoperiosteal flaps such as the Luebke-Ochsenbein flaps that place right-angle incisions apically to the dehiscence. But remember, horizontal incisions should always be made leaving at least 2 mm and more ideally 3 4 mm of attached gingiva [24–26]. Failure to respect this gingival attachment may lead to necrosis and sloughing defects of the soft tissue as the coronal segment is separated from sufficient blood supply [7, 27].

Care should also be taken to avoid incising directly over a bony defect. With the addition of *computed cone beam tomography (CBCT)* [28] and skilled interpretation in preoperative planning, the surgeon has tools to assess the size and shape of the lesion as well as predict where resulting margins will exist following the osteotomy with a high degree of fidelity. Periapical radiographs give excellent information regarding the extent of cortical bone destruction but significantly underestimate the measure of the less dense trabecular bone loss [29, 30]. The consequence of incision over the lesion is creating a pathway for organisms from the oral environment into the healing surgical wound postoperatively as well as compromising the blood supply to the repositioned flap. This significantly increases the risk of bacterial infiltration, postoperative pain, and gingival defects resulting from necrosis and sloughing [31]. To ensure sufficient solid bone under the margins of the mucoperiosteal flap, leave at least 5 mm of solid unaffected bone from the incision to outer edges of lesions or bony defects [31].

Vertical releasing incisions should be made in the shallow depressions between the roots of teeth extending to the mesial or distal line angle of the tooth serving as the outer border of the surgical operating field [7, 10, 19]. As previously discussed, one of the finer points is the surgeon should utilize the surgical operating microscope to help guide the incision perpendicular to the gingival margin and then gradually assume a trajectory coincident with the concavity parallel to the long axis of the tooth. The thicker gingiva in this region adds significant convenience for the endodontic surgeon. The thicker tissue provides easier manipulation and handling perioperatively. It more readily receives and retains sutures upon closing of the wound site at the conclusion of the procedure as well. An incision through the thin tissue over the bony eminence particularly in the region of the canines adds unnecessary difficulty to the procedure. As gingiva becomes thinner, it tears more easily and is more subject to localized ischemia and resulting necrosis, all of which make suturing far more challenging [32]. These challenges to the healing process may result in unsightly gingival fenestrations. Incisions at the mesial or distal line angles of border teeth provide additional convenience form for the surgeon while minimizing the risk of "black triangles" formed on necrosis due to splitting the papilla [27]. Generally, vertical releasing incisions join with the intrasulcular or horizontal incisions 1–2 teeth from the surgically treated tooth [33].

As previously mentioned, the endodontic surgeon should take note of the gingival biotype during preoperative planning as well to help determine the optimal placement of releasing incisions. In evaluating wound healing, it has been determined that a thin gingival biotype leads to a mean gingival recession of 0.32 mm which is significantly more than the gingival recession observed in cases with a thick biotype [34]. This is of particular importance in the esthetic zone within the smile line and should be considered in surgical planning of the flap design.

Maintaining the position of the incision between the roots of teeth within the concavity of the alveolus will also help to prevent incisions that are horizontal or too severely angled. In addition, improperly angled incisions will sever supraperiosteal blood vessels and collagen fibers that also travel roughly parallel to the long axis of the teeth attaching the crestal bone to gingiva [3, 7]. Compromised blood supply may lead to necrosis and sloughing of the affected gingiva. The impact of the severed collagen fibers becomes evident upon closure when the surgeon finds that they have contracted, and thus approximating the margins of the wound becomes difficult leading to undue stress on the suture sites increasing morbidity and scarring from healing by secondary intention [35].

When the clinical situation requires two vertical releasing incisions, it is important to ensure the width of the base of the flap is at least as long as the width of the separated free gingival margin. In order to produce esthetically pleasing outcomes, every attempt should be made to preserve as much blood supply as possible to the flap in order to optimize healing potential.

Once all incisions are made, reflecting the flap must be accomplished. This is a critical step in managing for esthetic surgical outcomes. Periosteal elevators are most commonly used for this purpose. These instruments need to be sharp and placed well with the bevel facing against the alveolar bone such that when controlled force is applied tangentially to the bone, the flap is lifted with mucosa, connective tissue, and periosteum as a single unit. Preoperative planning includes evaluation of the alveolar bone in the surgical field to identify exostoses or defects that will require special care on tissue reflection. Dull instruments, failure to press all the way to the bone, or erratic discontinuous movements may all lead to tearing of the tissue or leaving parts of the periosteum attached.

Reflection of the flap should begin by placing the periosteal elevator within the vertical releasing incision of full mucoperiosteal flaps a few millimeters apical to the junction of the horizontal releasing incision [20]. The elevator advances coronally under the periosteum to minimize traumatic forces as the surgeon separates the marginal gingiva and papillary tissues. This is due to the often fragile marginal gingiva and supracrestal root attachment fibers which may lead to loss of attachment [2, 20].

The damage resulting from elevation of the limited mucoperiosteal flaps is less critical as the

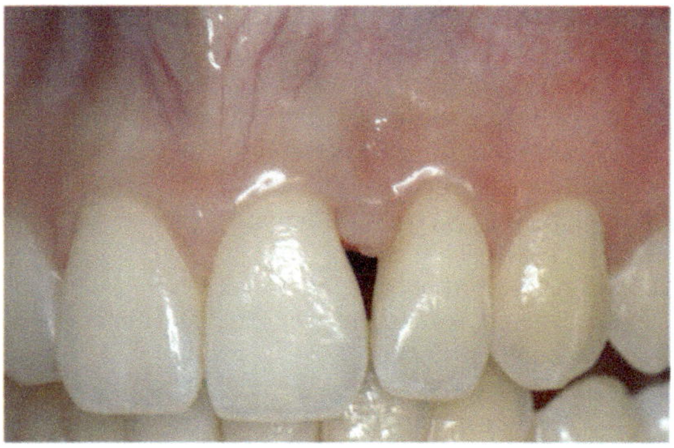

Fig. 7.6 Compromised esthetic results of poorly executed intrasulcular flap

marginal gingiva is left intact and margins of restorations are untouched [24, 26]; furthermore, the flap margin is often hidden beyond the smile line [26]. Nonetheless, it should still be avoided if at all possible to avert traumatizing a more delicate margin that may lead to shrinkage of the flap, delayed healing by secondary intention, and scar formation. Poor instrumentation on elevation of the flap increases the chances of postoperative pain, scarring, or soft tissue defects on healing [7, 27, 36] (Fig. 7.6).

Once the flap is surgically prepared, released, and reflected, it must be retracted. Blunt retractors must rest against the bone apical to the lesion to provide adequate visibility of the operating field while limiting the risk of crush injuries to the vasculature within the flap. Appropriate selection of retractors is important as retractors that are too small provide limited benefit and allow the flap to obscure the operating field, while retractors that are too large may traumatize the tissue. Furthermore, when the tissue is being retracted, remember to irrigate the periosteal surface of the flap with saline to prevent desiccation-related damage. Do not use sterile water as it is hypotonic to the cells [21].

Conclusion

While the measure of success in endodontic surgery was traditionally based on established objective criteria, postsurgical esthetic results are equally important. Esthetic outcomes in endodontic surgery have become much more viable in recent years due in large part to the introduction and utilization of the surgical operating microscope. Substantially improved visualization with improvement in micro instrumentation and flap design has enhanced the surgeon's ability to effectively manipulate the soft tissues thereby significantly improving the predictability of consistent positive esthetic outcomes. With CBCT becoming more commonplace, preoperative surgical planning has similarly improved. Ongoing research to understand additional variables in wound healing along with the clinical utilization of growth factors is promising [37]. These significant steps forward in technology have provided endodontic surgeons with excellent tools for the task at hand, but one must not overlook the importance of clinical experience and advanced training. Endodontists need to maintain the intellectual curiosity to look to related fields such as oral and maxillofacial surgery and periodontology which have provided new insights into how the surgeon can manage endodontic pathology while producing results that are pleasing not only when viewed on radiographs, but when the patient looks in the mirror.

References

1. Orstavik D. Reliability of the periapical index scoring system. Scand J Dent Res. 1988;96:108–11.
2. Jansson L, Sandstedt P, Laftman AC, Skoglund A. Relationship between apical and marginal healing in periradicular surgery. Oral Surg Oral Med Oral Pathol Oral Radiol Endod. 1997;83:596–601.
3. Schroeder HE, Listgarten MA. The gingival tissues: the architecture of periodontal protection. Periodontol 2000. 1997;13:91–120.
4. Bimstein E, Machtei E, Eidelman E. Dimensional differences in the attached and keratinized gingiva and gingival sulcus in the early permanent dentition: a longitudinal study. J Pedod. 1986;10:247–53.
5. Pilot T. Macro-morphology of the interdental papilla. Dtsch Zahnarztl Z. 1973;28:1220–1.
6. Tarnow D, Magner APF. The effect of the distance from the contact point to the crest of bone on the presence or absence of the interproximal dental papilla. J Periodontol. 1992;63:995–6.
7. Mormann W, Ciancio SG. Blood supply of human gingiva following periodontal surgery. A fluorescein angiographic study. J Periodontol. 1977;48:681–92.

8. Nobuto T, Yanagihara K, Teranishi Y, Minamibayashi S, Imai H, Yamaoka A. Periosteal microvasculature in the dog alveolar process. J Periodontol. 1989;60:709–15.
9. Klopper P, Muller JH, Van Hattum AH. Microsurgery and wound healing. Amsterdam: Expecta Medica; 1979.
10. Acland R. Practice manual for microvascular surgery. 2nd ed. St Louis: CV Mosby; 1989.
11. Tibbetts L. Principles and practice of periodontal microsurgery. Int J Microdent. 2009;1:13–24.
12. Barraquer JL. The history of microsurgery in ocular surgery. J Microsurg. 1980;1:288–99.
13. Jankovic J, Fahn S. Physiologic and pathologic tremors. Diagnosis, mechanism, and management. Ann Intern Med. 1980;93(3):460–5.
14. Elble RJ. Tremor: clinical features, pathophysiology, and treatment. Neurol Clin. 2009;27:679–95.
15. Sulzenbruck S, Hegele M, Rinkenaur G, Heuer H. The death of handwriting: secondary effects of frequent computer use on basic motor skills. J Mot Behav. 2011;43(3):247–51.
16. Daniel RK, Terzis JK. The operating microscope. In: Reconstructive microsurgery. Boston: Little Brown and Company; 1977. p. 3–23.
17. Chang BJ. Ergonomic benefits of surgical telescope systems: selection guidelines. J Calif Dent Assoc. 2002;30(2):161–9.
18. Kim S. Principles of endodontic microsurgery. Dent Clin North Am. 1997;41:481–97.
19. Velvert P, Peters CI. Soft tissue management in endodontic surgery. J Endod. 2005;1:4–16.
20. Gutmann JL, Harrison JW. Posterior endodontic surgery: anatomical considerations and clinical techniques. Int Endod J. 1985;18:8.
21. Harrison JW, Jurosky KA. Wound healing in the tissues of the periodontium following periradicular surgery. 1. The incisional wound. J Endod. 1991;17:425.
22. Harrison JW, Jurosky KA. Wound healing in the tissues of the periodontium following periradicular surgery. 2. The dissectional wound. J Endod. 1991;17:544.
23. Kohler CA, Ramjford SP. Healing in gingival mucoperiosteal flaps. Oral Surg. 1960;13:89.
24. Lang NP, Loe H. The relationship between the width of keratinized gingiva and gingival health. J Periodontol. 1972;43:623–7.
25. Tidwell E, Vreeland DL. Flap design for surgical endodontics. Oral Surg Oral Med Oral Pathol. 1982;54:461–5.
26. Luebke RG. Surgical endodontics. Dent Clin North Am. 1974;18:370–91.
27. Mormann W, Meier C, Firestone A. Gingival blood circulation after experimental wounds in man. J Clin Periodontol. 1979;6:417–24.
28. Patel S, Dawood A, Manocci F, Wilson R, Pitt Ford T. Detection of periapical bone defects in human jaws using cone beam computed tomography and intraoral radiography. Int Endod J. 2009;42(6):507–15.
29. Bender IB. Factors influencing the radiographic appearance of bony lesions. J Endod. 1982;8:161–70.
30. Lee S, Messer H. Radiographic appearance of artificially prepared periapical lesions confined to cancellous bone. Int Endod J. 1985;18:8.
31. Hooley JR, Whitacre RJ. A self-instructional guide to oral surgery in general dentistry. 2nd ed. Seattle: Stoma Press; 1980.
32. Tibbetts LS, Shanelec D. Current status of periodontal microsurgery. Curr Opin Periodontol. 1996;3:118–25.
33. Velvart P. Surgical retreatment. In: Bergenholtz G, Hørsted-Bindslev P, Reit C, editors. Textbook of endodontology. Oxford: Blackwell Munksgaard; 2003. p. 312–26.
34. Von Arx T, Salvi GE, Janner S, Jensen SS. Gingival recession following apical surgery in the esthetic zone: a clinical study with 70 cases. Eur J Esthet Dent. 2009;4:28–45.
35. Kon S, Caffesse RG, Castelli WA, Nasjleti CE. Revascularization following a combined gingival flap-split thickness flap procedure in monkeys. J Periodontol. 1984;55:345–51.
36. Hurzeler MB, Weng D. Functional and esthetic outcome enhancement of periodontal surgery by application of plastic surgery principles. Int J Periodontics Restorative Dent. 1999;19:36–43.
37. Hom DB, Thatcher G, Tibesar R. Growth factor therapy to improve soft tissue healing. Facial Plast Surg. 2002;18:41–52.

Periapical Osteotomy and Curettage

8

Igor Tsesis and Eyal Rosen

Abstract

Periapical osteotomy in endodontic surgery is aimed to provide adequate access for a proper surgical management of the apical part of the root. The osteotomy should be as small as possible but as large as necessary to accomplish the endodontic clinical objectives. Therefore, it is prudent to balance between the surgical needs and the case specific limitations, in order to achieve predictable clinical results with minimal associated risks for the patient.

Osteotomy produces heat depending on the drill design, the drilling technique, and the bone structure. Osteotomy based on light brushing motions using sharp high-speed burr, and copious irrigation, may prevent the risk of thermal osteonecrosis.

The possible damage to adjacent teeth during surgery varies from slight surface shaving to a complete root resection. Adjacent teeth should be evaluated before endodontic surgery. In case of damage to adjacent tooth during surgery, the tooth should be closely monitored, and in case of developing signs of pulp necrosis, root canal treatment should be performed.

Periapical curettage may jeopardize adjacent anatomical structures. Early curettage may also result in intraoperative excessive bleeding, and the final thorough curettage can be postponed to the end of the procedure when judged necessary.

The root canal anatomy is extremely complex and variable [1], and proper identification of the entire root end anatomy, such as identification of the root canal system ports of exit, is essential for the long-term prognosis of the endodontic surgery [1–4]. Therefore, the main goal of the osteotomy in endodontic surgery is to provide adequate access for proper surgical management of the apical part of the root [2–5].

Periapical wound healing following endodontic surgery includes repair or regeneration of the alveolar bone, periodontal ligament, and cementum [6], and it histologically depends on the nature of the wound and on the availability of

I. Tsesis, DMD (✉) • E. Rosen, DMD
Department of Endodontology,
Maurice and Gabriela Goldschleger School of Dental Medicine, Tel Aviv University, Tel Aviv, Israel
e-mail: dr.tsesis@gmail.com;
dr.eyalrosen@gmail.com

I. Tsesis (ed.), *Complications in Endodontic Surgery*,
DOI 10.1007/978-3-642-54218-3_8, © Springer-Verlag Berlin Heidelberg 2014

critical resources such as progenitor stem cells, growth and differentiation factors, and microenvironmental cues such as the extracellular matrix [6, 7]. The surrounding periodontal tissues are an essential reservoir of resources for the postsurgical bony healing process [6, 8]. A conservative osteotomy compared to a large osteotomy would better preserve those critical local resources and would facilitate improved conditions for the periapical wound healing process [2, 6, 7]. Thus, in small periapical bony defects following conservative osteotomy, resident osteoblasts, PDL cells, and cementoblasts are capable of restoring the damaged periapical tissues. However, if the size of the osseous defect is too large, osseous regeneration of the wound will not occur, and the defect might heal by fibrous connective tissue repair [6, 8, 9].

The geometry of the surgical bony defect is also significant for the potential for improved wound healing following the surgical procedure. Large bony defects, and through-and-through lesions, compared to four-wall defects, may compromise the potential for periodontal regeneration (by the formation of new bone, cementum, and periodontal ligament tissues), due to undesired proliferation of gingival connective tissue or migration of oral epithelium into the defect [6, 10, 11]. Refer to the Guided Tissue Regeneration (see Chap. 16) for additional details.

Although it seems that the size of the periapical bony defect does not directly affect the long-term prognosis of the surgical procedure, the smaller the osteotomy, the faster would be the expected healing process [2–5, 12]. Rubinstein et al. found that small lesion healed within 6.4 months, while large lesions healed within 11 months [12]. Thus, a large osteotomy may lead to delayed healing and complicate the postoperative evaluation process.

Too small osteotomy may provide insufficient access for thorough inspection of the root end anatomy, thus leading to missing of root anatomy and ensuing improper surgical management of the root end, therefore, jeopardizing the long-term outcome of the procedure [1–4].

Enlarged osteotomy, especially if directed towards the coronal margin, may result in excessive removal of healthy bone around the cervical part of the tooth, thus potentially leading to compromised periodontal attachment and even to perio-endo communication and an ensuing compromised long-term prognosis of the tooth [2, 13].

A large osteotomy may also increase the risk of complications that are related to damage to adjacent anatomical structures, such as nerve bundles, blood vessels, maxillary sinus involvement, and damage to adjacent teeth. Refer to nerve injury, (see Chaps. 10, 11, 13)

An inherent preconceived risk with the traditional endodontic surgery was potential damage to nerve bundles because of excessive osteotomies [14]. The large osteotomies led to an increased risk of direct trauma to nerve bundles or to indirect nerve damage by edema or hematoma from damage to major blood vessels. This potential problem has been overcome with the use of surgical operating microscope and refined microsurgical instruments and ultrasonic tips. With the modern microsurgical techniques, the size of the osteotomy significantly decreased, to just 4–5 mm in diameter, large enough to allow the surgical manipulations such as the ability of an ultrasonic tip of 3 mm in length to freely prepare the root end [2]. Thus, the potential for osteotomy ensuing nerve injury decreased significantly.

In order to help locating the lesion and identify the involved root when there is no fenestration of the lesion (intact cortical bone) and when the apical bone is dense, the surgeon should inspect the operating field for the presence of root eminences in the cortical plate and evaluate the angle of the crown to the root. Probing of the bone at the apical region with sharp explorer may be helpful. The evaluation of the approximated root length based on periapical radiographs and measuring the length of the radiographic crown and estimating the length of the root relatively to the length of the crown can help to estimate the position of the lesion and reducing the required osteotomy size. If the cortical bone plate is thin or absent, curettes may be used to expose the apex of the root. A CBCT can be helpful in estimation of the width of the cortical plate.

In conclusion, the osteotomy should be as small as possible but as large as necessary to accomplish the clinical objectives. Therefore, it is recommended that the osteotomy would be planed ahead of time, while balancing between the surgical needs and the anatomical and case-specific hazards and limitations, in order to achieve predictable clinical results with minimal associated risks for the patient.

Thermal Osteonecrosis During Drilling

Drilling of bone generates heat [15, 16]. The bone itself is a poor conductor of heat [17]. In certain cases, the temperature raise may be damaging and even fatal to the bone tissue. Excessive frictional heat generated during osteotomy preparation causes interruption of blood flow, inactivation of alkaline phosphatase and decreased osteoclastic and osteoblastic activity, dehydration, and desiccation, with resulting osteocytic degeneration and osteonecrosis [15, 16].

The threshold level for heat-induced cortical bone necrosis was found to be tissue temperature raise to over 47 °C (116.6 °F) for at least 1 min [18]. In endodontic surgery, the problem is possibly aggravated by the temporary decrease in bone blood supply due to the local anesthesia rendering it more sensitive to heat injury [19]. Therefore, it is critical to reduce the heat generation in the bone during the drilling for the osteotomy.

The factors that may influence the amount of heat generated during the osteotomy can be related to the drill design, the drilling technique, and to the bone structure.

There are various controversial reports in the literature regarding various burr designs and related heat generation during osteotomy, and many drill design characteristics were evaluated in the context of heat generation during osteotomy, including flute design, point design, point angle, diameter, and the drill material composition [20].

Drills wore out during repeated drilling and sterilization, therefore reducing the sharpness of the drill and causing increased heat production [20]. Thus, ideally, a new drill should be used for each surgery.

The proper drilling technique is essential for the prevention of thermal osteonecrosis. Controversial reports have been published regarding the effect of the speed of the osseous drilling on heat generation [20]. There are wide variations in the definitions of high and low speeds of drilling. While some authors claimed that high-speed cutting effects on bone are similar to or even less than those observed at lower-speed ranges [21], others recommended that the drill rotational speed should be reduced as much as possible [22].

It was found that independent increase of either the drilling speed or the drilling load increased the temperature in the bone. However, increasing both the speed and the load together allowed for more efficient cutting with no significant increase in temperature [23]. Thus, there is no evidence that support a use of a low-speed handpiece over the use of a high speed, and it seems that the speed of drilling by itself has no significant influence on heat generation.

While there are no recommendations regarding the optimal cooling system to be used in endodontic surgery, cooling is essential for preventing the thermal osteonecrosis of the bone. The irrigation enhances elimination of debris, thus indirectly causing reduction of friction, and the lubrication causes reduction in friction [20].

Cooling may also pose risk of infection spreading and may pose a risk of serious intra-surgical complications such as emphysema. Subcutaneous emphysema is a rare complication of endodontic surgery and was reported for cases when air turbine handpiece was used [24]. Emphysema occurs when air is injected into the subcutaneous/submucous layer of the tissue and requires a combination of a compressed air procedure, together with a communication between the oral cavity and deeper tissue producing dissection [24, 25]. Ideally, a drill should be positioned so that the air is directed away from the surgical field; however, many dentists use drills that have an air-and-water-cooled burr. The resulting dispersion can direct some of the air and water directly into the wound and into the potential spaces of the neck [26]. When tissue emphysema occurs, antibiotic therapy combined with close patient observation is necessary. If an airway distress appears, a prompt patient hospitalization is imperative.

The cortical bone is the hardest part of the bone, and the duration of bone drilling depends on the cortical bone thickness. The hardness of cortical bone correlates to bone mineral density (BMD). Higher BMD would lead to higher bone temperature with the same combination of drilling parameters [27]. The thickness of a rabbit cortical bone is 1.5 mm with average duration of drilling of 5 s; cortical bone thickness of human femur is 6–6.5 mm with an average duration of drilling of 18 s [28].

Apart from the thermal damage, drilling of bone can also cause micro damage to the bone. Small cracks accumulate in the mineralized matrix of bone which can cause osteocyte apoptosis [29]. However, unlike root dentine, the bone constantly goes through a remodeling process that is aimed to eliminate these micro bone cracks

In conclusion, the safest preparation of the osteotomy site in endodontic surgery with the least risk of thermal osteonecrosis would be by the application of light brushing motions using a sharp new high-speed burr and copious irrigation.

The use of ultrasonic energy has been proposed as an adjunct in endodontic surgery [30–35]. The primary advantage of ultrasonic osteotomy is the precise, clean, and smooth cutting capability with excellent visibility [36]. While ultrasonic provides a more conservative and controlled osseous incision [37], Metzger et al. observed that rotary burr produced regular bone edges, whereas the piezoelectric device produced loosened bone edges. The average surface roughness was significantly higher for the samples prepared with the piezoelectric device than for those prepared with the rotary bur [38].

Damage to Adjacent Teeth

The possible damage to adjacent teeth during surgery varies from slight surface shaving to a complete root resection. These complications were reported to happen not only during endodontic surgery, but are quite often in many other surgical procedures, such as Caldwell-Luc approaches to the maxillary sinus, cystectomies, and biopsies in the vicinity of root apices, and is most commonly perhaps during removal or exposure of impacted teeth [39]. Therefore, adjacent teeth should be evaluated before endodontic surgery. The pulpal condition should be checked using vitality tests, and the presence of periapical radiolucencies or signs of root resorption should be noted (Fig. 8.1a–g).

The influence of root resection on the vital pulp has been evaluated in animal studies. Some authors reported severe pulp damage with resulting fibrotic changes or complete replacement of the pulp with new tissue [39] root resorption and pulp necrosis [40]; others reported that the pulp remained vital [41]. When the injury is not extensive and the pulp chamber is not involved, healing of PDL without long-term damage can be expected. If inadvertent transection of only one root occurred in multi-rooted teeth, the vitality of the remainder of the tooth may be assured by collateral circulation [39, 41].

In case of damage to adjacent tooth during bone cutting, the tooth should be closely monitored, and in case of developing signs of pulp necrosis, root canal treatment should be performed.

Periapical Curettage

Periapical curettage is a surgical procedure to remove diseased or reactive tissue and/or foreign material around the root [42]. At the same time, curettage may help attaining access to the surgical site and visualization of root end anatomy. Ideally, if the pathological tissue is removed in one piece, there is less bleeding and less dissemination of the infection into adjacent bone and soft tissues (Fig. 8.2a, b). Moreover, in cases when a biopsy is indicated, controlled complete removal of the tissue in one piece without crashing or tearing facilitates histological examination and final diagnosis.

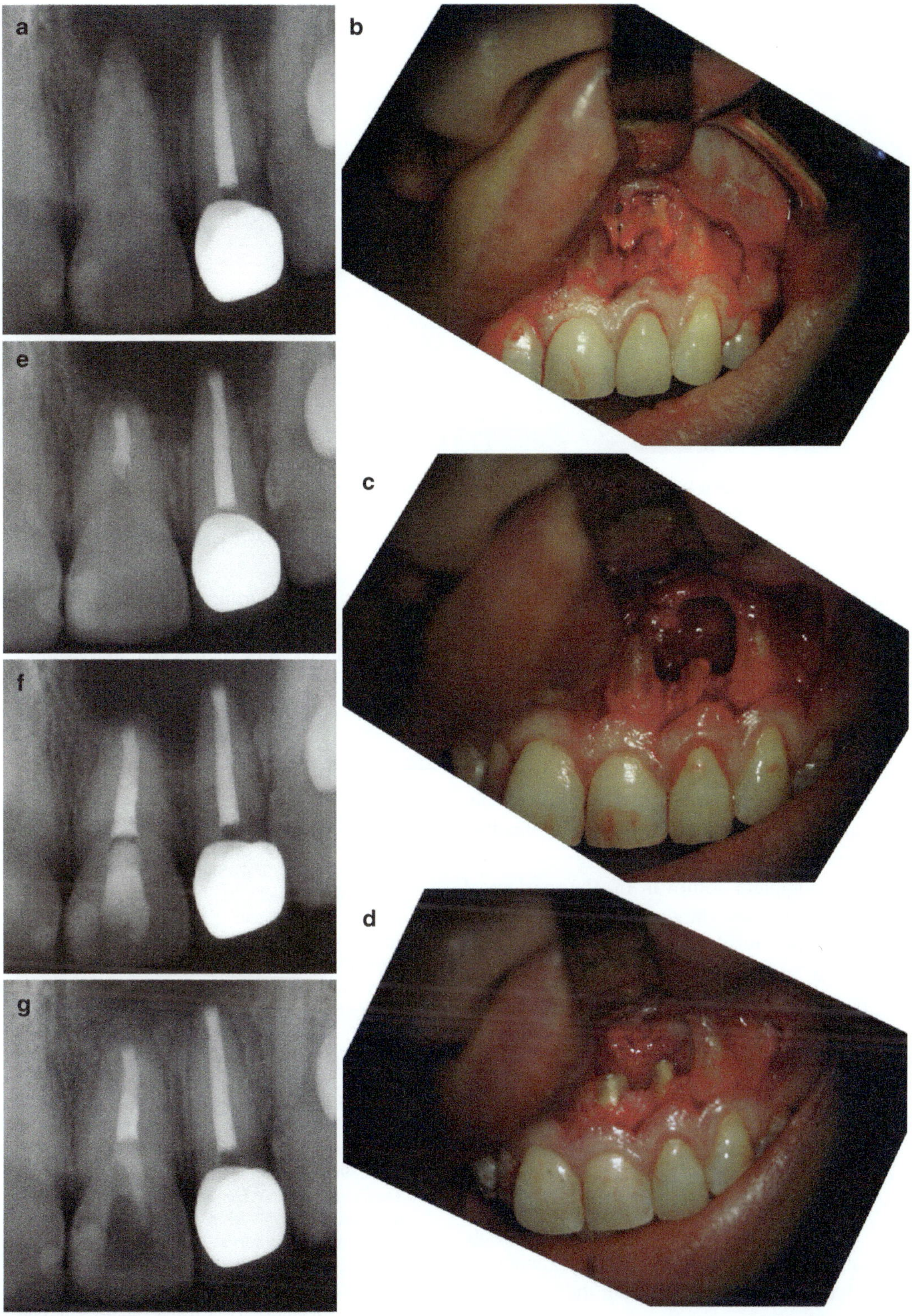

Fig. 8.1 A large periapical lesion related to the second maxillary incisor, the first incisor tested vital. (**a**) Preoperative radiograph. (**b**) Intraoperative photograph following flap elevation, a large osseous defect is exposed. (**c**) Following curettage of the granulation tissue, the apex of the first incisor is exposed, and its neurovascular bundle is severed. (**d**) Root end preparation and filling performed on both maxillary incisors. (**e**) Immediate postoperative radiograph with root end filling on both incisors. (**f**) Orthograde root canal treatment of the first incisor completed 1 week following the surgery. (**g**) Incomplete healing (scar) 1 year following the surgery

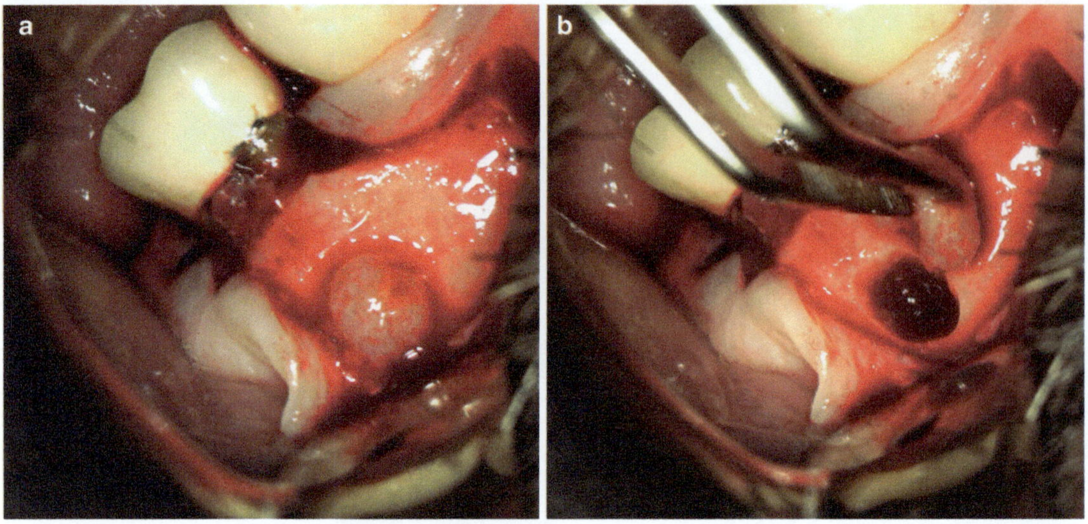

Fig. 8.2 Periapical curettage in endodontic surgery. (**a**) Bone fenestration with granulation tissue following flap elevation. (**b**) Periapical curettage demonstrating a complete removal of the pathological tissue in one piece

In the majority of cases, the pathological periapical tissues are reactive responses to irritants from the root canal. Therefore, it is not necessary to completely curette all the inflamed periradicular tissues during surgery, since this granulation-like tissue will be incorporated into the new granulation tissue as part of the healing process [43]. Overzealous curettage may jeopardize adjacent anatomical structures, resulting in bleeding and impeded healing.

For a complete removal of the periapical pathological tissues, larger osteotomy should be created thus resulting in larger bone cavity that should heal, which can influence both the postoperative quality of life, the flap reposition, together with the healing time, and eventually the outcome of the procedure [44].

It has been stated in the literature that complete curettage should be performed early in the surgery to prevent bleeding during root end management [2, 5, 44]. While in theory it seems a logical assumption, in reality in most of the cases, it is much easier to achieve good hemostasis using appropriate technique (see Chap. 11) on ischemic granulation tissue than on healthy bone lining the osteotomy site. In addition, a granulation tissue may limit the dissemination of debris and foreign materials that are released during the root end preparation and prevent the contamination of bone or adjacent anatomical structures such as maxillary sinus. The final thorough curettage can be performed at the end of the procedure when judged necessary.

References

1. Vertucci FJ. Root canal anatomy of the human permanent teeth. Oral Surg Oral Med Oral Pathol. 1984;58(5):589–99.
2. Kim S, Kratchman S. Modern endodontic surgery concepts and practice: a review. J Endod. 2006;32(7):601–23.
3. Tsesis I, Faivishevsky V, Kfir A, Rosen E. Outcome of surgical endodontic treatment performed by a modern technique: a meta-analysis of literature. J Endod. 2009;35(11):1505–11.
4. Tsesis I, Rosen E, Taschieri S, Telishevsky Strauss Y, Ceresoli V, Del Fabbro M. Outcomes of surgical endodontic treatment performed by a modern technique: an updated meta-analysis of the literature. J Endod. 2013;39(3):332–9.
5. Tsesis I, Rosen E, Schwartz-Arad D, Fuss Z. Retrospective evaluation of surgical endodontic treatment: traditional versus modern technique. J Endod. 2006;32(5):412–6.
6. Tsesis I, Rosen E, Tamse A, Taschieri S, Del Fabbro M. Effect of guided tissue regeneration on the outcome of surgical endodontic treatment: a systematic review and meta-analysis. J Endod. 2011;37(8):1039–45.

7. Lin L, Chen MY, Ricucci D, Rosenberg PA. Guided tissue regeneration in periapical surgery. J Endod. 2010;36(4):618–25.
8. Grzesik WJ, Narayanan AS. Cementum and periodontal wound healing and regeneration. Crit Rev Oral Biol Med. 2002;13(6):474–84.
9. Andreasen JO, Rud J. Modes of healing histologically after endodontic surgery in 70 cases. Int J Oral Surg. 1972;1(3):148–60.
10. Pecora G, De Leonardis D, Ibrahim N, Bovi M, Cornelini R. The use of calcium sulphate in the surgical treatment of a 'through and through' periradicular lesion. Int Endod J. 2001;34(3):189–97.
11. Taschieri S, Del Fabbro M, Testori T, Saita M, Weinstein R. Efficacy of guided tissue regeneration in the management of through-and-through lesions following surgical endodontics: a preliminary study. Int J Periodontics Restorative Dent. 2008;28(3):265–71.
12. Rubinstein RA, Kim S. Short-term observation of the results of endodontic surgery with the use of surgical operation microscope and Super-EBA as root end filling material. J Endod. 1999;25:43–8.
13. Kim E, Song JS, Jung IY, Lee SJ, Kim S. Prospective clinical study evaluating endodontic microsurgery outcomes for cases with lesions of endodontic origin compared with cases with lesions of combined periodontal-endodontic origin. J Endod. 2008;34(5):546–51.
14. Kratchman SI. Endodontic microsurgery. Compendium. 2007;28(6):324–31.
15. Heinemann F, Hasan I, Kunert-Keil C, Gotz W, Gedrange T, Spassov A, et al. Experimental and histological investigations of the bone using two different oscillating osteotomy techniques compared with conventional rotary osteotomy. Ann Anat. 2012;194(2):165–70.
16. Lavelle C, Wedgwood D. Effect of internal irrigation on frictional heat generated from bone drilling. J Oral Surg. 1980;38(7):499–503.
17. Biyikli S, Modest MF, Tarr R. Measurements of thermal properties for human femora. J Biomed Mater Res. 1986;20(9):1335–45.
18. Eriksson AR, Albrektsson T. Temperature threshold levels for heat-induced bone tissue injury: a vital-microscopic study in the rabbit. J Prosthet Dent. 1983;50(1):101–7.
19. Stropko JJ, Doyon GE, Gutmann JL. Root-end management: resection, cavity preparation, and material placement. Endod Topics. 2005;11:131–51.
20. Augustin G, Zigman T, Davila S, Udilljak T, Staroveski T, Brezak D, et al. Cortical bone drilling and thermal osteonecrosis. Clin Biomech (Bristol, Avon). 2012;27(4):313–25.
21. Moss RW. Histopathologic reaction of bone to surgical cutting. Oral Surg Oral Med Oral Pathol. 1964;17:405–14.
22. Davidson SR, James DF. Drilling in bone: modeling heat generation and temperature distribution. J Biomech Eng. 2003;125(3):305–14.
23. Brisman DL. The effect of speed, pressure, and time on bone temperature during the drilling of implant sites. Int J Oral Maxillofac Implants. 1996;11(1):35–7.
24. Durukan P, Salt O, Ozkan S, Durukan B, Kavalci C. Cervicofacial emphysema and pneumomediastinum after a high-speed air drill endodontic treatment procedure. Am J Emerg Med. 2012;30(9):2095 e3-6.
25. Peñarrocha M, Ata-Ali J, Carrillo C, Peñarrocha M. Subcutaneous emphysema resulting from surgical extraction without elevation of a mucoperiosteal skin flap. J Clin Exp Dent. 2011;3(3):265–7.
26. Barkdull TJ. Pneumothorax during dental care. J Am Board Fam Pract. 2003;16(2):165–9.
27. Karaca F, Aksakal B, Kom M. Influence of orthopaedic drilling parameters on temperature and histopathology of bovine tibia: an in vitro study. Med Eng Phys. 2011;33(10):1221–7.
28. Eriksson RA, Albrektsson T, Magnusson B. Assessment of bone viability after heat trauma. A histological, histochemical and vital microscopic study in the rabbit. Scand J Plast Reconstr Surg. 1984;18(3):261–8.
29. Noble B. Bone microdamage and cell apoptosis. Eur Cell Mater. 2003;6:46–55.
30. Rashad A, Kaiser A, Prochnow N, Schmitz I, Hoffmann E, Maurer P. Heat production during different ultrasonic and conventional osteotomy preparations for dental implants. Clin Oral Implants Res. 2011;22(12):1361–5.
31. Gonzalez-Garcia A, Diniz-Freitas M, Somoza-Martin M, Garcia-Garcia A. Ultrasonic osteotomy in oral surgery and implantology. Oral Surg Oral Med Oral Pathol Oral Radiol Endod. 2009;108(3):360–7.
32. Beziat JL, Bera JC, Lavandier B, Gleizal A. Ultrasonic osteotomy as a new technique in craniomaxillofacial surgery. Int J Oral Maxillofac Surg. 2007;36(6):493–500.
33. Su YC. [Development and clinical application of ultrasonic osteotomy in dentistry]. Shanghai Kou Qiang Yi Xue. 2007;16(1):1–7.
34. Taschieri S, Del Fabbro M, Testori T, Francetti L, Weinstein R. Endodontic surgery with ultrasonic retrotips: one-year follow-up. Oral Surg Oral Med Oral Pathol Oral Radiol Endod. 2005;100(3):380–7.
35. Taschieri S, Testori T, Francetti L, Del Fabbro M. Effects of ultrasonic root end preparation on resected root surfaces: SEM evaluation. Oral Surg Oral Med Oral Pathol Oral Radiol Endod. 2004;98(5):611–8.
36. Happe A. Use of a piezoelectric surgical device to harvest bone grafts from the mandibular ramus: report of 40 cases. Int J Periodontics Restorative Dent. 2007;27(3):241–9.
37. Torrella F, Pitarch J, Cabanes G, Anitua E. Ultrasonic ostectomy for the surgical approach of the maxillary sinus: a technical note. Int J Oral Maxillofac Implants. 1998;13(5):697–700.
38. Metzger MC, Bormann KH, Schoen R, Gellrich NC, Schmelzeisen R. Inferior alveolar nerve transposition–an in vitro comparison between piezosur-

gery and conventional bur use. J Oral Implantol. 2006;32(1):19–25.
39. Hitchcock R, Ellis 3rd E, Cox CF. Intentional vital root transection: a 52-week histopathologic study in Macaca mulatta. Oral Surg Oral Med Oral Pathol. 1985;60(1):2–14.
40. Yoshida S, Oshima K, Tanne K. Biologic responses of the pulp to single-tooth dento-osseous osteotomy. Oral Surg Oral Med Oral Pathol Oral Radiol Endod. 1996;82(2):152–60.
41. Yaghmaiee M, Yavari AS, Mashhadiabbas F, Bahrami A, Farnia P, Sharifi D, et al. Histological assessment of pulp condition after apical vital root transection in one root of multirooted teeth in dogs: a preliminary study. J Endod. 2007;33(9):1061–5.
42. AAE. Glossary of endodontic terms. 8th ed. Chicago: AAE; 2012.
43. Lin LM, Gaengler P, Langeland K. Periradicular curettage. Int Endod J. 1996;29(4):220–7.
44. Tsesis I, Shoshani Y, Givol N, Yahalom R, Fuss Z, Taicher S. Comparison of quality of life after surgical endodontic treatment using two techniques: a prospective study. Oral Surg Oral Med Oral Pathol Oral Radiol Endod. 2005;99(3):367–71.

Complications in Root-End Management

9

Stefano Corbella, Massimo Del Fabbro, Eyal Rosen, and Silvio Taschieri

Abstract

Root-end management is a fundamental part of endodontic surgery. It involves a root resection, preparation for the root-end cavity, and obturation of the apical root canal. This phase is critical for the resolution of the periapical pathosis, allowing periradicular tissue regeneration including the formation of a new attachment apparatus.

The management of the root end can be divided into different phases (apex resection, retrograde cavity preparation, and apical sealing). In each phase, several complications can occur due to inadequate planning of the procedure, inappropriate technique, or anatomical characteristics of the site. The success of the entire endodontic surgery may be severely influenced by the occurrence of an adverse event during the root-end management.

Complication prevention and early identification can allow an adequate management of such event, allowing a successful procedure.

S. Corbella, DDS, PhD (✉)
Department of Biomedical, Surgical and Dental Sciences, Dental Clinic, IRCCS Istituto Ortopedico Galeazzi, University of Milan,
Via Riccardo Galeazzi, 4, 20161 Milan, Italy
e-mail: stefano.corbella@gmail.com

M. Del Fabbro, BSc, PhD • S. Taschieri, MD, DDS
Department of Biomedical, Surgical and Dental Science, Centre for Research in Oral Health,
IRCCS Istituto Ortopedico Galeazzi, University of Milan,
Via Riccardo Galeazzi, 4, 20161 Milan, Italy
e-mail: massimo.delfabbro@unimi.it; silvio.taschieri@fastwebnet.it

E. Rosen, DMD
Department of Endodontology, Maurice and Gabriela Goldschleger School of Dental Medicine,
Tel Aviv University, Tel Aviv, Israel
e-mail: dr.eyalrosen@gmail.com

Introduction

Root-end management is a fundamental part of endodontic surgery. It involves a root resection, preparation for the root-end cavity, and obturation of the apical root canal. This phase is critical for the resolution of the periapical pathosis, allowing periradicular tissue regeneration including the formation of a new attachment apparatus.

The management of the root end can be divided into different phases (apex resection, retrograde cavity preparation, and apical sealing). In each phase, several complications can occur due to inadequate planning of the procedure, inappropriate technique, or anatomical characteristics of the site. The success of the entire

I. Tsesis (ed.), *Complications in Endodontic Surgery*,
DOI 10.1007/978-3-642-54218-3_9, © Springer-Verlag Berlin Heidelberg 2014

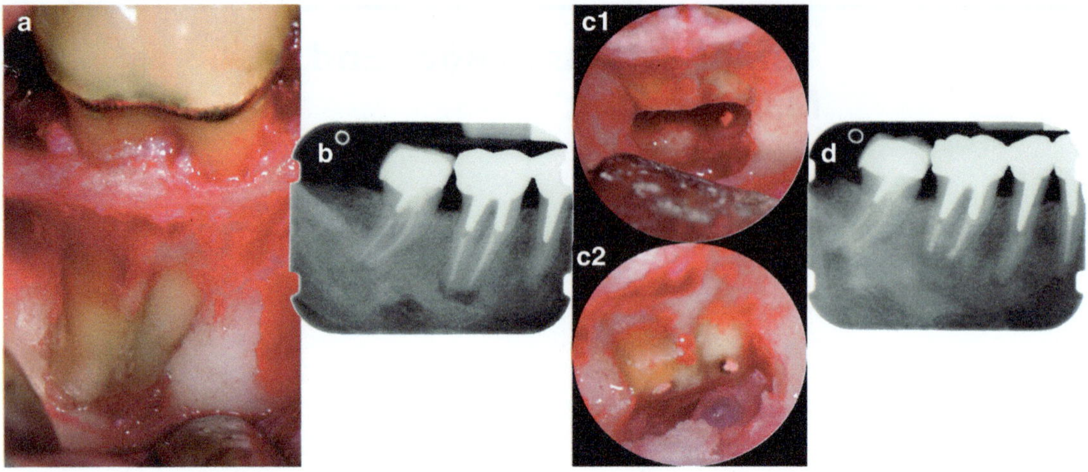

Fig. 9.1 Surgical endodontic treatment of the first mandibular molar

endodontic surgery may be severely influenced by the occurrence of an adverse event during the root-end management.

Complication prevention and early identification can allow an adequate management of such event, allowing a successful procedure (Fig. 9.1).

A knowledge of all the possible complications and their clinical and radiological signs, together with the application of techniques for their management, is fundamental to successfully perform an adequate root-end management.

Apex Resection

The resection of the root end was traditionally recommended in order to remove the contaminated apical part of the root canal and to provide access for retrograde cavity preparation [1, 2]:

- Most canal aberrations and anomalies are within the apical 3 mm of the root; this is the least amount of root end that should be removed [3].
- Apex resection is fundamental for the visualization of apical foramen and to provide access to retrograde preparation.

But, in some cases, the benefits of root resection could be questionable:

- Apicoectomy results in the exposure of an oval canal shape, which may, combined with root shortening, result in increased leakage [4] (Fig. 9.2).
- Reduction of the crown-to-root ratio may compromise the survival of the tooth in the long run [3, 5].
- In cases with long posts, the root resection may compromise the preparation of the retrograde cavity and may result in insufficient space for a retrograde sealing material.
- Resection of the root apex may expose the periapical tissues' infected dentinal tubules and canal irregularities included in this part of the root, which may cause endodontic surgery to fail [2].

Abrasion of the root apex can be an alternative to the direct cut of the apical portion. Abrasion allows a better control of the length of the portion that is excised and can help to correct small variability in bevel angle. Moreover, abrasion is an easier technique to perform than apex resection, because it can limit the possibility of an undesirable migration of the resected apex into the sinus cavity, when there is communication of the lesion with the maxillary sinus.

Bevel

When the apical end of a root is removed, the remaining surface of the root is described as having been "beveled" [6]. The shape and direction of the bevel can strongly influence both success rate of the whole procedure and the incidence of complications that may occur.

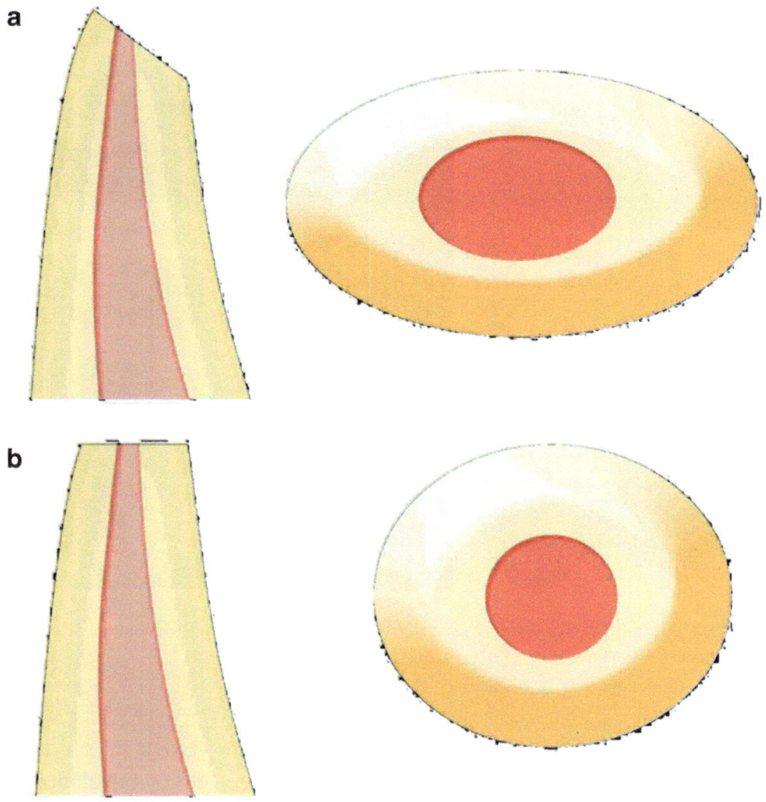

Fig. 9.2 The figure shows the difference between an oblique cutting angle (**a**) and a 90° one (**b**). An oblique cutting angle causes the exposure of a larger area, containing dentinal tubules (**a**). A 90° cutting angle results in a round shape of the root-end and a minimal exposure of dentinal canals (**b**)

Historically, a long bevel was proposed in order to obtain a better visualization, especially in posterior regions, of the root end and an easier access while preparing the retrograde cavity. However, nowadays, several drawbacks can be evaluated and considered while using a large bevel which has to be avoided due to the improvements in technique and instruments available. Main complications and drawbacks can be:

- Increased leakage due to the exposure and opening of a large area of the dentinal canals that create an access to the root canal that cannot be sealed [7] (Fig. 9.2).
- A risk of leaving a lingual part of the root untreated and missing the root canal anatomy (Fig. 9.3).
- An attempt to remove enough apical root can cause an excessive shortening of the root and damage to the crown-to-root ratio, shortening the remaining portion of the root.
- The shape of the root end becomes more oval than round, when resecting the apex with an angle different from 90°; this can create more difficulties in sealing a higher risk of leakage.

Crown-to-Root Ratio

Crown-to-root ratio is defined as the physical relationship between the portion of the tooth within the alveolar bone and the portion not within the alveolar bone, as determined radiographically [8]. While an ideal crown-to-root ratio of 1:2 has been suggested for a tooth to serve as an abutment, it is rarely observed in practice. The original guidelines for crown-to-root ratio in the selection of abutments were found to be exceptionally conservative and treatment limiting, and 1:1 ratio might be adequate in cases with a carefully designed occlusion and controlled periodontal inflammation [9].

Various clinical procedures have been reported to directly affect the crown-to-root ratio such as

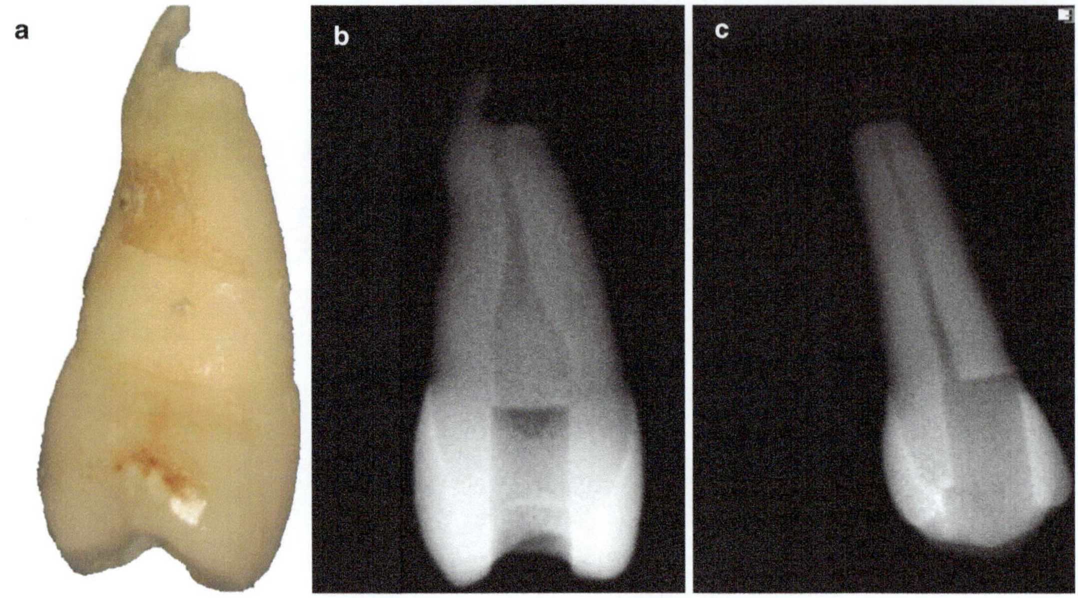

Fig. 9.3 Incomplete root-end resection (**a**). While it is seen on the mesio-distal radiograph (**b**), the incomplete root-end resection is not visible on a bucco-lingual radiograph (**c**)

abutment preparation for overdentures, surgical crown lengthening, and forced eruption [5].

Endodontic surgery cuts off the apical root and may result in an unfavorable crown-to-root ratio.

While most roots have a conical shape, molars have root trunk portion with wider surface area than just conical root portion. Thus, on these teeth the loss of apical root is less significant for alveolar bone support [10].

The most common cause of increased crown-to-root ratio is marginal periodontitis [11]. Cervical bone support is the most important to sustain the stresses from occlusal load. Therefore, periodontal bone loss is detrimental to the prognosis of abutment tooth. On the contrary, apical root resection is not as harmful as periodontal bone loss because the occlusal stress concentrates on the cervical area, not on the apical area [10].

However, from an anatomical point of view, the amputation of the apex, which decreases the longitudinal distance between alveolar bone margin and resected root end, can increase the risk of endo-perio communication, increasing the risk of infection spread.

The preservation of an adequate crown-to-root ratio should be considered essential in endodontic surgery. The use of a minimum bevel allows a greater preservation of the tooth structure than a larger bevel does. However, it should be taken into consideration that the main goal of endodontic surgery remains the regeneration of periapical tissues after the removal of the infectious periapical *noxa*. As reported, the aim of preserving tooth structure must not compromise the goal of endodontic surgery [12].

Missed Canals and Anatomy

Missed multiple canals or missed complete roots are among the most severe complications because it may compromise the success of the procedure due to persistence of pathogens in contact with the tooth surrounding the tissues.

This occurrence can be caused by an inadequate root resection or incomplete visualization of the anatomy both in planning and in surgical phases. Missing root canal anatomy is strictly linked to the anatomy of the tooth or of the root that has to be treated (Fig. 9.4).

It is known that many variations can be observed in the root canal anatomy of the tooth, as described by Vertucci [13]. In his publications the authors described a number of different root

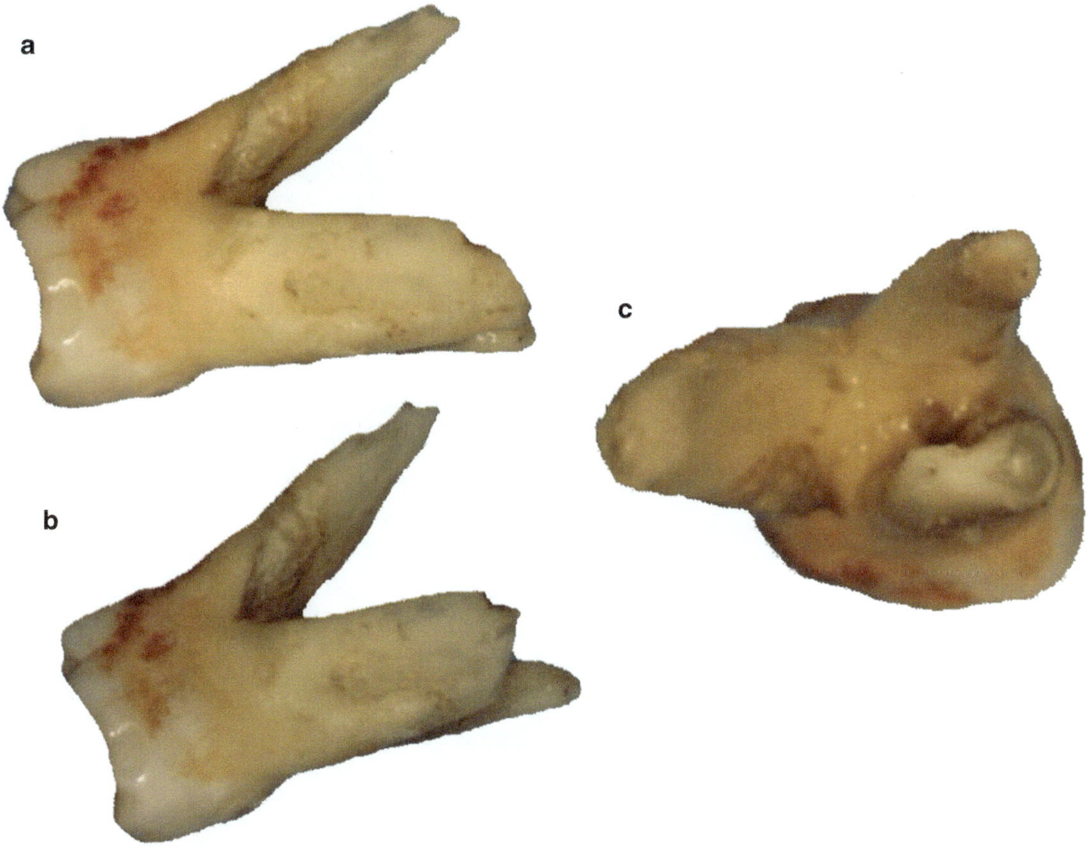

Fig. 9.4 Figures show that an not sufficient root-end resection can cause the missing of the root canal anatomy (**a**, **b**). In this case, a maxilllary molar, second mesiobuccal canal became visible only when appropriate root-end resection was performed (**c**)

canal anatomical features, classifying them on the basis of the number of canals and isthmus or communications among them (Fig. 9.5).

So, the shape of the root canal end after resection can be different on the basis of the position of the resection plane, affecting the three-dimensional sealing procedure. A deep knowledge of root canal anatomy allows an appropriate planning of the procedure and, during the surgery, can reduce the risk of missing root anatomy.

Retrograde Cavity Preparation

Tridimensional Filling and Sealing

The preparation of the root-end cavity aims to create the conditions for a tridimensional obturation of the root end, eliminating the pathways of the source of infection from the root canal into periradicular tissues.

The ideal root-end cavity preparation should be at least 3–5 mm deep Black class-I cavity, with walls parallel to the long axis of the root [14], and should incorporate the root canal anatomy and retain the retrograde filling material [15].

Several complications can occur during root-end preparation due to inadequate instrumentation or visualization of the surgical site:

- Inadequate cleaning of the canal due to inappropriate instrumentation and irrigation of the root end can lead to unsuccessful healing, with the persistence of infectious microorganisms; it can follow an incorrect angulation of the endodontic tip, leaving a portion of the canal unprepared and contaminated.

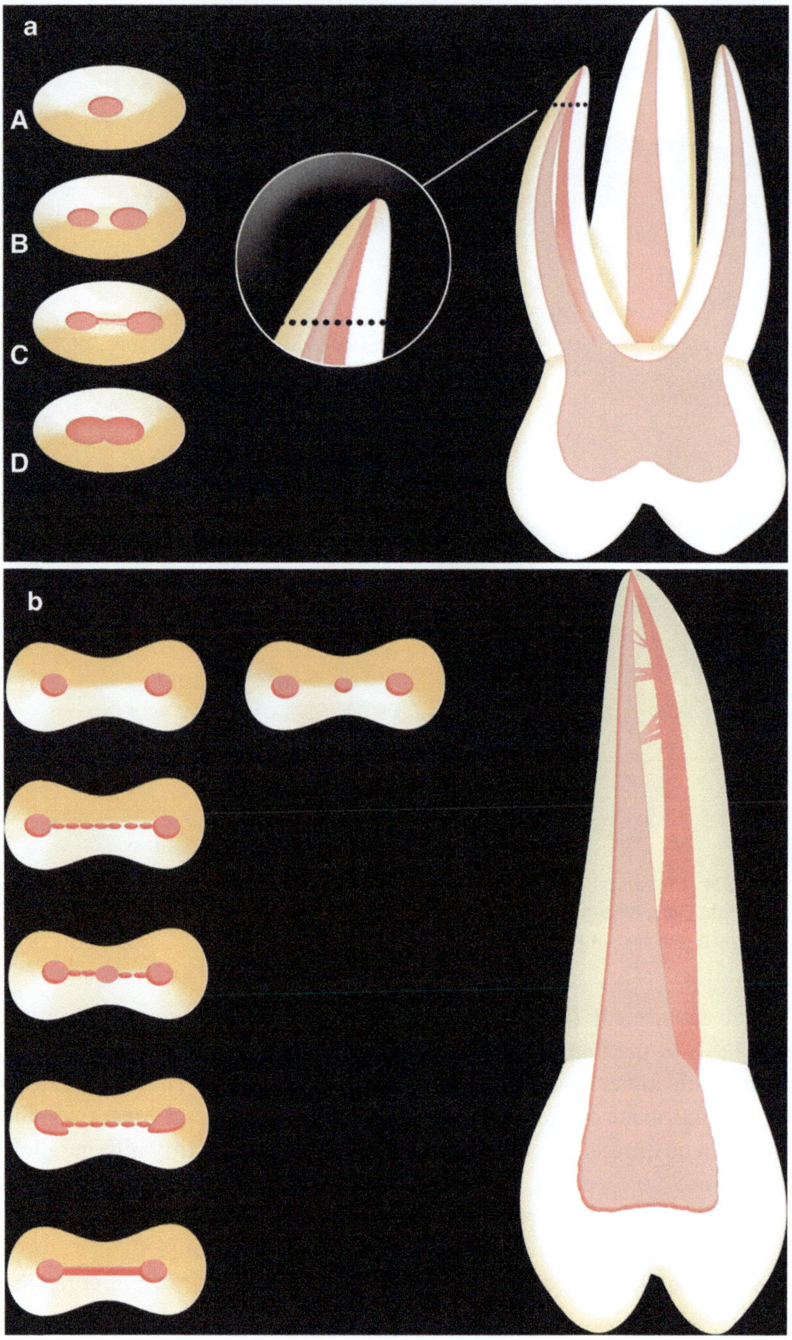

Fig. 9.5 (**a**) Mesiobuccal root of a maxillary molar. Different position of the cutting plane results in variable anatomy of the root-end. In the Figures A to D some examples of anatomy are proposed from coronal to apical portion of the root. (**b**) Maxillary premolar. Different position of the cutting plane results in variable anatomy of the root-end. Some examples of anatomy are proposed from coronal to apical portion of the root

- Deviation of the preparation from the long axis of the tooth, caused by an inadequate angulation of the endodontic tip.
- Root perforation due to inadequate visualization and deviations of the path of the preparation from the root canal (Fig. 9.6).
- Missed canals and anatomy because of inappropriate use of visualization devices.
- Hemorrhage of the surrounding tissue can limit the possibility of an adequate and complete view of the root-end anatomy. The use of hemostatic agents can help in cases of excessive bleeding.

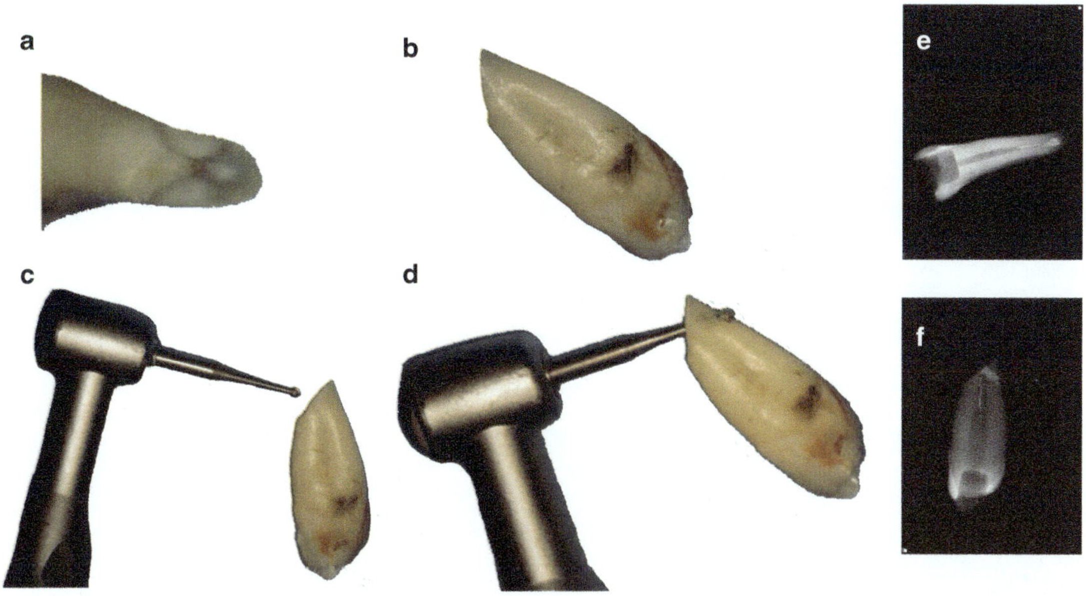

Fig. 9.6 The figure shows a clinical situation when a 45° angle of resection was used (**a**, **b**). In figure (**b**) and (**c**) an inadequate visualization together with an inappropriate use of the device can cause a perforation (palatal) due to the angulation. In figure (**e**) and (**f**) it is evident that the perforation is visible only through a radiograph in mesio-distal direction

Some complications can occur also depending on the instruments used for root-end preparation. The use of burs can be associated to an inadequate visualization of the site. Moreover the angulation of the burs cannot be completely controlled, and the high abrasive power may cause perforations or deviation from the long axis of the tooth that cannot easily be cleaned and sealed.

However, also the use of ultrasonic endodontic tips may have several drawbacks that should be considered. Fracture of the tip can occur while cleaning the canal, and usually the fractured portion can be removed easily even with the use of magnification devices (Fig. 9.7). Dentinal crack may follow the preparation of the root ends due to the effects of ultrasonic instrumentation on dentinal structures. Fractures must be detected, prepared through removal, and sealed as a lateral canal. Transportations and root perforations can occur also with ultrasonic instrumentation although they are less frequent than when using burs.

Many advantages of ultrasonic preparation have to be considered. A better and safer preparation can be achieved with ultrasonic tips, with a better alignment (parallelism) of the root-end cavity with the long axis of the root canal. Moreover the preparation of complex anatomical situations can be achieved with less risks of perforation and of missing anatomy [16].

The ultrasonic cavities produced more parallel walls and deeper depths for retention. In addition, the ultrasonic tips followed the direction of the canals more closely than those prepared by burs. Scanning electron microscopic examination of the cavity walls showed presence of cleaner surfaces of root-end cavities prepared by ultrasonic tips than those made with burs [17].

Ultrasonic diamond-coated tips preparation is easier and faster, but the tips should be used cautiously to avoid over-preparation or perforation of the root end [18].

Several simple indications may help a safe and effective use of ultrasonic endodontic tips. First, the lighter the touch, the more efficient the cutting will be, while the use of a greater pressure may cause fracture of the tips and perforations. Then the correct amount of water is very important. In fact, if too much spray is used, visibility and cutting efficiency are both decreased. On the contrary, if too little water is used, the necessary

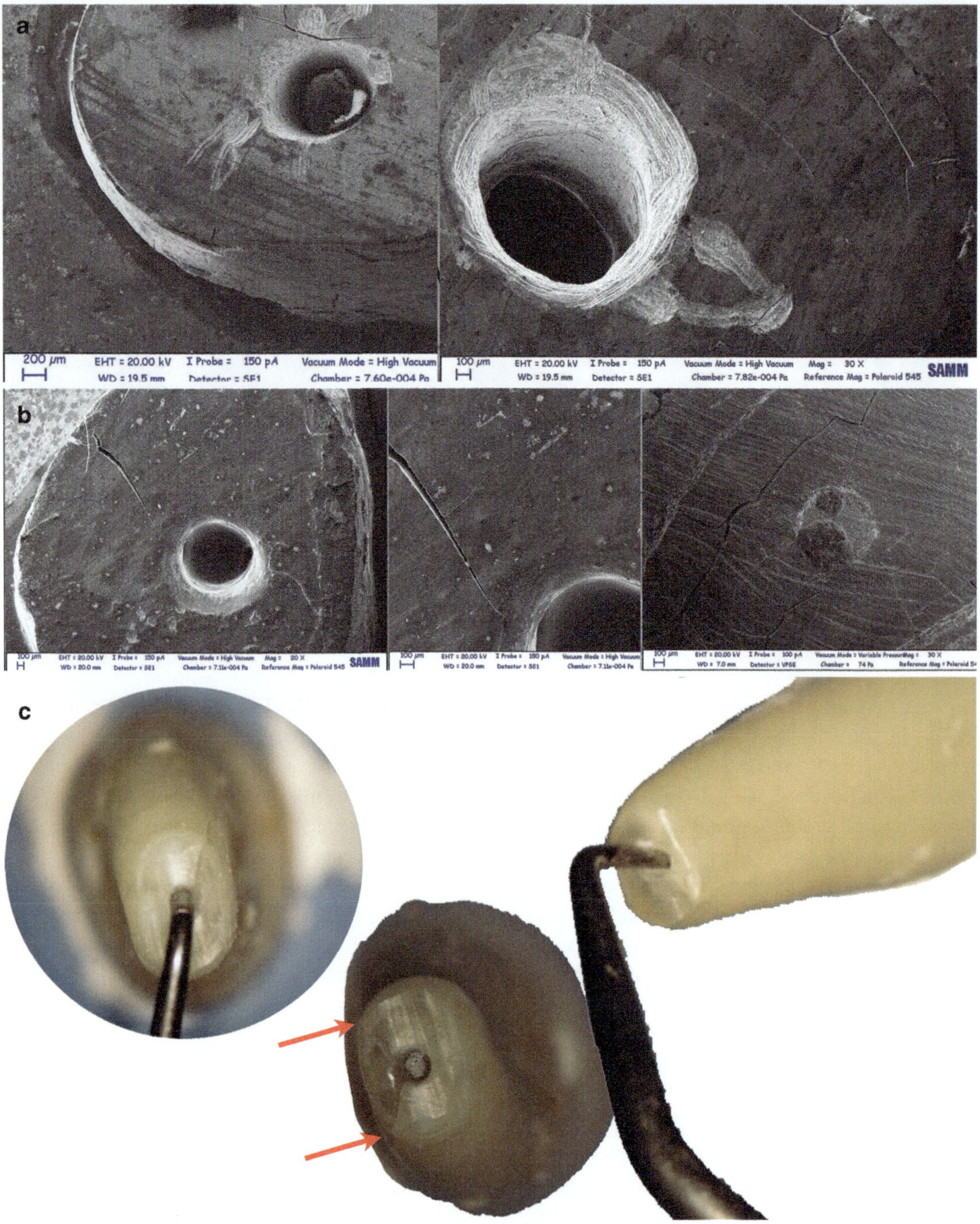

Fig. 9.7 (**a**) SEM analysis of a root-end; dentinal cracks are visible on the surface and should be adequately treated. (**b**) SEM analysis of a root-end; dentinal cracks can go from the external surface of the root, directing to the root canal. (**c**) The use of ultrasonic tips may cause dentinal cracks due to the preparation. The crack has to be treated as an accessory canal before sealing

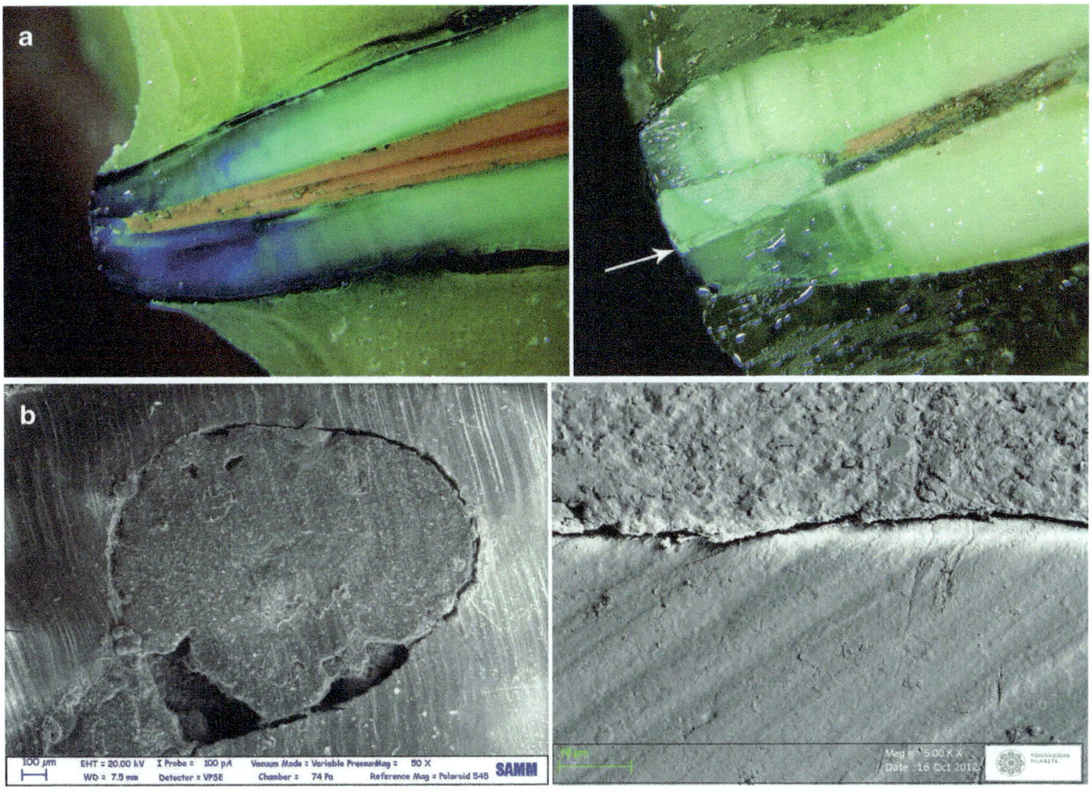

Fig. 9.8 (**a**) Sealing of the root-end after resection and removal of the root canal guttapercha. (**b**) SEM analysis of the sample in (**a**). the filler is in contact with the internal root canal wall

amount of cooling and rinsing of the debris will not occur. This can cause overheating of the root dentin [6].

Retrograde Obturation

A three-dimensional filling of the prepared apical portion of the resected root is the last phase of root-end management. The purpose of root-end filling is to seal the canal in order to prevent bacteria and their by-products that remain in the root canal from entering the periapical tissue. In any case, a toxic product is unacceptable as a root-end filling material.

If the previous phases were performed correctly, a proper apical seal can be obtained with consequent success of the whole endodontic surgery. However, in certain cases complications that influence the sealing ability may occur.

Inadequate placement and compaction of the root-end filling material due to misuse of instruments and an insufficient visualization of the root-end cavity are the main causes of an inappropriate obturation. The sealing material should be plugged carefully, and plugging must be repeated several times using small quantity of materials, to achieve a better control of the procedure (Fig. 9.8). Magnification devices (surgical microscope or endoscope) should be always used during the procedure to have a complete visualization of the root end. "Blind" procedures must be avoided. In cases of doubtful filling, intraoperative radiographs should be used to have the certainty of three-dimensional filling, while most of the sealing materials are radiopaque (Fig. 9.9).

Excessive bleeding, or wetting of the cavity, can preclude the possibility of an adequate filling due to the limits of adequate visualization and to the impossibility of a three-dimensional filling

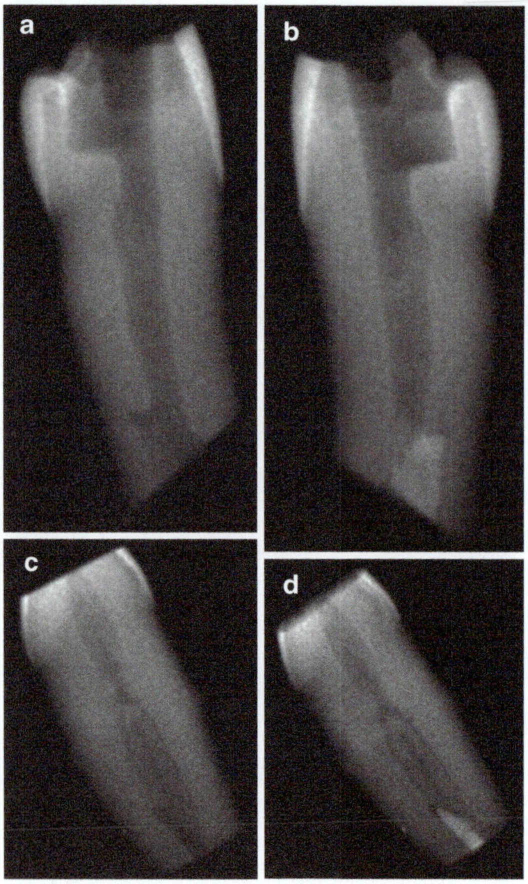

Fig. 9.9 (**a–d**) it can be observed that a non-axial preparation of retrograde cavity may lead to incomplete and inadequate sealing of the root canal system

due to the hydrophobic characteristics of the sealing material. To obtain a correct filling, root-end cavity should be dried carefully through the use of paper points, and bleeding from the surrounding tissues (periodontal ligament and bone) should be stopped using hemostatic agents (collagen, bone wax, tranexamic acid, and others). Only when the cavity is dried and bleeding is controlled can the filling procedure begin.

After completing the filling, finishing burs, curettes, and cotton pellet can be useful in finishing the sealing material, reducing the possibility of further migration of the material in the surrounding tissues and eliminating sealing in excess. Moreover, the presence of extruded material could prevent an adequate visual control of the sealing that must always follow the root-end management procedure.

The biocompatibility has been claimed to be one of the most important requirements of any root-end filling material [19].

As long as root-end filling remains confined within the root canal, it seems that a degree of its biocompatibility does not play a significant role in the outcome or possible adverse effects and complications of endodontic surgery.

As a rule, the root-end filling materials should be confined to the root canal; thus, a maximal contact surface should not exceed the diameter of apical preparation. At this interface, the interaction between the material and periapical tissues occurs. With some materials, a fully reconstituted periodontal ligament with a newly formed cementum over the resected root end and the root-end filling material were demonstrated in certain cases, though unpredictably [19, 20]. While theoretically the ultimate goal of any surgical treatment is an achievement of complete tissue regeneration, in practice, the clinical significance of the reconstruction of the normal anatomy of cementum in contact with fractions of millimeters of interface of root-end filling remains unclear.

But, in case of inadvertent extrusion of root-end filling material into periapical tissues, the biocompatibility becomes an issue.

Many materials are used for root canal sealing. Amalgam was mostly used in the past and was considered as the material of choice in traditional endodontic surgery. Amalgam has several drawbacks, including corrosion and dimensional changes, amalgam tattoos, and some issues concerning biocompatibility. Many authors showed that amalgam causes the presence of a persistent inflammation at the root end, with unfavorable tissue response [21–23]. The biocompatibility of amalgam also depends on the composition of the alloy. As an example, the presence of zinc is associated to cytotoxic reactions [23].

Zinc oxide-eugenol (ZOE) cements have biologic properties that can influence their biocompatibility. Eugenol is the main cytotoxic component in ZOE cements [24]. Also zinc demonstrates a cytotoxic effect. As regards ethoxybenzoic acid (EBA) as SuperEBA cement, the major cytotoxic component is represented by liquid eugenol, even though it rapidly dissolves over time [25]. Moreover the relatively low solubility of SuperEBA if compared to other ZOE cements is responsible for the higher biocompatibility [23]. Also observed was a better cellular response to ZOE cements (SuperEBA in particular) than amalgam, with the absence of an inflammatory reaction, as seen in histologic studies [26].

Mineral Trioxide Aggregate (MTA) is one of the most commonly used materials in three-dimensional root-end sealing. The biocompatibility of MTA was widely demonstrated by scientific literature [23]. Moreover, MTA has the ability of favoring hard tissue deposition and periodontal ligament formation when used as a retrograde filler [27]. Currently, MTA should be considered the most biocompatible material for retrograde filling. Glass-ionomer cements were also used as sealing materials in endodontic surgery. An intense inflammatory response was demonstrated by in vitro studies, even though the inflammation can disappear over time [23, 28]. Composite resin demonstrated an inhibitory effect on cell growth and was not able to induce the production of cytokines [29].

Conclusion

Root-end management could be complicated by several occurrences that may prevent the successful healing of the periapical lesion after periradicular surgery. A deep knowledge of all the possible complications may help the surgeon both in the prevention of such occurrences, through the adoption of safer procedures, and in their management. Most of the occurrences can be managed without aborting the whole procedure, and, if adequate protocols of management are adopted, the success rate may not be influenced.

References

1. Kim S, Kratchman S. Modern endodontic surgery concepts and practice: a review. J Endod. 2006;32: 601–23.
2. Lin S, Platner O, Metzger Z, Tsesis I. Residual bacteria in root apices removed by a diagonal root-end resection: a histopathological evaluation. Int Endod J. 2008;41:469–75.
3. Roy R, Chandler NP, Lin J. Peripheral dentin thickness after root-end cavity preparation. Oral Surg Oral Med Oral Pathol Oral Radiol Endod. 2008;105:263–6.
4. Kontakiotis EG, Lagoudakos TA, Georgopoulou MK. The influence of root-end resection and root-end cavity preparation on microleakage of root filled teeth in vitro. Int Endod J. 2004;37:403–7.
5. Grossmann Y, Sadan A. The prosthodontic concept of crown-to-root ratio: a review of the literature. J Prosthet Dent. 2005;93:559–62.
6. Stropko JJ, Doyon GE, Gutmann JL. Root-end management: resection, cavity preparation, and material placement. Endod Topics. 2005;11:131–51.
7. Gilheany PA, Figdor D, Tyas MJ. Apical dentin permeability and microleakage associated with root end resection and retrograde filling. J Endod. 1994;20:22–6.
8. The glossary of prosthodontic terms. J Prosthet Dent. 2005;94:10–92.
9. Penny RE, Kraal JH. Crown-to-root ratio: its significance in restorative dentistry. J Prosthet Dent. 1979;42: 34–8.
10. Cho SY, Kim E. Does apical root resection in endodontic microsurgery jeopardize the prosthodontic prognosis? Restor Dent Endod. 2013;38:59–64.
11. McGuire MK. Prognosis versus actual outcome: a long-term survey of 100 treated periodontal patients under maintenance care. J Periodontol. 1991; 62:51–8.
12. Gutmann JL, Harrison JW. Surgical endodontics. Boston: Blackwell Scientific Publications; 1991.
13. Vertucci FJ. Root canal anatomy of the human permanent teeth. Oral Surg Oral Med Oral Pathol. 1984;58:589–99.
14. Del Fabbro M, Tsesis I, Rosano G, Bortolin M, Taschieri S. Scanning electron microscopic analysis of the integrity of the root-end surface after root-end management using a piezoelectric device: a cadaveric study. J Endod. 2010;36:1693–7.
15. Torres-Lagares D, Rodriguez-Martos R, Castellanos-Cosano L, Yanez-Vico R, Segura-Egea JJ, Gutierrez-Perez JL. Confocal microscopy: a valid approach to evaluate the three-dimensional characteristics of root-end cavities. Med Oral Patol Oral Cir Bucal. 2013;18:e542–6.
16. Lin CP, Chou HG, Kuo JC, Lan WH. The quality of ultrasonic root-end preparation: a quantitative study. J Endod. 1998;24:666–70.
17. Wuchenich G, Meadows D, Torabinejad M. A comparison between two root end preparation techniques in human cadavers. J Endod. 1994;20:279–82.
18. Peters CI, Peters OA, Barbakow F. An in vitro study comparing root-end cavities prepared by diamond-coated and stainless steel ultrasonic retrotips. Int Endod J. 2001;34:142–8.
19. Regan JD, Gutmann JL, Witherspoon DE. Comparison of Diaket and MTA when used as root-end filling materials to support regeneration of the periradicular tissues. Int Endod J. 2002;35:840–7.
20. Torabinejad M, Hong CU, Lee SJ, Monsef M, Pitt Ford TR. Investigation of mineral trioxide aggregate for root-end filling in dogs. J Endod. 1995;21:603–8.

21. Chong BS, Pitt Ford TR, Kariyawasam SP. Short-term tissue response to potential root-end filling materials in infected root canals. Int Endod J. 1997;30:240–9.
22. Chong BS, Ford TR, Kariyawasam SP. Tissue response to potential root-end filling materials in infected root canals. Int Endod J. 1997;30:102–14.
23. Chong BS, Pitt Ford TR. Root-end filling materials: rationale and tissue response. Endod Topics. 2005;11: 114–30.
24. Hume WR. Effect of eugenol on respiration and division in human pulp, mouse fibroblasts, and liver cells in vitro. J Dent Res. 1984;63:1262–5.
25. Bruce GR, McDonald NJ, Sydiskis RJ. Cytotoxicity of retrofill materials. J Endod. 1993;19:288–92.
26. Pitt Ford TR, Andreasen JO, Dorn SO, Kariyawasam SP. Effect of super-EBA as a root end filling on healing after replantation. J Endod. 1995;21:13–5.
27. Thomson TS, Berry JE, Somerman MJ, Kirkwood KL. Cementoblasts maintain expression of osteocalcin in the presence of mineral trioxide aggregate. J Endod. 2003;29:407–12.
28. DeGrood ME, Oguntebi BR, Cunningham CJ, Pink R. A comparison of tissue reactions to Ketac-Fil and amalgam. J Endod. 1995;21:65–9.
29. Apaydin ES, Shabahang S, Torabinejad M. Hard-tissue healing after application of fresh or set MTA as root-end-filling material. J Endod. 2004; 30:21–4.

Endodontic Surgical Complications Related to Maxillary Sinus Involvement

10

Silvio Taschieri, Stefano Corbella, and Massimo Del Fabbro

Abstract

The maxillary sinuses are large aerial cavities superior to the oral cavity, which have important implications on oral surgery in general and on endodontic surgery in particular. In cases of maxillary tooth necrosis and infection, microorganisms might be in contact with structures of the maxillary sinus such as Schneiderian membrane, either due to direct contact between the infected tooth apex and the membrane or due to expansion of the bony lesion into the maxillary sinus.

Hence, cases of maxillary tooth infection may lead to sinusitis, a complication with important implications for patients, which should be taken into consideration while planning treatment for tooth infection.

For endodontic surgery, when a periapical lesion involves the maxillary sinus, removal of the infection should be performed carefully, in order to avoid perforation of the sinus membrane or limit its extension. The sinus cavity must be protected during the apical third preparation and while sealing, for avoiding the extrusion of the filling material into the cavity.

As endodontic surgery may involve the maxillary sinus, adequate considerations and measures should be taken while planning and executing the surgery.

S. Taschieri, MD, DDS (✉)
M. Del Fabbro, BSc, PhD
Department of Biomedical, Surgical and Dental Science, Centre for Research in Oral Health, IRCCS Istituto Ortopedico Galeazzi, University of Milan, Via Riccardo Galeazzi, 4, 20161 Milan, Italy
e-mail: silvio.taschieri@fastwebnet.it; massimo.delfabbro@unimi.it

S. Corbella, DDS, PhD
Department of Biomedical, Surgical and Dental Science, Dental Clinic, IRCCS Istituto Ortopedico Galeazzi, University of Milan, Via Riccardo Galeazzi, 4, 20161 Milan, Italy
e-mail: stefano.corbella@gmail.com

Maxillary Sinus Anatomy and Physiology

The maxillary sinus (or antrum of Highmore) is the largest among the paranasal cavities. The average dimensions of the adult maxillary sinus are 2.5–3.5 cm wide, 3.6–4.5 cm high, and 3.8–4.5 cm deep [1]. Its estimated volume is approximately 12–15 cc [2].

The sinus cavity is an aerial cavity of a triangular pyramid shape, with three walls: a superior wall that corresponds to the floor of the orbit, a

I. Tsesis (ed.), *Complications in Endodontic Surgery*,
DOI 10.1007/978-3-642-54218-3_10, © Springer-Verlag Berlin Heidelberg 2014

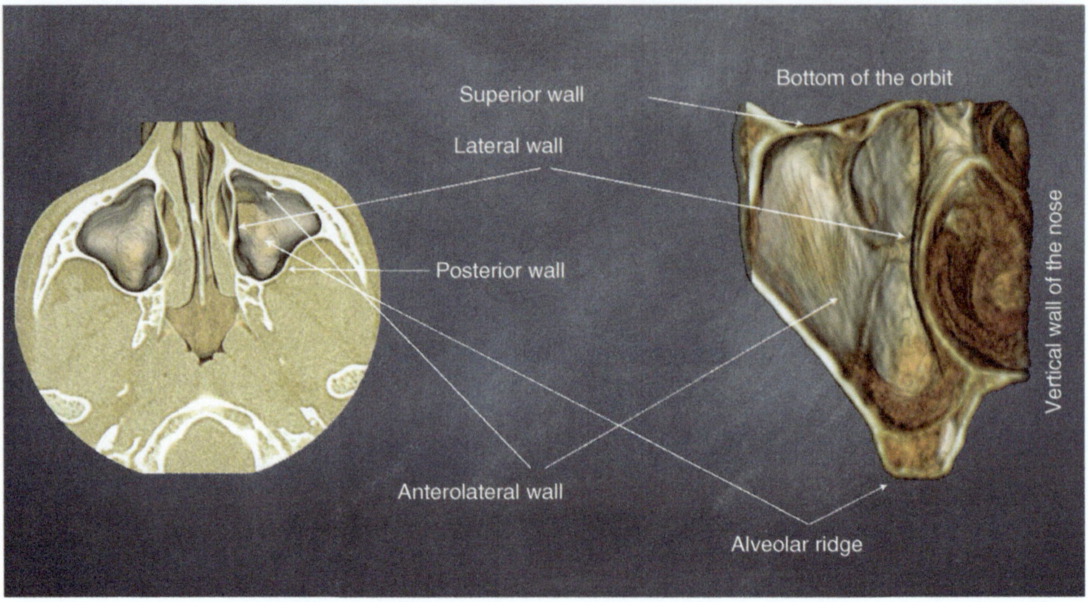

Fig. 10.1 The sinus cavity is an aerial cavity of a triangular pyramid shape whose medial base corresponds to the lateral vertical wall of the nose and whose apex extends within the zygomatic process of the maxillary bone

posterior wall that corresponds to the maxillary tuberosity and is located near the infratemporal and pterygopalatine fossae, and an anterolateral wall which is depressed because of the presence of the canine eminence (Fig. 10.1).

The maxillary sinus bony cavity is internally lined by a mucous membrane, named Schneiderian membrane, which is covered by a pseudostratified columnar ciliated epithelium. The sinus epithelium has similar characteristics to the respiratory epithelium, but with less vascularization than the nasal epithelium. The antral mucosa is thinner and less vascular than nasal mucosa [1]. The membrane is of variable thickness, ranging between 0.13 and 0.5 mm.

A natural opening from the maxillary sinus (maxillary ostium) is located anterosuperiorly on the medial wall of the sinus. It is the only sinus drainage pathway, and it drains into the middle meatus. The ostium has a mean diameter of 2.4 mm [3] (Fig. 10.2).

The ciliated cells of the maxillary mucosa are able to beat about 8–20 times per second, in a specific direction, resulting in a pattern of mucus flows, which often moves material against gravity to the sinus' exit. Thus, mucus may travel around the entire sinus cavity prior to exiting through the ostium and draining out.

Non-ciliated cells of the maxillary mucosa are characterized by microvilli that cover the apical aspect of the cell and serve to increase the surface area of the epithelium in order to improve air humidification and warming.

Serous and mucinous glands are located under the basal membrane and produce thick or thin mucus in response to the autonomic nervous system (parasympathetic system) [4]. The sinus' mucus is composed mostly of water (96 %), but also contains immunoglobulins and additional factors. It constitutes the most important mechanism of protection of the nasal-sinus apparatus.

The maxillary vascular network is extensive, guaranteeing a high amount of blood flow, which have important surgical implications (Fig. 10.3).

The venous drainage of the maxillary sinus occurs via the facial vein, the sphenopalatine vein, and the pterygoid plexus. The fact that the venous drainage of the sinus may occur both via typical pathways as the jugular veins and via the ethmoidal and frontal sinuses up to the cavernous sinus implies a risk of cerebral infection following

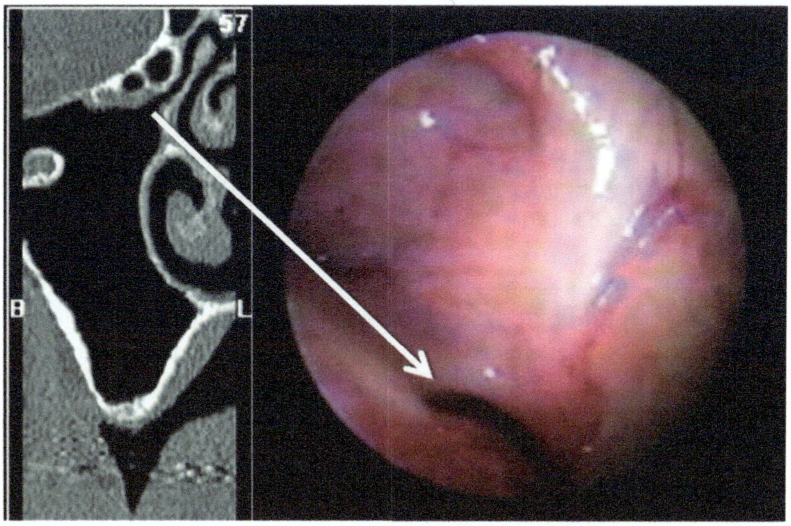

Fig. 10.2 Computed tomography scan (*left side*) and an endoscopic view (*right side*) of the maxillary sinus ostium (*arrow*)

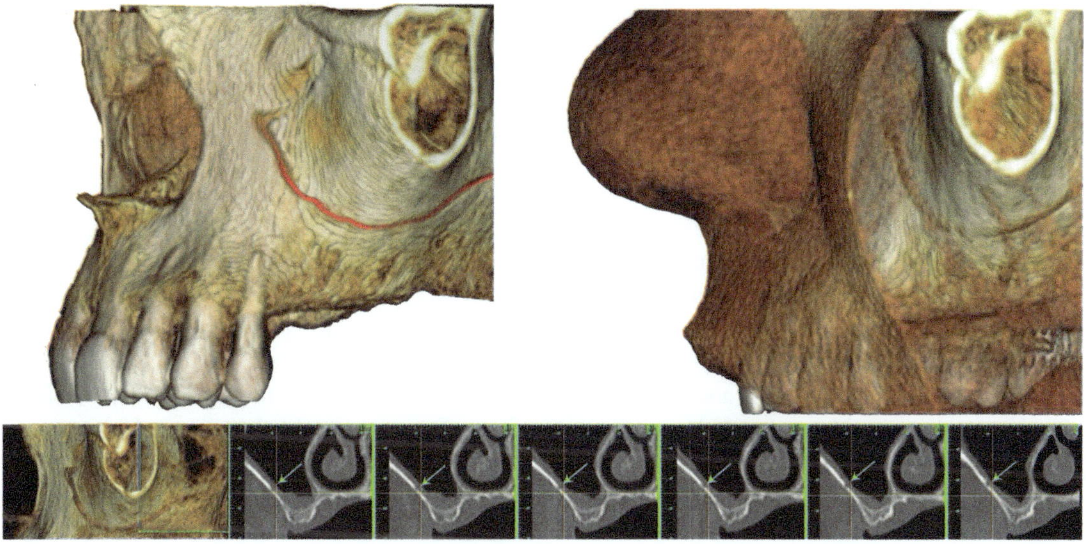

Fig. 10.3 Computed tomography scan 3D view of the lateral wall of the maxillary sinus which shows the point of emergence of the infraorbital artery (IOA) and the point of anastomosis between the IOA and the alveolar antral artery (AAA) as well as the route of the AAA. The *arrow* identifies the CT image of AAA

maxillary sinus contamination. Spread of infection via this route is a serious complication of maxillary sinus infections [5].

The maxillary sinus nerve supply is via the maxillary branch of the trigeminal nerve, coming directly from the posterior middle superior nerves (in the posterior wall) and anterior superior alveolar nerves (anterior wall), the infraorbital nerve (superior or orbital wall), the anterior palatine nerve, and the lateral branches of the sphenopalatine nerve (medial or nasal wall) [6].

The alveolar nerves travel within the anterior wall of the sinus and innervate the related teeth [7]. Thus, it may be difficult to distinguish between pain of a dental origin and pain originating from the maxillary sinus.

The maxillary sinus plays several roles in the human body, such as reducing the relative weight of the cranium, insulating sensitive structures, providing immunological defense, and more. Still, the function of the paranasal sinuses remains partially unknown. It is suggested that the main functional structure of the nasal fossa and paranasal sinuses is the mucosal lining, which helps the removal of inhaled particles [8].

Morphological Features of Upper Maxillary Roots in Relation to the Maxillary Sinus, Periapical Infections, and Sinusitis

Many bacterial and fungal species, such as *Streptococcus*, *Candida* (especially *C. albicans*), and *Propionibacterium* may be involved in the etiology of persistent periapical infections [9]. Cultural studies showed that one of the most common bacterial species found in this type of lesions is *Enterococcus faecalis* [10–12].

In patients with chronic rhinosinusitis with nasal polyposis (CRS with NP), the presence of a complex bacterial contamination has been demonstrated. This contamination may cause damage to the mucosa, resulting in an inflammatory process, which may lead to a hyperplastic process. *Staphylococcus* species, *Streptococcus viridans*, *Pseudomonas aeruginosa*, *Enterococcus faecalis*, and *Corynebacterium* [13], and even Fungi, may be associated with cases of chronic hyperplastic sinusitis (CHS).

It is important to note that many microorganisms were found both in the maxillary sinus and in endodontic infections, for example, *Staphylococcus epidermidis*, *Staphylococcus aureus*, *Klebsiella* spp., and Streptococci [14].

Microorganisms that may contaminate the extraradicular tissues are the few bacterial species able to survive outside the root canals in an immune-hostile environment. For example, *Actinomyces* (*A. israelii* and *A. radicidentis*) that elude the host immune system response by avoiding the phagocytic mechanism through bacterial aggregation [14]. Infection of the sinus caused by *Actinomyces* may therefore be difficult to treat because of the characteristics of resistance of these microorganisms [15, 16].

Intimate anatomic relationship may exist between the roots of the first and second maxillary molars and the maxillary sinus, sometimes with only a thin layer of cancellous bone separating the sockets of these maxillary molars and the floor of the sinus cavity. In many cases the molar roots may even protrude into the sinus cavity [8]. The root tip may touch or overlap the sinus floor, and the root apices may project into the floor of the sinus causing small elevations or prominences [17]. The mean distance between the maxillary posterior teeth and the floor of the maxillary sinus is about 2 mm.

Periapical periodontitis may result in maxillary sinusitis of dental origin with resultant inflammation and thickening of the mucosal lining of the sinus in areas adjacent to the involved teeth (Fig. 10.4a, b). Melen et al. reported that the frequency of sinusitis of dental origin varied considerably, ranging between 4.6 and 47 % of all sinusitis cases [18]. Studies showed that sinus mucosal hyperplasia is present in approximately 80 % of maxillary teeth with periapical pathology [19]. The closer the apex of a pulpally involved tooth to the floor of the sinus, the more likely and the greater the impact on the sinus tissues [20].

In a study performed on cadavers in 1943, Bauer [21] reported a direct extension of dental sepsis into the sinus and presented examples of pulpally involved teeth with histologically evident extension of the disease into the maxillary sinus. The same study also revealed microscopically the "diseased areas," showing the destruction of the bone separating the sinus from the teeth, with particular loss of the cortical bone normally found in the sinus floor. Other changes were found in the sinus mucosa, such as swelling with inflammation, cyst formation, hypertrophy, and even transformation of the mucosa to granulation tissue, hyalinization, or complete necrosis [21].

Sinusitis may follow endodontic surgery in the absence of previous inflammation of the sinus mucosa. The resected apex, the root canal filler (most frequently gutta-percha), and/or the retrograde filler may migrate into the maxillary sinus cavity, inducing a foreign body reaction by the respiratory mucosa, leading to a sinusitis. Moreover, oral pathogens may directly infect the maxillary mucosa by migrating from the oral

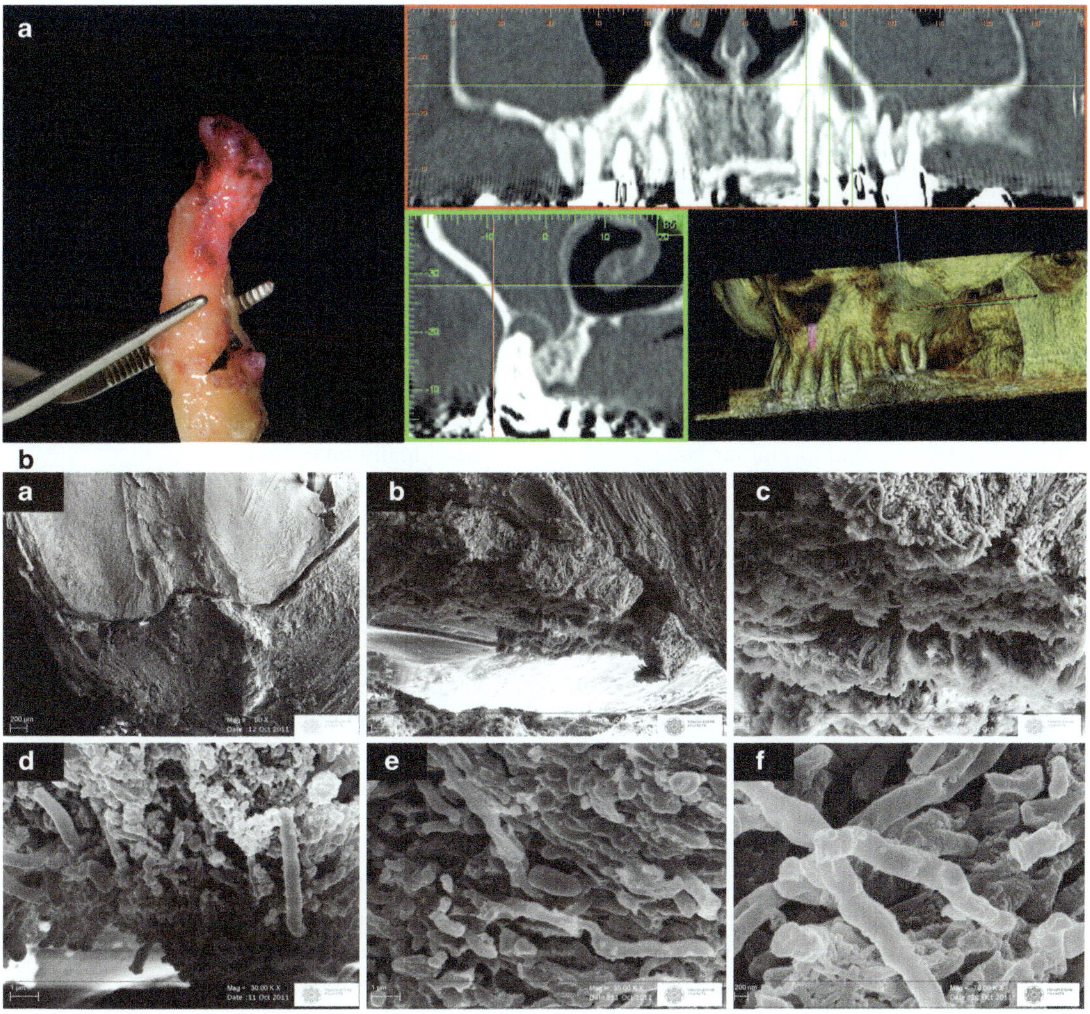

Fig. 10.4 (**a**) Computed tomography views of a maxillary premolar tooth with persistent periapical endodontic lesion and the tooth soon after extraction showing the apical lesion attached to the root apex. (**b**) A sequence of SEM images at different magnification of a section passing through the apical foramen of treated tooth. (**a**: Apical third of the root canal system showing a pathological tissue attached to the apex, **b**, **c**, **e**: Bacterial biofilm in contact with the apical wall of the root surface extending to the external root surface, d: bacterial biofilm at higher magnification showing intertwining bacterial filaments appears to be mainly constituted by *E. Coli*). A pathologic tissue is attached to the apex. Bacterial biofilm protrudes through the apical foramen

environment or from the periapical lesion area into the sinus. Another mechanism of sinusitis following periapical surgery is the obstruction of the ostium due to postoperative swelling of the maxillary sinus mucosa with complete impairment of the function of the mucociliary cleansing system, even in the absence of membrane perforation and direct communication between the sinus and oral cavities [22].

Sinusitis (or rhinosinusitis) is defined as an inflammation of the mucous membrane that lines the paranasal sinuses and is classified to several categories based on chronology of the disease:

1. Acute: a new infection that may last up to four weeks and can be subdivided symptomatically into severe and non-severe.
2. Recurrent acute: four or more separate episodes of acute sinusitis that occur within one year.
3. Subacute: an infection that lasts between four and 12 weeks and represents a transition between acute and chronic infection.

4. Chronic rhinosinusitis: the signs and symptoms last for more than 12 weeks.
5. Acute exacerbation of chronic sinusitis: the signs and symptoms of chronic rhinosinusitis exacerbate but return to baseline after treatment.

The typical signs and symptoms of sinusitis are headache and facial pain, or a constant dull pressure (dull pain), or ache over the affected sinuses [4]. This pain is typically localized in the involved sinus and may change when the affected person bends over or lies down or during mastication. A feeling of "fullness" around the first molar-second premolar area is often present [23].

Sinusitis may be accompanied by thick nasal discharge and may contain pus (purulent) and/or blood. Nasal discharge is considered a significant sign of sinus infection.

Severe acute or subacute sinusitis rarely produces fever. However, as said before, severe fulminant sinusitis may produce high fever.

Some authors correlated the time course of disease development to the degree of infection [5, 24–26].

In periapical chronic inflammation, the disease develops slowly, with no significant infection, and its spreading within the sinus may be slow and with minimal impact. On the contrary, acute infectious pulpal disease is much more rapidly spreading and destructive, involving the adjacent sinus within a short time. There have been reported cases of rapid spread of dental infections through the maxillary sinus leading to subsequent periorbital cellulitis, blindness, and even life-threatening cavernous sinus thrombosis, exemplifying the serious potential complications of endo-antral syndrome (EAS) [5, 24–26].

The clinical examination of a patient with suspected maxillary sinus disease should include extraoral tapping on the anterior and lateral walls of the sinus over the prominence of the cheekbones and/or palpation intraorally of the lateral surface of the maxilla between the canine fossa and the zygomatic buttress. If there is dental involvement, the teeth will be moderately or extremely sensitive to palpation and/or percussion. The pain typically radiates to all posterior teeth in the quadrant, so that all these teeth usually become tender to percussion [23].

Selden termed endo-antral syndrome (EAS) as the spread of pulpal disease beyond the confines of the dental supporting tissues into the maxillary sinus [27–29] and underlined five radiographic features characterizing EAS [29]:

1. Pulpal disease in a tooth whose apex approximates the floor of the maxillary sinus
2. Periapical radiolucencies on pulpally involved teeth
3. Radiographic loss of the lamina dura defining the inferior border of the maxillary sinus over the pulpally involved tooth
4. A faintly radiopaque mass bulging into the sinus space above the apex of the involved tooth, connected neither to the tooth nor to the lamina dura of the tooth socket (representing localized swelling and thickening of the sinus mucosa)
5. Variable degrees of radiopacity of the surrounding sinus space (comparison to the contralateral sinus is often helpful)

Clinical cases do not always present with all five features; thus, diagnostic and therapeutic decisions may be challenging.

In cases with maxillary sinus pathologies with doubtful differential diagnosis or with severe signs and symptoms of sinusitis, consultation with an ear, nose, and throat (ENT) specialist is strictly recommended.

Therapeutic Decision Making

In cases of maxillary sinusitis following endodontic surgery, a pharmacological approach may be considered in the short term, but only in cases with clean serum exudate and without presence or migration of a bone graft in the sinus cavity [30]. The drug therapy consists of amoxicillin and clavulanic acid 1 gr TID and metronidazole 500 mg TID per os for 7–10 days or levofloxacin 400 mg BID per os for 7–10 days in patients allergic to penicillin. In cases of a massive sinus infection, with or without migration of a bone graft, after ENT consultation a surgical approach should be considered [30].

In the past, several studies suggested that after the disease was addressed, the first-choice treatment would be tooth extraction, as the sinus inflammatory reactions had disappeared after extraction of the affected teeth [21, 31].

However, scenarios of maintaining the teeth and regression of sinus hyperplasia of dental origin in the mucosa of maxillary sinus have been documented by many other clinical studies [28, 29, 32]. These studies should be considered before choosing tooth extraction as the treatment alternative.

Endodontic Surgery and Sinus-Related Complications

Oberli et al. [17] evaluated a possible correlation between radiographic findings and presence of an oroantral communication (OAC). They analyzed the correlation between the positions of the root tip and the periapical lesion versus the sinus floor and the presence of an oroantral communication (OAC). While the perforation of the maxillary sinus during periapical surgery could not be predicted from the periapical radiographs, the following radiographic classification was proposed: (a) class I apices, where there is a distance between the root tip and the sinus floor; (b) class II apices, where the root tip touches the sinus floor; and (c) class III apices, where the root tip overlaps the sinus floor. The same classification was applied for the periapical lesions: (a) class I lesions, where there is a distance between the lesion and the sinus floor; (b) class II lesions, where the lesion touches the sinus floor; and (c) class III lesions, where the lesion overlaps the sinus floor.

In terms of clinical relevance, class I lesions show a high probability of leaving the sinus unharmed after periapical surgery, while for class III lesions (lesions seen inside the sinus cavity) perforation of the membrane may be unavoidable [17].

The outline of the lesions was described as either well defined or blurred. A well-defined outline means a sharp traceable radiopaque line. A blurred outline of the lesion means an unclear radiographic border of the lesion, which makes it impossible to trace the lesion accurately or to classify it.

The thin layer of bone covering the root is seen as a fusion of the lamina dura and the floor of the sinus [33]. In some cases with chronic periapical periodontitis, this line can be well defined and easy to trace, although in others the radiopaque line appears less defined or blurred.

A periapical radiograph may fail to show the lamina dura covering the root apex in areas with defective bony covering and it is not adequate in cases of large lesions. However, panoramic radiography provides an extensive overview of the sinus floor and its relationship with the teeth roots. It allows determination of the size of periapical lesions and cysts as well as radiodense foreign bodies [23]. But, both methods may not provide a clear visualization of the real dimensions and position of the lesion, due to intrinsic limitations.

Eberhardt et al. [20] stated that "standard dental radiographs, including panoramic radiograph and pluridirectional tomography, present a 2-dimensional image and as such are inadequate and/or impractical for precise morphometric assessment of osseous relationships. Because of the projection angle between the x-ray and the periapical film, it is difficult to detect whether a root tip overlapping the floor of the maxillary sinus is anatomically protruding into the maxillary sinus or is just being projected into it."

The use of 3D radiographic techniques as computerized tomography (CT) and cone-beam CT should be considered in order to adequately diagnose the anatomical relationships between the lesion and the maxillary sinus, to prevent invasion into the sinus lumen during surgery, and to plan the surgical procedure and timing [17]. The 3D radiographic techniques allow to obtain a three-dimensional view of the surgical field. Specific computer programs enable to achieve sound knowledge of dental and skull anatomical features, to define the real extent of the periapical lesion, and to determine the exact location of foreign bodies inside the sinus.

High-resolution axial and coronal CT and MRI (magnetic resonance imaging) are the most accurate noninvasive imaging techniques for the paranasal sinuses and adjacent structures and areas [33, 34]. The use of CBCT is considered an essential step for adequate planning of endodontic surgery when the lesion is near anatomic noble structure as maxillary sinus because of its ability to detect anatomical variations [35, 36]. The accuracy of CBCT in reproducing the three-dimensional anatomy allows the evaluation of cortical bone thickness and even of the relations between the tooth lesion and other structures as the maxillary sinus [17, 36–38]. Presurgical assessment using CBCT may also be useful for evaluating the features of the mesiobuccal root of permanent first molars, aimed at performing adequate root-end management and root-end filling of all canal orifices and detecting isthmi.

Furthermore, in the presurgical assessment, CBCT is useful to detect the presence of pathological findings in the maxillary sinus cavity, due to its relevant specificity and sensitivity [39–41].

Moreover, some studies reported that CBCT may be beneficial for the diagnosis of the relations between maxillary sinusitis and dental infection in the posterior maxilla, thus allowing pre-assessment of the chances of sinusitis resolution after adequate endodontic treatment [42, 43].

Radiologic maxillary sinusitis (RMS) is defined as the presence of unilateral or bilateral opacification reflecting air–fluid levels within the maxillary sinuses in a paranasal computerized tomography scan.

Another noninvasive imaging technique that has been introduced as a diagnostic screening tool for sinus pathology is A-mode ultrasound. A back wall echo is obtained when fluid or a large polyp carries ultrasound waves to the posterior bony wall that reflects an echo [44]. Ultrasound has been compared with radiography for the detection of secretions in sinuses as confirmed by trephination or sinus puncture [45]. In adults, ultrasound was found to be 90 % accurate and radiography 82 %. If the radiographic scan is abnormal, ultrasound is not a replacement for radiographic studies, which are necessary to differentiate fluid, polyps, thick mucosa, and tumors [45].

Root-End Management

The surgical approach may depend on the ENT diagnosis; if the sinus physiology is not altered, endodontic surgery can be performed as usual. In other cases, a treatment plan combining functional endoscopic sinus surgery technique and endodontic surgery (FESS) may be considered.

The proximity of the maxillary posterior teeth apices to the maxillary sinus raises special considerations during endodontic surgery due to a possible oroantral communication.

The frequency of membrane perforation during upper maxillary molar endodontic surgery has been reported as varying between 9.6 % (in a retrospective investigation by Oberli in 2007 [17]) and 50 % [46].

Hauman et al. reported in their review article (2002) [23] that a small Schneiderian membrane perforation during oral surgical procedures involving the maxillary sinus is not detrimental to the clinical outcome of the treatment. Furthermore, Oberli et al. in 2007 [17] concluded that an intraoperative OAC (oroantral communication) should not be considered a severe surgical accident if certain precautions had been taken [47].

However, the impact of a perforation on the sinus physiology in terms of alterations in of the sinus' function and the time needed for recovery of its functionality has never been assessed [38].

It has been suggested that trauma to the Schneiderian membrane, such as a perforation, may transiently and unpredictably inhibit ciliary activity [48] and also predispose the sinus to altered mucous composition due to a possible bacterial infection.

As a general rule the physiological status of the sinus should be verified prior to the surgical procedure [48], identifying any previous nasal trauma or surgery, nasal respiratory obstruction, and recurrent or chronic naso-sinusal diseases.

Management of Sinus Injury During Root-End Preparation

Garcia et al. showed that when sinus membrane perforations were smaller than 5–6 mm, no specific treatment was needed, as they did not lead to any particular complications in the postsurgical period (Figs. 10.5a–f and 10.6) [49].

In the course of surgical management of the root apex, cases of maxillary sinus membrane perforation may bear the risk of displacement of bacteria from either the infected periapical tissue, the resected root tips, or the bony drilling debris into the sinus [23].

When the lesion is inside the sinus cavity (class III Oberli), perforation of the membrane is unavoidable. Thus, in such cases, it is of utmost importance that a meticulous technique is used to ensure that foreign material (resected tooth apex, bony drilling debris, endodontic filling material) or bacteria from the infected periapical tissue do not enter the sinus. In order to avoid sinus mucosal thickening and signs of sinusitis [50], it was described as a method in which a hole is drilled in the root apex to secure the root tip with a suture before apicectomy, thus enabling the removal of the inflammatory lesion with the root tip. They recommended the use of a gauze to isolate the area and to prevent retro-preparation debris and retro-fill materials from entering the sinus. Garcia et al. [49] used a gauze to block the maxillary sinus and avoid the penetration of foreign bodies, but in their case, the sinus lining was not perforated.

In a recent article [38], an iatrogenic perforation of the Schneiderian membrane was isolated using an absorbable hemostatic gelatin sponge. Spongostan is a gelatin-based sponge that stimulates the intrinsic clotting pathway by promoting platelet activation and subsequent release of thromboplastin and thrombin. Spongostan is indicated for hemostasis in surgical procedures (excluding ophthalmic), when control of capillary, venous, and arteriolar bleeding by pressure, ligature, and other conventional procedures is ineffective or impractical and it shows a high capability of arresting bleeding. It may be recommended for the management of perforation of the Schneiderian membrane instead of using a gauze.

In another study of the same author [51], the sponge was removed after the root-end management, and the surgical site was embedded using pure platelet-rich plasma (P-PRP) supernatant, a P-PRP clot was applied over the perforation, and another clot was used to fill the bone cavity. Finally, P-PRP supernatant was gently injected at the suture site, using an atraumatic needle, in order to accelerate the wound healing as it was done also in other studies [52–55]. In these works, P-PRP was able to seal the perforation in an effective way. In fact, the conclusion of these

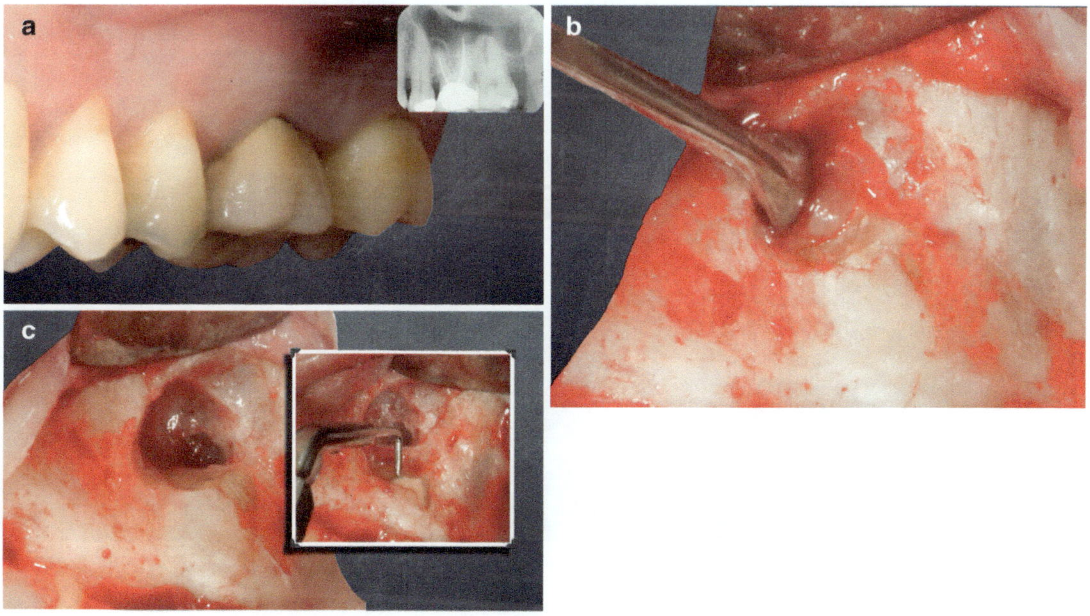

Fig. 10.5 (**a–f**) A step-by-step case of endodontic surgery of a first upper maxillary tooth with periapical lesion close to the maxillary sinus. Perforation to the sinus. An endoscope was used to explore both the root-end bevel and the sinus membrane integrity

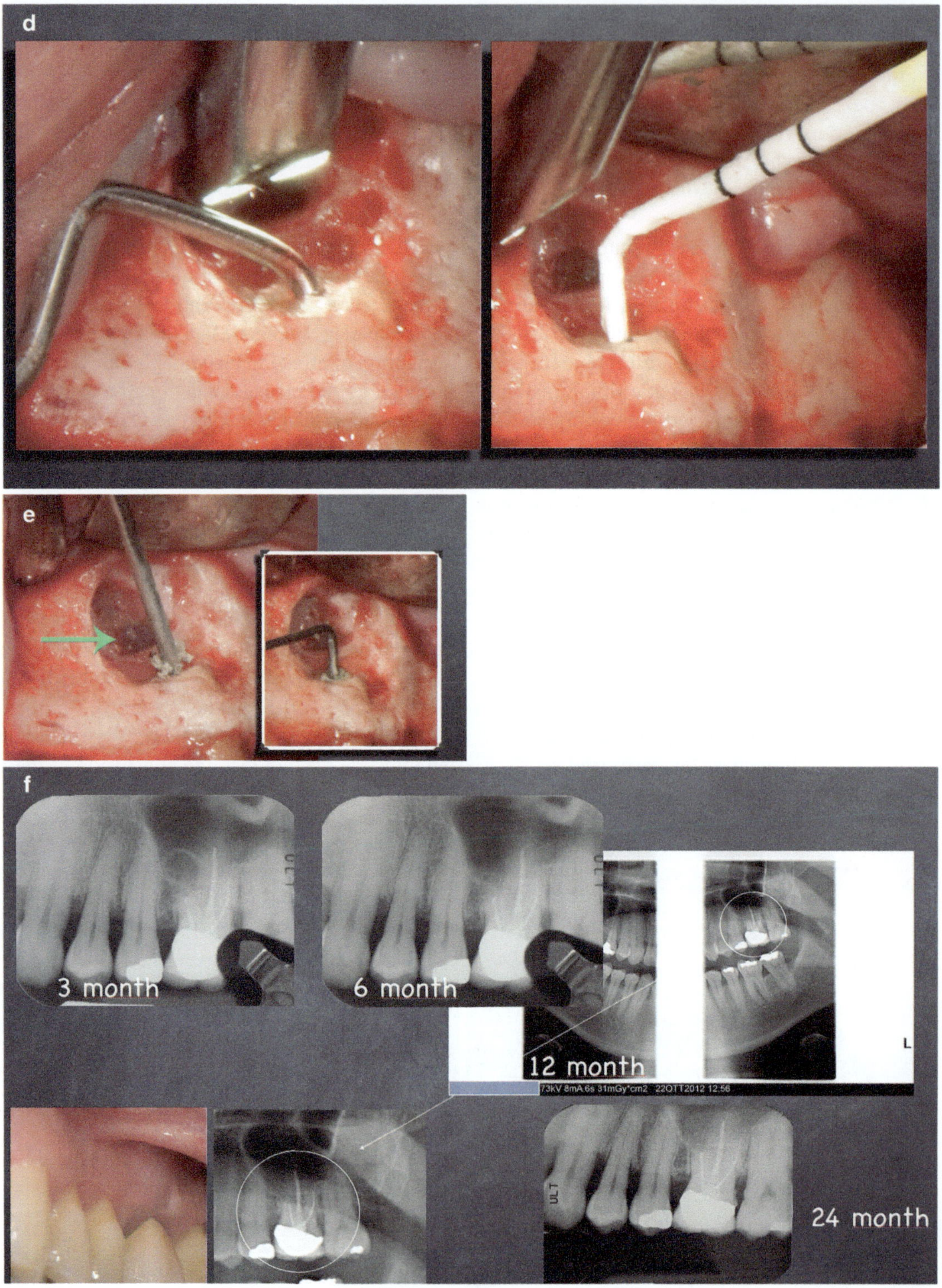

Fig. 10.5 (continued)

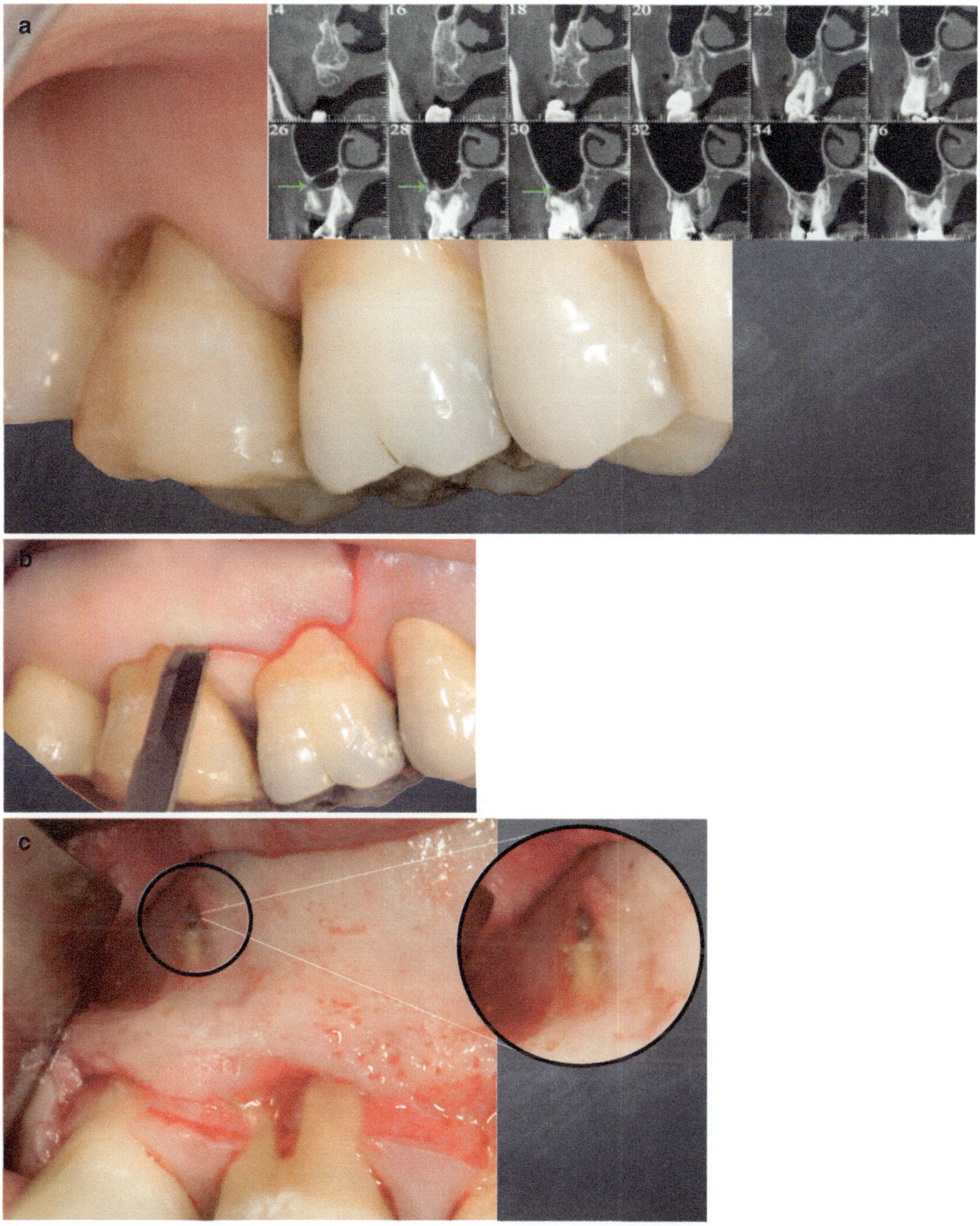

Fig. 10.6 A step by step case of endodontic surgery of a first upper maxillary tooth with close periapical lesion proximity to the maxillary sinus. Two apical roots were involved. Perforation to the sinus. An endoscope was used to explore both the root and the sinus cavity. An absorbable hemostatic gelatine sponge was placed into the bone access to shield the membrane perforation during root-end cavity management. The sponge was removed after root-end management and a autologus platelets clot was used to fill the bone cavity, in order to temporary close the perforation and enhancing the Sinus membrane repair

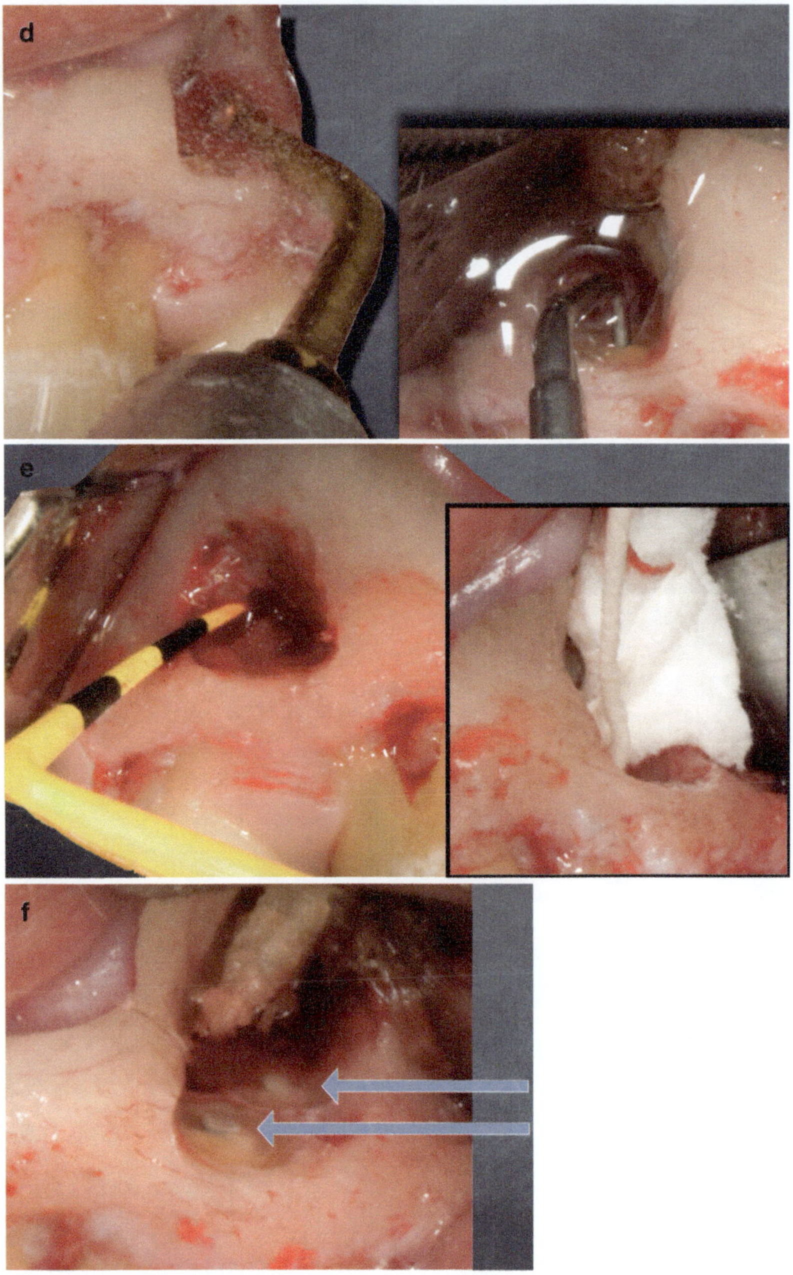

Fig. 10.6 (continued)

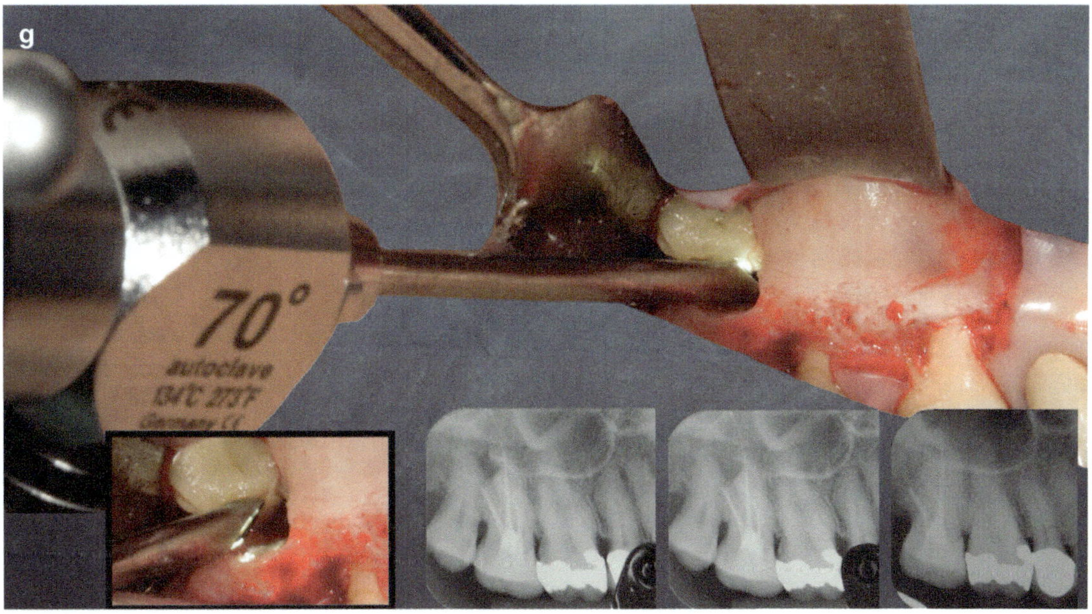

Fig. 10.6 (continued)

studies underlined that, in general, a small sinus membrane perforation (less than 6 mm) during endodontic surgery did not cause severe complications. The use of platelet concentrates could be effective in reducing the negative impact on patients' quality of life by decreasing pain and postsurgical effects as swelling.

One of the most favorable aspects of the use of P-PRP in endodontic surgery is that some of the platelet-derived components have the capability to reduce the inflammatory response after surgery, thus positively affecting the postoperative quality of life of the patients. The anti-inflammatory properties may be explained by both the suppression of proinflammatory chemokines as IL-1 and the observed antimicrobial effect [54]. Considering these aspects, it is reasonable to consider that the properties of PRP had a main role in significantly reducing the most common postoperative symptoms as pain and swelling as observed in the majority of patients treated.

In case of postsurgical acute sinusitis, the patient should be referred to the ENT specialist.

Endoscopy as a Multipurpose Magnification Device

The use of an endoscope can be helpful in both sinus surgery and root-end management [56–59]. Transalveolar access via an already existing connection between the oral cavity and the antrum (e.g., when the antrum is artificially exposed during apicectomy) is the least invasive access to the sinus in this type of clinical case.

This access to the sinus is possible due to the flexibility of the endoscope in the surgical field and the ease of changing the magnification degree. Thus, the endoscope (30°and 70°angle view) is useful during root-end management by eliminating the need for a change of magnification device during surgery, resulting in shorter surgical time. Conversely, when using a microscope, any movement of the microscope itself or of the patient, while increasing the magnitude, will cause the surgical field to become out of focus. In the authors' experience, a microscope is useful, but when using an endoscope the depth of field is similar to that of the naked eye. Using an endoscope, the surgeon can examine the morphological aspects of the root from almost any direction in a short time. This takes longer using a microscope and it is sometimes very difficult or impossible, especially in the posterior region of the jaws, unless beveling the root-end more than 45°, which increases the possibility of root-end filling bacterial leakage [60].

Furthermore, by using an endoscope, it is also possible to see behind the roots and ascertain the presence of a periradicular lesion, and it is especially useful for exploring the sinus cavity, thus obtaining a sound knowledge of the surgical field. The rod-lens system of the endoscope allows good visualization, even in the presence of irrigation fluids. The surgeon may use retrotips with sterile water irrigation in order to avoid overheating and at the same time to have the lens cleaned.

Conclusion

The maxillary sinus is a complex anatomical structure with major implications in endodontic surgery of the first and second maxillary molars, which are important for both planning and execution of the surgical procedure.

The infraction of the Schneiderian membrane during endodontic surgery may be unavoidable but can be adequately addressed by appropriate surgical procedures.

Moreover, pathology of the sinus may be derived from an odontogenic infection and might limit the effects of the endodontic surgery.

Accurate preoperative planning, including the use of modern radiographic techniques, allows a safe approach to endodontic lesions in case of endodontic lesions invading the maxillary sinus, limiting the surgical complications and the postoperative adverse sequelae.

References

1. van den Bergh JP, ten Bruggenkate CM, Disch FJ, Tuinzing DB. Anatomical aspects of sinus floor elevations. Clin Oral Implants Res. 2000;11:256–65.
2. Chanavaz M. Maxillary sinus: anatomy, physiology, surgery, and bone grafting related to implantology–eleven years of surgical experience (1979–1990). J Oral Implantol. 1990;16:199–209.
3. Gaudy J-F. Anatomie clinique. 2nd ed. Rueil-Malmaison: Cahiers de Protheses; 2007.
4. Bailey B, Johnson J, Newlands S. Head & neck surgery – otolaryngology. Philadelphia: Lippincott Williams & Wilkins; 2006.
5. Robbins KT, Tarshis LM. Blindness: a complication of odontogenic sinusitis. Otolaryngol Head Neck Surg. 1981;89:938–40.
6. Watzek G, Bernhart T, Ulm C. Complications of sinus perforations and their management in endodontics. Dent Clin North Am. 1997;41:563–83.
7. Wallace JA. Transantral endodontic surgery. Oral Surg Oral Med Oral Pathol Oral Radiol Endod. 1996;82:80–3.
8. Gutmann JL, Harrison JW. Surgical endodontics. Boston: Blackwell Scientific Publications; 1991.
9. Siqueira Jr JF, Rocas IN. Diversity of endodontic microbiota revisited. J Dent Res. 2009;88:969–81.
10. Molander A, Reit C, Dahlen G, Kvist T. Microbiological status of root-filled teeth with apical periodontitis. Int Endod J. 1998;31:1–7.
11. Pinheiro ET, Gomes BP, Ferraz CC, Sousa EL, Teixeira FB, Souza-Filho FJ. Microorganisms from canals of root-filled teeth with periapical lesions. Int Endod J. 2003;36:1–11.
12. Sundqvist G, Figdor D, Persson S, Sjogren U. Microbiologic analysis of teeth with failed endodontic treatment and the outcome of conservative re-treatment. Oral Surg Oral Med Oral Pathol Oral Radiol Endod. 1998;85:86–93.
13. Zernotti ME, Angel Villegas N, Roques Revol M, Baena-Cagnani CE, Arce Miranda JE, Paredes ME, et al. Evidence of bacterial biofilms in nasal polyposis. J Investig Allergol Clin Immunol. 2010;20:380–5.
14. Figdor D, Gulabivala K. Survival against the odds: microbiology of root canals associated with post-treatment disease. Endod Topics. 2011;18:62–77.
15. Gocmen G, Varol A, Goker K, Basa S. Actinomycosis: report of a case with a persistent extraoral sinus tract. Oral Surg Oral Med Oral Pathol Oral Radiol Endod. 2011;112:e121–3.
16. Vorasubin N, Wu AW, Day C, Suh JD. Invasive sinonasal actinomycosis: case report and literature review. Laryngoscope. 2013;123:334–8.
17. Oberli K, Bornstein MM, von Arx T. Periapical surgery and the maxillary sinus: radiographic parameters for clinical outcome. Oral Surg Oral Med Oral Pathol Oral Radiol Endod. 2007;103:848–53.
18. Melen I, Lindahl L, Andreasson L, Rundcrantz H. Chronic maxillary sinusitis. Definition, diagnosis and relation to dental infections and nasal polyposis. Acta Otolaryngol. 1986;101:320–7.
19. Matilla K. Roentgenological investigations of the relationship between periapical lesions and conditions of the mucous membrane of the maxillary sinuses. Acta Odontol Scand. 1965;23:42–6.
20. Eberhardt JA, Torabinejad M, Christiansen EL. A computed tomographic study of the distances between

the maxillary sinus floor and the apices of the maxillary posterior teeth. Oral Surg Oral Med Oral Pathol. 1992;73:345–6.
21. Bauer WH. Maxillary sinusitis of dental origin. Am J Orthod Oral Surg. 1943;29:133–51.
22. Bertrand B, Eloy P. Relationship of chronic ethmoidal sinusitis, maxillary sinusitis, and ostial permeability controlled by sinusomanometry: statistical study. Laryngoscope. 1992;102:1281–4.
23. Hauman CH, Chandler NP, Tong DC. Endodontic implications of the maxillary sinus: a review. Int Endod J. 2002;35:127–41.
24. Albin R, Wiener J, Gordon R, Willoughby JH. Diagnosis and treatment of pansinusitis: report of case. J Oral Surg. 1979;37:604–7.
25. Gold RS, Sager E. Pansinusitis, orbital cellulitis, and blindness as sequelae of delayed treatment of dental abscess. J Oral Surg. 1974;32:40–3.
26. Jarrett 2nd WH, Gutman FA. Ocular complications of infection in the paranasal sinuses. Arch Ophthalmol. 1969;81:683–8.
27. Selden HS. The interrelationship between the maxillary sinus and endodontics. Oral Surg Oral Med Oral Pathol. 1974;38:623–9.
28. Selden HS. The endo-antral syndrome: an endodontic complication. J Am Dent Assoc. 1989;119(397–8):401–2.
29. Selden HS. Endo-Antral syndrome and various endodontic complications. J Endod. 1999;25:389–93.
30. Testori T, Drago L, Wallace SS, Capelli M, Galli F, Zuffetti F, et al. Prevention and treatment of postoperative infections after sinus elevation surgery: clinical consensus and recommendations. Int J Dent. 2012;2012:365809.
31. Ericson S, Welander U. Local hyperplasia of the maxillary sinus mucosa after elimination of adjacent periapical osteitis. A follow-up study. Odontol Revy. 1966;17:153–9.
32. Nenzen B, Welander U. The effect of conservative root canal therapy on local mucosal hyperplasia in the maxillary sinus. Odontol Revy. 1967;18:295–302.
33. White SC, Pharoah MJ. Oral radiology – principles and practice. 4th ed. St. Louis: Mosby, Year Book, Inc.; 2000.
34. Perez CA, Farman AG. Diagnostic radiology of maxillary sinus defects. Oral Surg Oral Med Oral Pathol. 1988;66:507–12.
35. Patel S. New dimensions in endodontic imaging: Part 2. Cone beam computed tomography. Int Endod J. 2009;42:463–75.
36. Rigolone M, Pasqualini D, Bianchi L, Berutti E, Bianchi SD. Vestibular surgical access to the palatine root of the superior first molar: "low-dose cone-beam" CT analysis of the pathway and its anatomic variations. J Endod. 2003;29:773–5.
37. Patel S, Dawood A. The use of cone beam computed tomography in the management of external cervical resorption lesions. Int Endod J. 2007;40:730–7.
38. Taschieri S, Fabbro MD, Corbella S, Weinstein T, Rosano G, Tsesis I. Endoscopic minimally invasive management of a periradicular lesion invading the maxillary sinus. J Oral Sci. 2011;53:533–8.
39. Maillet M, Bowles WR, McClanahan SL, John MT, Ahmad M. Cone-beam computed tomography evaluation of maxillary sinusitis. J Endod. 2011;37:753–7.
40. Bornstein MM, Wasmer J, Sendi P, Janner SF, Buser D, von Arx T. Characteristics and dimensions of the Schneiderian membrane and apical bone in maxillary molars referred for apical surgery: a comparative radiographic analysis using limited cone beam computed tomography. J Endod. 2012;38:51–7.
41. Ritter L, Lutz J, Neugebauer J, Scheer M, Dreiseidler T, Zinser MJ, et al. Prevalence of pathologic findings in the maxillary sinus in cone-beam computerized tomography. Oral Surg Oral Med Oral Pathol Oral Radiol Endod. 2011;111:634–40.
42. Cymerman JJ, Cymerman DH, O'Dwyer RS. Evaluation of odontogenic maxillary sinusitis using cone-beam computed tomography: three case reports. J Endod. 2011;37:1465–9.
43. Brullmann DD, Schmidtmann I, Hornstein S, Schulze RK. Correlation of cone beam computed tomography (CBCT) findings in the maxillary sinus with dental diagnoses: a retrospective cross-sectional study. Clin Oral Investig. 2012;16:1023–9.
44. Revonta M. Ultrasound in the diagnosis of maxillary and frontal sinusitis. Acta Otolaryngol Suppl. 1980;370:1–55.
45. Landman MD. Ultrasound screening for sinus disease. Otolaryngol Head Neck Surg. 1986;94:157–64.
46. Persson G. Periapical surgery of molars. Int J Oral Surg. 1982;11:96–100.
47. Ericson S, Finne K, Persson G. Results of apicoectomy of maxillary canines, premolars and molars with special reference to oroantral communication as a prognostic factor. Int J Oral Surg. 1974;3:386–93.
48. Pignataro L, Mantovani M, Torretta S, Felisati G, Sambataro G. ENT assessment in the integrated management of candidate for (maxillary) sinus lift. Acta Otorhinolaryngol Ital. 2008;28:110–9.
49. Garcia B, Martorell L, Marti E, Penarrocha M. Periapical surgery of maxillary posterior teeth. A review of the literature. Med Oral Patol Oral Cir Bucal. 2006;11:E146–50.
50. Jerome CE, Hill AV. Preventing root tip loss in the maxillary sinus during endodontic surgery. J Endod. 1995;21:422–4.
51. Taschieri S, Corbella S, Tsesis I, Del Fabbro M. Impact of the use of plasma rich in growth factors (PRGF) on the quality of life of patients treated with endodontic surgery when a perforation of sinus membrane occurred: a comparative study. Oral Maxillofac Surg. 2014;18:43–52.
52. Del Fabbro M, Bortolin M, Taschieri S, Weinstein R. Is platelet concentrate advantageous for the surgical treatment of periodontal diseases? A systematic review and meta-analysis. J Periodontol. 2011;82:1100–11.
53. Del Fabbro M, Bortolin M, Taschieri S, Weinstein RL. Effect of autologous growth factors in maxillary

sinus augmentation: a systematic review. Clin Implant Dent Relat Res. 2013;15:205–16.
54. Del Fabbro M, Ceresoli V, Lolato A, Taschieri S. Effect of platelet concentrate on quality of life after periradicular surgery: a randomized clinical study. J Endod. 2012;38:733–9.
55. Anitua E, Sanchez M, Nurden AT, Nurden P, Orive G, Andia I. New insights into and novel applications for platelet-rich fibrin therapies. Trends Biotechnol. 2006;24:227–34.
56. Held SA, Kao YH, Wells DW. Endoscope–an endodontic application. J Endod. 1996;22:327–9.
57. von Arx T, Frei C, Bornstein MM. [Periradicular surgery with and without endoscopy: a prospective clinical comparative study]. Schweiz Monatsschr Zahnmed. 2003;113:860–5.
58. von Arx T, Montagne D, Zwinggi C, Lussi A. Diagnostic accuracy of endoscopy in periradicular surgery - a comparison with scanning electron microscopy. Int Endod J. 2003;36:691–9.
59. Taschieri S, Del Fabbro M, Testori T, Weinstein R. Microscope versus endoscope in root-end management: a randomized controlled study. Int J Oral Maxillofac Surg. 2008;37:1022–6.
60. Gagliani M, Taschieri S, Molinari R. Ultrasonic root-end preparation: influence of cutting angle on the apical seal. J Endod. 1998;24:726–30.

Bleeding in Endodontic Surgery 11

Eyal Rosen and Igor Tsesis

Abstract

Modern endodontic surgery is a highly predictable treatment for teeth with apical periodontitis. While mild hemorrhage during the surgical procedures is common, severe bleeding during endodontic surgery due to an insult to a major blood vessel is relatively rare and may lead to serious systemic complications such as airway compromise, cardiovascular effects, and worsening of the mental status of the patient, and if not controlled may even lead to death. Elderly patients and patients with systemic diseases may be more susceptible to complications following severe blood loss. In addition, in patients with systemic bleeding disorders, excessive bleeding may occur even if only relatively small blood vessels were damaged during the surgical procedure.

Adequate bleeding control is essential for the success of periapical surgery, since it improves visualization of the surgical site, minimizes the operating time, and enables the dry field for retrograde filling material placement. Even mild hemorrhage during endodontic surgery may cause complications during the surgical procedure and may even jeopardize the prognosis of the treatment.

Careful treatment planning and surgical technique, combined with knowledge of the surgical anatomy and recognition of possible hemorrhage related complications, are essential in order to prevent bleeding during endodontic surgery. In addition, a thorough clinical evaluation and anamnesis should be preformed prior to the surgical procedure in order to reveal patients with potential systemic risks of excessive uncontrolled bleeding.

Introduction

Modern endodontic surgery is a highly predictable treatment for teeth with apical periodontitis [1, 2]. However, an insult to blood vessels during the surgical procedure may lead to hemorrhage, a relatively common surgical complication [3–7].

E. Rosen, DMD (✉) • I. Tsesis, DMD
Department of Endodontology, Maurice and Gabriela Goldschleger School of Dental Medicine, Tel Aviv University, Tel Aviv, Israel
e-mail: dr.eyalrosen@gmail.com; dr.tsesis@gmail.com

I. Tsesis (ed.), *Complications in Endodontic Surgery*,
DOI 10.1007/978-3-642-54218-3_11, © Springer-Verlag Berlin Heidelberg 2014

While severe hemorrhage in the oral cavity is not frequent, it may present serious systemic complications, resulting in a drop of blood pressure, heart rate increase, and worsening of the mental status of the patient, and if not controlled even may lead to death [5, 8]. Generally the loss of up to 15 % of blood volume does not cause serious systemic effects and once the hemorrhage is controlled does not require additional medical intervention [5, 8]. Elderly patients and patients with systemic diseases may be even more susceptible to complications following severe blood loss. In addition, in patients with systemic bleeding disorders, excessive bleeding may occur even if only relatively small blood vessels were damaged during the surgical procedure [5, 8].

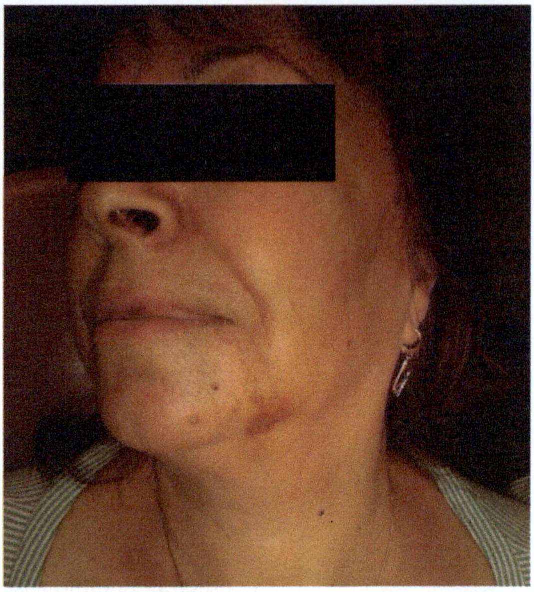

Fig. 11.1 Facial hematoma following endodontic surgery of the mandibular premolar

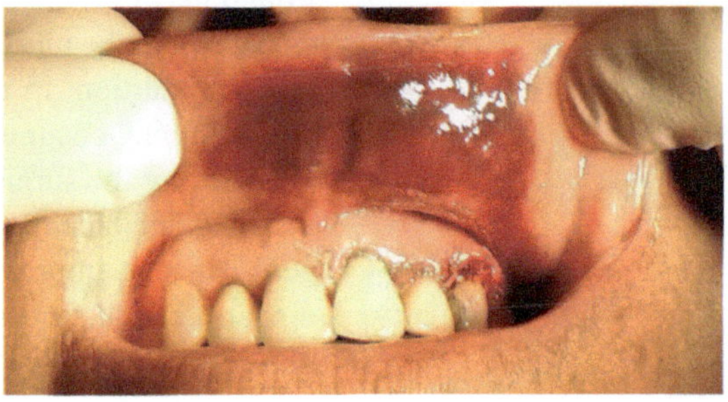

Fig. 11.2 Ecchymosis of the oral mucosa at the upper lip region following endodontic surgery of the maxillary incisors

Only few dental procedures have the potential to result in life-threatening bleeding [5, 8]. For severe hemorrhage to occur, an insult to a major blood vessel is usually required and is quite rare to happen during minor surgical procedures such as endodontic surgery [5, 8]. Blood loss during endodontic surgical procedures on average was found to range from 10 to 50 ml, and the duration of the surgical procedures had an exponential influence on the total blood loss [9]. The immediate danger for a healthy patient with severe postoperative hemorrhage in the oral cavity is airway compromise. Excessive bleeding that is not controlled by local measures in the dental office should be referred to the nearest hospital emergency department so the hemorrhage would be managed appropriately, and the airway can be secured [8].

In some cases when the bleeding is not perforating the oral mucosa or the skin, the bleeding may result in the formation of hematoma. *Hematoma* is a localized collection of blood that leaked from blood vessels into oral mucosa or adjacent facial tissues and may cause its discoloration (Fig. 11.1). In rare cases excessive hematoma, especially in the floor of the mouth, may lead to potentially life-threatening scenario, requiring close monitoring and continual airway assessment [10].

Ecchymosis is an extravasation of blood into subcutaneous tissue or mucosa (Fig. 11.2) [11–13].

Ecchymosis or *mucosal petechiae* are quite unpredictable. The inflammatory reaction after surgery and subsequent fragility of the capillaries may be a major contributor to ecchymosis and petechiae development [11]. Although both are transient symptoms, skin ecchymosis is unaesthetic. Therefore, its prevention is useful [12]. Skin ecchymosis can be induced by a problem in the production of coagulation factors by the liver, inadequate reticuloendothelial clearance of fibrin degradation products, and decreased production of platelets, which promote secondary fibrinolysis [13]. Ecchymosis can last for up to 2 weeks presenting an esthetic problem and generally requires no treatment.

Mild hemorrhage is relatively common during endodontic surgery, and although it is usually not life threatening, it may cause complications during the surgical procedure and may even jeopardize the prognosis of the treatment [4]. Adequate bleeding control is essential for the success of periapical surgery, since it improves visualization of the surgical site, minimizes the operating time, and enables the dry field for retrograde filling material placement [4, 7].

This chapter will discuss the local and systemic considerations of the prevention, diagnosis, and management of bleeding-related complications in endodontic surgery.

Systemic Considerations

Hemostasis may be defined as the process whereby bleeding is controlled [14]. Biologically, hemostasis is a tightly regulated process that maintains the blood flow through the vasculature simultaneously as a thrombotic response to tissue damage occurs [6, 7]. The hemostatic process is extremely complex and for simplicity may be classified to a primary phase, initiated at time of injury and ends with the formation of an unstable soft plug, and an ensuing secondary phase that starts by the initiation of the full-scale coagulation cascade that ends in the formation of a stable fibrin clot [6, 7]. Impairment in one or more of the hemostasis cascade components may lead to bleeding disorder and an increased potential for bleeding-related complications during surgery [3–7, 15, 16].

Bleeding during or following minor surgical procedures of the oral cavity is not rare and fortunately, in healthy patients, is usually self-limiting and manageable [3]. However, a small sector of the general population has an increased risk of bleeding due to inherited bleeding disorders, and even more common are patients with hemostatic impairments that are secondary to underlying disease or medication [3]. In those population groups, even a relatively minor surgical procedure may precipitate an excessive and prolonged bleeding incident [3], impaired wound healing, and increase risk of infection [3]. It has been reported that while the incidence of postoperative bleeding following minor oral surgical procedures is within the range of 0.2 and 3.3 %, in patients under chronic anticoagulation therapy, the occurrence of postoperative bleedings is much more prevalent and ranges between 8.6 and 32.1 % [5].

Identification of patients with bleeding disorder is a key objective of the preoperative anamnesis and evaluation, in order to prevent surgical complications. The practitioner needs to be familiar with the different categories of bleeding disorders, their clinical manifestation, and most importantly, their clinical relevance to the planned surgical procedure [3, 5–7]. In general, bleeding disorders may be divided for simplicity to platelets disorders, inherited coagulation disorders, and acquired coagulation abnormalities.

Platelet Disorders

There is a number of platelet-related defects, both inherited and acquired, that may be grossly divided as defects in the number of platelets (i.e., "thrombocytopenia") or of platelet function, though some platelet disorders are characterized by both decreased number and impaired platelet function [3, 5].

Normal blood platelet levels are usually within the range of 150–400 × 10^9/L, and thrombocytopenia leading to increased bleeding is rarely clinically significant unless platelet counts are less than 50 × 10^9/L [3, 5]. On the other hand, platelet function disorders, such as adhesion or aggregation defects, may lead to surgical bleeding and may require preparation prior to surgery, such as platelet transfusion [3, 5].

Drug-induced platelet defects posses potential significant adverse effects on platelet number and function. Heparin, aspirin, some nonsteroidal anti-inflammatory drugs (NSAIDs) such as ibuprofen, and even some over-the-counter medical products may attenuate platelet activity [3, 5].

Inherited Coagulation Disorders

Von Willebrand disease (VWD) results from quantitative or qualitative defects in VW factor, a key protein in hemostasis, and is the most common inherited bleeding disorder, affecting up to 1 % of the general population [3]. The clinical manifestations of VWD are easy bruising, epistaxis, menorrhagia, and operative bleeding [3].

Hemophilia is an inherited bleeding disorder caused by deficiencies of either factor VIII (termed: "hemophilia A") or factor IX ("hemophilia B") [3, 5]; both types are not clinically distinguishable [3, 5]. The prevalence of hemophilia is 1 in 5,000 males [3, 5]. Hemophilia patients are characterized by easy bruising, excessive post-trauma bleeding, spontaneous muscle and joint hemorrhage, and excessive bleeding following surgical procedures [3, 5].

Additional congenital coagulation deficiencies are extremely rare [3, 5]. Thus, although factor XI deficiency in the Ashkenazi Jewish population has a prevalence of 1 in 1,000, the prevalence of other factors deficiencies is in the range of 1 in 0.5–1 per million [3, 5]. Usually, with possible some exceptions, the bleeding manifestations in these disorders are less severe than in hemophilia patients [3, 5].

Acquired Coagulation Abnormalities

Patients on chronic anticoagulation therapy are at increased risk of bleeding during surgical procedures [3, 5], and the risk of bleeding is relative to the intensity and duration of the anticoagulation therapy [3, 5].

Warfarin is a relatively common anticoagulation agent indicated usually for prevention of thromboembolism [3, 5]. Warfarin is a vitamin K antagonist, and its effect is monitored by the *international normalized ratio* (*INR*; a standardization of the prothrombin time assay). The therapeutic INR may vary depending on the clinical indication, but is usually within the range of 2.0–3.0 for most patients [3, 5].

The management of patients who are receiving warfarin and require endodontic surgery is a relatively common clinical difficulty, and when indicated, warfarin treatment interruption is clinically simple since it requires just waiting until the anticoagulant effect wears off and resume it when there is adequate hemostasis. However, it requires a complex decision because of thromboembolic risks during anticoagulant interruption [17]. Case selection of patients on warfarin is therefore very important, and patients with coexisting medical problems (such as liver disease, renal disease, and thrombocytopenia or who are taking antiplatelet drugs) in certain cases should NOT have a surgical dental procedure in the primary care setting [18].

The risk of significant bleeding in patients on oral warfarin with stable INR levels in the therapeutic range is low. However, the risk of thrombosis if warfarin treatment is discontinued may be increased. Thus, oral anticoagulants should not be routinely discontinued in patients requiring endodontic surgery, and the matter should be discussed with the patient's hematologist, particularly when the INR levels are high or when the INR levels are unstable [18].

In patients receiving warfarin, an INR check shortly prior to surgery is recommended. Perry et al. [18] recommended that in patients receiving long-term warfarin and who are stably anticoagulated, an INR check 72 h prior to surgery is recommended to allow sufficient time for dose modification if necessary to ensure a safe INR on the day of surgery [18]. Douketis [17] recommended an INR check 1 day prior to an elective surgery.

It is important to note that the commonly used NSAIDs should be avoided in patients receiving warfarin because of their antiplatelet action and the risk of over anticoagulation and hemorrhage [17].

When the risk for bleeding during or following the surgery is significant, in certain cases warfarin interruption is indicated. In addition, for patients with significant risk of thromboembolism following warfarin interruption, anticoagulation bridging may be required [17]. Bridging anticoagulation for warfarin interruption consists of warfarin stop about a week prior to surgery and start of heparin bridging [17]. The decision if and how to interrupt an anticoagulation treatment and whether to adopt an anticoagulation bridging protocol is a complex decision that requires consultation with the patient's primary physician [17, 18].

Heparin is a cofactor of the naturally occurring anticoagulant antithrombin, accelerating inhibition of the serine proteases of the coagulation cascade [3, 5], and has a short half-life (about 1 h, for "unfractionated" heparin) [3, 5]. Heparin is given by intravenous bolus followed by infusion to maintain its therapeutic levels. However, low molecular weight heparin (LMWH) possesses a longer half-life than unfractionated heparin and can be delivered daily subcutaneously [3, 5]. Usually, most patients on long-term heparin therapy do not require laboratory monitoring. However, when monitoring is indicated, an anti-Xa assay is used [3, 5].

It is important to note that sometimes the preoperative anamnesis and the routine clinical evaluation may not reveal an underlying clinically significant bleeding disorder [5]. Thus, in case of unexplained prolonged and difficult-to-manage intraoperative bleeding or in case of recurrent postoperative bleedings, the surgeon should always consider the possibility of an undetected underlying systemic bleeding disorder [3, 5, 17, 18].

The possibility of intra- or postoperative bleeding always exists when a surgical procedure is undertaken, especially in patients receiving anticoagulation therapy or with an underlying systemic bleeding disorder [3, 5, 17, 18]. A thorough preoperative evaluation and anamnesis are needed in order to screen for potential bleeding disorders. Before surgery, and especially in patients with systemic bleeding disorders, the practitioner is required to ask himself or herself several key questions before he or she performs the surgical procedure [3, 5, 17, 18]:

- What is the exact bleeding disorder, including the severity of the disorder, its current and updated status, and its clinical relevance to the planned surgical procedure?
- Do I have all necessary means (including knowledge, clinical settings, and equipment) to manage any potential bleeding during or following the surgical procedure?
- Is the potential benefit to my patient outweighs the potential risks associated with bleeding?

It is also recommended to communicate with the patient's primary physician in order to obtain complete and up-to-date information on the patient's condition and recommendations regarding required special adjustments in the management of the patient before and following the surgery [3, 5, 17, 18].

Local Considerations

Achieving proper hemostasis is an essential principle of surgery, and achieving adequate hemostasis in bone is particularly important during endodontic surgery [19].

Prevention and management of bleeding during surgery is a complex and multilayered process that includes preoperative, intraoperative, and postoperative considerations [7].

The surgeon's actions play a significant role in achieving surgical hemostasis [6, 7, 16]. Thus, proper preoperative evaluation, integration of relevant anatomical and systemic consideration into the treatment planning, and most importantly adequate surgical procedures are the key for achieving appropriate bleeding control during surgery [7].

Anatomical Considerations

It is common to speculate that different arteries supply certain specific regions of the periodontium and of the dentition. However, in fact, there are abundant anastomoses present between the different arteries. Thus, the entire system of blood vessels, rather than a specific group of vessels, should be regarded as the supplying source of the soft and hard tissue of the jaws [20–23].

The anatomy of the major blood vessels of the maxillofacial region is relevant to the risk of *severe* hemorrhage and massive hematomas [5, 7, 8, 10]. Thus, the treatment planning and all the surgical procedures, such as flap design and osteotomy, should respect the anatomical structure of the blood perfusion system of the periodontium, in order to minimize potential complications such as surgical bleeding.

Mandible

Anastomoses of the sublingual and submental arteries are responsible for the arterial blood supply of the floor of the mouth. The submental artery is a branch of the facial artery. The sublingual artery (2 mm in average diameter) arises from the lingual artery and is found coronal to the mylohyoid muscle [20]. A vascular wound after surgical procedure is usually attributed to perforations of the lingual cortical plate. Pressure by the expanding hematomas may displace the tongue and floor of the mouth both superiorly and posteriorly [21] and may lead to extensive bleeding into the submandibular space, resulting in a life-threatening acute airway obstruction [22]. Consequently, if the hemorrhage spreads in the soft tissues of the floor of the mouth, it may require emergency treatment to achieve airway by intubation or even tracheostomy [8, 10, 21, 22].

Accordingly, bleeding risks are one of the reasons why lingual approach for surgical endodontic procedures is not recommended and why care should be taken not to perforate cortical plate.

Maxilla

The location of the surgery may potentially affect the risk of bleeding and amount of blood loss during surgery, both by influencing the operating time and by virtue of anatomical variations in vascularity. Selim et al. [9] measured the amount of blood loss during endodontic surgery in different tooth locations and reported that palatal surgery of maxillary molars led to a rate of blood loss almost three times the average for all teeth, and the maxillary first premolar showed blood loss almost double the average for all teeth [9]. These anatomical effects on the risk of bleeding should be taken under consideration, and a palatal approach is not recommended for endodontic surgery.

Local Anesthesia

The goals of local anesthesia during surgical endodontic treatment is to achieve profound anesthesia and patient comfort, together with proper hemostasis by administrating a local anesthesia agent with vasoconstrictor [3, 6, 7, 15, 16].

The use of adrenergic vasoconstrictors may pose several risks of complications, such as systemic effects (that may be clinically significant especially for certain medically compromised patients), adverse effect on bleeding due to intramuscular injection [15], increased postoperative pain and delayed wound healing because of local ischemia with subsequent tissue acidosis and accumulation of inflammatory mediators [23], and risk of an ischemic necrosis of surgical flaps infiltrated with the adrenergic vasoconstrictor [23]. Further aspects are discussed in a separate chapter (see Chap. 5).

Several sympathomimetic-amine vasoconstrictor hemostatic agents were recommended for periradicular surgery, including epinephrine, norepinephrine, and phenylephrine [4, 6, 7, 24, 25].

Epinephrine is both an α- and a β-adrenergic receptor agonist. α receptors are present in the oral mucosa, submucosa, bone, and periodontium and when bounded produce vasoconstriction. β receptors are present in skeletal muscles and when bounded cause increased heart rate and cardiac output, and vasodilation [4, 6, 7, 24, 25].

Epinephrine is most commonly used in a concentration of 1:80,000 (12.5 mg/ml), and it was proposed to be used even in higher, 1:50,000 concentration in endodontic surgery for improved hemostasis [15]. However, for the majority of cases, 1:100,000 epinephrine concentration should be sufficient to achieve hemostasis, and the clinical difference between the two concentrations is undetectable [23].

Epinephrine possesses an effective hemostatic effect in endodontic surgery; however, when epinephrine is injected intraosseously, it may cause transient tachycardia and increased heart rate [24, 25]. Thus, it may cause adverse systemic effects, determined based on the selected application method [24, 25].

Occasionally, a secondary bleeding phase is observed after an infiltration of local anesthetic with vasoconstrictor. This phenomenon is explained with the *reactive hyperemia* process ("*the rebound phenomenon*") [26]. Reactive hyperemia is the transient increase in organ blood flow that occurs following a brief period of ischemia. This term is used to describe a delayed beta-adrenergic effect that follows the hemostasis produced by the injection of vasopressor amines, and this "rebound" occurs from a shift from an alpha (vasoconstriction) to a beta (vasodilation) vascular response [27].

Following the injection of a vasopressor amine, tissue concentration of the vasopressor gradually decreases to a level that no longer produces an alpha-adrenergic vasoconstriction, and the restricted blood flow slowly returns to normal, but then rapidly increases to a rate well beyond normal flow as a beta-adrenergic effect occurs [28]. This effect occurs due to local ischemia and tissue hypoxia resulting in a buildup of metabolic waste and acidosis caused by sustained vasoconstriction [27, 28].

The reactive hyperemia may last for hours and it is usually impossible to reestablish hemostasis by additional injections. Also, when operating on inflamed tissue, the alpha-adrenergic response is limited and the rebound phenomenon may occur more rapidly [28]. Thus, during endodontic surgery, especially if a long surgical procedure is anticipated, the more complicated or hemostasis-dependent procedures (such as root-end management) should be done first, and the less hemostasis-dependent procedures should be accomplished in a descending order of degree of difficulty, reserving the periradicular curettage and biopsy for last [27, 28].

Flap Design

The gingiva receives its blood supply through supra-periosteal blood vessels which depending on the specific region may be branches of the sublingual artery, mental artery, buccal artery, facial artery, greater palatine artery, infraorbital artery, and posterior superior dental artery. The supra-periosteal blood vessels anastomose with blood vessels from the alveolar bone. The free gingiva receives its blood supply from several sources: supra-periosteal blood vessels, the blood vessels of the periodontal ligament, and the blood vessels of the alveolar bone [23].

The supra-periosteal blood vessels of the attached gingival extend from the alveolar mucosa, parallel to the long axis of the teeth, and superficial to the periosteum [7]. The anatomical structure of the gingival apparatus and its blood supply may lead to excessive bleeding during surgery and additional surgical complications [7]. Vertical relaxing incision together with full thickness mucoperiosteal flap design maintains the intra-flap vasculature unharmed, thus, reducing the risk of bleeding [7, 15].

Further aspects are discussed in a separate chapter (see Chap. 6).

Osteotomy and Root-End Management

Bleeding control is essential for the precise and delicate micromanagement of the apical root part during endodontic surgery and is especially crucial during the osteotomy and root-end management phases of the surgical procedure [1, 2, 4, 7, 15].

The alveolar bone is prone to diffuse bleeding as a result of surgical drilling or curettage, and bleeding of cancellous bone is a common concern during the osteotomy phase in endodontic surgery [7, 29]. The blood perfusion of the alveolar bone is available by blood vessels in Haversian canals (canals containing a blood vessel surrounded by concentric, mineralized lamellae to form "osteon") and connecting vessels in Volkmann's canals (canals through which blood vessels, lymphatics, and nerve fibers pass from the alveolar bone to the periodontal ligament). The compact bone (alveolar bone proper), which lines the tooth socket, is perforated by numerous Volkmann's canals [23].

Controlling bleeding of bone using the traditional methods of soft-tissue hemostasis, such as manual compression or ligation, is not as effective because oozing blood often emanates continuously from a wide bone area [7, 29]. In endodontic surgery the osteotomy is usually performed in a pathological bony site with highly vascularized granulation tissue, thus, predisposes to even a greater risk of bleeding [1, 2, 4, 7, 15]. A controversy exists whether it is advisable to completely curate all granulomatous tissue as soon as possible before root-end preparation or to postpone the curettage to a later phase of the surgery, after the root end is properly managed [1, 2, 4, 7, 15]. These aspects will be discussed in a separate chapter. When appropriate hemostasis techniques are used, bleeding control can be achieved as well with the granulation tissue in situ [7, 15].

Technical and Therapeutic Means to Control Bleeding During Surgery

Adequate case selection, treatment planning, surgical technique, and postoperative management should minimize the risk of excessive bleeding [7, 15]. However, during surgery minor bleeding is still common and should be managed appropriately in order to prevent it from jeopardizing achieving the treatment goals and in order to prevent further escalation. Bleeding may be controlled by a variety of technical means such as digital compression, gauze tamponade, cauterization, suturing of the bleeding vessel (ligation), and adjunct topical hemostatic agents [4, 6, 7, 15, 16, 19, 30, 31].

Electrocauterization

Electrocauterization is the process of obliterate tissue using heat conduction from a probe heated by electric current, and historically cauterization was used to stop heavy bleeding. The procedure can be used to stop small vessels bleeding or for cutting soft tissue [30, 31]. Electrosurgery has been used in dentistry for more than half a century and is used both in a cutting mode (as replacement for traditional scalpel) and in a coagulating mode. The coagulation mode is typically used on surgically exposed surfaces and results in a coagulum that sloughs off within hours or days [30]. However, electric coagulation current should be used only when the other methods are ineffective and the need for hemostasis outweighs the considerably increased risk of necrosis and infection following electrosurgery [31].

Ligation

The principle of *ligation*, attributed to Hippocrates and Galen, found its modern use in the 1970s. Ligation of the blood vessel is the treatment of choice for excessive acute hemorrhage, while sometimes it may be difficult due to limited or impossible access [32].

Topical Hemostatic Agents

The properties of an ideal topical hemostatic agent are as follows: rapid and effective effect; effective contact with the bleeding surface; acceptable adverse-event profile; reliable; easy to handle; simple to prepare; multiple, versatile delivery options; active; and compatible with the patient's own physiology [3, 4, 6, 7, 15, 16, 19].

It should be noted that some hemostatic agents should be completely removed from the surgical site following their application, and some are self-degradable. However, most hemostatic agents, if not all of them, posses a dual tissue effect, a desired hemostatic effect and tissue reaction adverse effects [3, 4, 6, 7, 15, 16, 19], with potential foreign-body reaction development, chronic inflammation, infection, and granuloma formation [3, 4, 6, 7, 15, 16, 19].

Bone wax was introduced as a hemostatic agent more than a century ago by Sir Victor Horsley in 1892 [19]. Since then, bone wax has been used for many years and is considered easy to handle, though remnants of the material may cause adverse tissue reactions [4]. Bone wax is a nonabsorbable hemostatic agent, is composed of 88 % beeswax and 12 % isopropyl palmitate, and is known to cause retarded bone healing and predisposition to infection (chronic inflammation with foreign-body reaction). Thus, it is not recommended for use in endodontic surgery [4, 6, 7, 19].

Ferric sulfate is a necrotizing agent (pH = 0.8–1.6), causing protein coagulation, and requires complete removal following its use. If not removed it may cause impaired healing and acute inflammation and necrosis of surrounding tissues [4, 6, 7, 19].

Cotton Pellets

Sympathomimetic-amine vasoconstrictors, such as epinephrine, norepinephrine, and phenylephrine, have been utilized for hemorrhage control during surgery. A concern exists about their systemic adverse effects [24, 25]. However, topical application (on cotton pellets) produces adequate hemostasis with no evidence of cardiovascular changes. It is believed that the topically positioned pellets, saturated with epinephrine, cause an immediate local vasoconstriction, thus little absorption of epinephrine into the systemic circulation [4, 6, 7, 24, 25].

Cotton pellets containing particles of cellulose-containing materials that are left in the periapical area following surgery can cause persistent apical periodontitis ("cellulose granuloma") [33]. Ludlow et al. presented a case of a

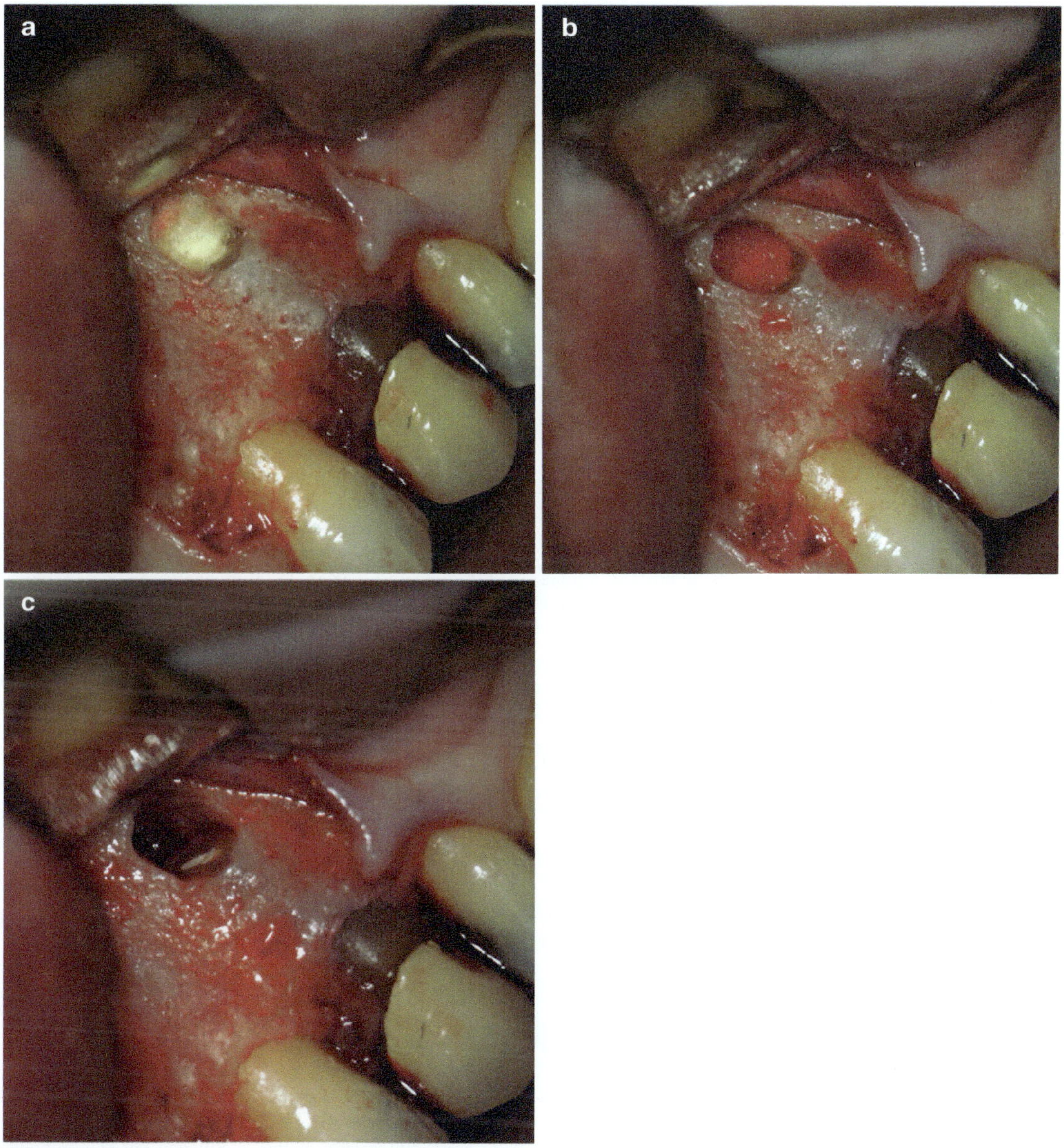

Fig. 11.3 (**a–c**) Cotton pellets used for hemostasis in endodontic surgery. (**a**) A cotton pellet placed during endodontic surgery; The cotton pellet (**b**) was removed (**c**), after hemostasis establishment

foreign-body reaction to cotton fibers left under the surgical flap following endodontic surgery [34]. Thus, cotton pellets should be removed during the surgery and not forgotten (Fig. 11.3a–c).

In conclusion, careful and adequate treatment planning and surgical technique, combined with knowledge of the surgical anatomy and recognition of possible hemorrhage related complications, are essential in order to prevent and control bleeding during endodontic surgery [8]. In addition, a thorough clinical evaluation and anamnesis should be preformed prior to the surgical procedure in order to reveal patients with potential systemic risks of excessive uncontrolled bleeding [5, 8].

References

1. Tsesis I, Rosen E, Taschieri S, Telishevsky Strauss Y, Ceresoli V, Del Fabbro M. Outcomes of surgical endodontic treatment performed by a modern technique: an updated meta-analysis of the literature. J Endod. 2013;39(3):332–9.
2. Tsesis I, Faivishevsky V, Kfir A, Rosen E. Outcome of surgical endodontic treatment performed by a modern technique: a meta-analysis of literature. J Endod. 2009;35(11):1505–11.
3. Israels S, Schwetz N, Boyar R, McNicol A. Bleeding disorders: characterization, dental considerations and management. J Can Dent Assoc. 2006;72(9):827.
4. Penarrocha-Diago M, Maestre-Ferrin L, Penarrocha-Oltra D, von Arx T. Influence of hemostatic agents upon the outcome of periapical surgery: dressings with anesthetic and vasoconstrictor or aluminum chloride. Med Oral Patol Oral Cir Bucal. 2013;18(2): e272–8.
5. Reich W, Kriwalsky MS, Wolf HH, Schubert J. Bleeding complications after oral surgery in outpatients with compromised haemostasis: incidence and management. Oral Maxillofac Surg. 2009;13(2):73–7.
6. Samudrala S. Topical hemostatic agents in surgery: a surgeon's perspective. AORN J. 2008;88(3):S2–11.
7. Witherspoon DE, Gutmann JL. Haemostasis in periradicular surgery. Int Endod J. 1996;29(3):135–49.
8. Moghadam HG, Caminiti MF. Life-threatening hemorrhage after extraction of third molars: case report and management protocol. J Can Dent Assoc. 2002;68(11):670–4.
9. Selim HA, el Deeb ME, Messer HH. Blood loss during endodontic surgery. Endod Dent Traumatol. 1987;3(1):33–6.
10. Goldstein BH. Acute dissecting hematoma: a complication of oral and maxillofacial surgery. J Oral Surg. 1981;39(1):40–3.
11. De Paepe A, Malfait F. Bleeding and bruising in patients with Ehlers-Danlos syndrome and other collagen vascular disorders. Br J Haematol. 2004;127(5):491–500.
12. Kim JC, Choi SS, Wang SJ, Kim SG. Minor complications after mandibular third molar surgery: type, incidence, and possible prevention. Oral Surg Oral Med Oral Pathol Oral Radiol Endod. 2006;102(2): e4–11.
13. Peters KA, Triolo PT, Darden DL. Disseminated intravascular coagulopathy: manifestations after a routine dental extraction. Oral Surg Oral Med Oral Pathol Oral Radiol Endod. 2005;99(4):419–23.
14. American association of Endodontics. Glossary of endodontic terms. Chicago: 2003.
15. Kim S, Kratchman S. Modern endodontic surgery concepts and practice: a review. J Endod. 2006;32(7): 601–23.
16. Sileshi B, Achneck HE, Lawson JH. Management of surgical hemostasis: topical agents. Vascular. 2008;16 Suppl 1:S22–8.
17. Douketis JD. Perioperative management of patients who are receiving warfarin therapy: an evidence-based and practical approach. Blood. 2011;117(19):5044–9.
18. Perry DJ, Nokes TJC, Heliwell PS. Guidelines for the management of patients on oral anticoagulants requiring dental surgery. British Society for Haematology. London; 2011.
19. Gupta G, Prestigiacomo CJ. From sealing wax to bone wax: predecessors to Horsley's development. Neurosurg Focus. 2007;23(1):E16.
20. Romanos GE, Gupta B, Crespi R. Endosseous arteries in the anterior mandible: literature review. Int J Oral Maxillofac Implants. 2012;27(1):90–4.
21. Kalpidis CD, Setayesh RM. Hemorrhaging associated with endosseous implant placement in the anterior mandible: a review of the literature. J Periodontol. 2004;75(5):631–45.
22. Goodacre CJ, Kan JY, Rungcharassaeng K. Clinical complications of osseointegrated implants. J Prosthet Dent. 1999;81(5):537–52.
23. Lindhe J, Lang NP, Karring T. Clinical periodontology and implant dentistry. 5th ed. Oxford: Blackwell Publishing Ltd; 2008.
24. Vickers FJ, Baumgartner JC, Marshall G. Hemostatic efficacy and cardiovascular effects of agents used during endodontic surgery. J Endod. 2002;28(4):322–3.
25. Vy CH, Baumgartner JC, Marshall JG. Cardiovascular effects and efficacy of a hemostatic agent in periradicular surgery. J Endod. 2004;30(6):379–83.
26. Lindorf HH. Investigation of the vascular effect of newer local anesthetics and vasoconstrictors. Oral Surg Oral Med Oral Pathol. 1979;48(4):292–7.
27. Morrow SG, Rubinstein RA. Endodontic surgery. In: Ingle JI, Bakland LK, editors. Endodontics. 5th ed. Hamilton: BC Decker Inc; 2002.
28. Gutmann JL, Harrison JW. Surgical endodontics. Boston: Blackwell Scientific Publications; 1991.
29. Sherman R, Chapman WC, Hannon G, Block JE. Control of bone bleeding at the sternum and iliac crest donor sites using a collagen-based composite

combined with autologous plasma: results of a randomized controlled trial. Orthopedics. 2001;24(2):137–41.

30. Livaditis GJ. Comparison of monopolar and bipolar electrosurgical modes for restorative dentistry: a review of the literature. J Prosthet Dent. 2001;86(4):390–9.
31. Soballe PW, Nimbkar NV, Hayward I, Nielsen TB, Drucker WR. Electric cautery lowers the contamination threshold for infection of laparotomies. Am J Surg. 1998;175(4):263–6.
32. Bouloux GF, Perciaccante VJ. Massive hemorrhage during oral and maxillofacial surgery: ligation of the external carotid artery or embolization? J Oral Maxillofac Surg. 2009;67(7):1547–51.
33. Nair PN. Pathogenesis of apical periodontitis and the causes of endodontic failures. Crit Rev Oral Biol Med. 2004;15(6):348–81.
34. Ludlow MO, Brenneise CV, Haft RT. Chronic pain associated with a foreign body left under the soft tissue flap during periapical surgery. J Endod. 1994;20(1):48–50.

Pain, Swelling, and Surgical Site Infection

12

Eyal Rosen and Igor Tsesis

Abstract

Pain and swelling are common side effects of endodontic surgery, and their intensity depends on the degree of the surgical damage to the tissue.

The pain and swelling are associated with inflammatory responses that are part of the typical wound healing process. Infection of the surgical site may complicate the postoperative sequel, aggravate the symptoms, and may require further pharmacologic and surgical interventions.

Several possible factors may affect the risk and intensity of postsurgical side effects, including patient-related factors and the surgical technique, and this chapter will review methods to prevent and manage postoperative side effects.

Introduction

Surgical procedures commonly produce side effects, and the intensity of those side effects depends on the degree of tissue damage [1–5]. Pain and swelling are common side effects following surgical endodontic treatment [6–9], and traditionally, approximately two-thirds of the patients require analgesics during the postoperative period [6–9].

Postoperative pain and swelling are related to the inflammatory response to the trauma induced during the surgery, and these reactions have several functions: defend the body organ, removal of necrotic or dying tissue, and repair and regeneration promotion [10]. *Inflammation* is defined as "the cellular and vascular response of tissues to injury" [11]. Histologically, following an injury damaged cells dispense their contents into extracellular spaces, and chemical mediators that regulate the inflammatory response are released. These mediators cause inflammatory changes such as vasodilatation and increased vascular permeability, which cause edema. All these inflammatory processes can proceed with or without concomitant surgical site infection [10, 12–14].

Surgical site infection (*infection*) can be defined as "invasion and proliferation of pathogenic microorganisms in body tissues following a surgical procedure and the reaction of the tissues to their presence." These tissue reactions include

E. Rosen, DMD (✉) • I. Tsesis, DMD
Department of Endodontology, Maurice and Gabriela Goldschleger School of Dental Medicine, Tel Aviv University, Tel Aviv, Israel
e-mail: dr.eyalrosen@gmail.com; dr.tsesis@gmail.com

I. Tsesis (ed.), *Complications in Endodontic Surgery*,
DOI 10.1007/978-3-642-54218-3_12, © Springer-Verlag Berlin Heidelberg 2014

also inflammatory reactions [11]. Thus, following surgery, inflammation may occur due to the surgical tissue injury alone (*noninfectious post-surgical inflammation* (*NIPSI*)) or as a result of the tissue injury combined with infection (*infectious post-surgical inflammation* (*IPSI*)).

The traditional signs of inflammation are the following: *dolor* (pain), *calor* (heat), *rubor* (redness), *tumor* (swelling), and *functio laesa* (loss of function) [12]. Infection also usually includes at least one of the following signs and symptoms: pain or tenderness, localized swelling, redness, or heat [13–15]. In addition, *NIPSI* may cause pathological conditions (such as edema development) that may provide favorable conditions for an ensuing contamination and infection of the surgical site with subsequent *IPSI*. Thus, the clinical diagnosis between *NIPSI* and *IPSI* may be difficult [8, 12–14].

The management of *NIPSI* is usually palliative (e.g., the use of anti-inflammatory medication protocol) and usually bares no or little long-term and systemic risks. On the other hand, *IPSI* may bare significant systemic risks and sometimes may require more aggressive treatment modalities (e.g., antibiotic therapy, with\without surgical drainage). Thus, the difficulty to differentially diagnose between *IPSI* and *NIPSI* presents a clinical dilemma to the practitioner [8, 10, 12–14].

This chapter would review pain swelling and infection as possible complications of endodontic surgery.

Pain and Swelling Definitions and Sequel

Pain is defined as "an unpleasant sensory and emotional experience associated with actual or potential damage or described in terms of such damage" [16]. Pain perception is a highly subjective experience modulated by multiple physical and psychological factors [17, 18]. In addition, pain measurement is burdened with hazards and opportunities for errors [18, 19], and different scales and methods have been used to assess pain after endodontic therapy [18, 19], including visual analog scale (VAS) that is considered a valid and reliable ratio scale to measure pain [18, 19].

Swelling may begin minutes to hours after the surgical procedure and is the consequence of two processes: hemorrhage and edema. These can continue for several days, depending upon the tissue injury severity. The *edema*, defined as "an accumulation of fluid in a tissue [11]," does not emerge equally in all directions from the site of injury [10]. In addition, after an injury, the bleeding usually stops within several minutes because of clotting. Therefore, the swelling is usually caused by edema [1, 3, 6–10].

The maximum severity of pain is usually reported during the first 24 postoperative hours, similar to results found in studies on the extraction of impacted third molars, and between 40 and 76 % of patients present either no or moderate pain [1]. The maximum swelling is presented between the first and second postoperative day, and between 45 and 66 % of patients present either no or moderate swelling [1].

Pain and Swelling Risk Factors

Several possible factors affecting the risk and\or intensity of postsurgical symptoms were reported, including the type of surgical technique (traditional versus modern surgical technique [1, 6, 9, 20]), poor oral hygiene [21], smoking [21], preoperative medication [8], local anesthesia type [22], type of root-end filling material [23], and the patient's age or gender [21].

The Surgical Technique

Endodontic surgery is usually performed in teeth with persistent periradicular pathosis [9]. The traditional technique of endodontic surgery ("traditional technique") consisted of root-end resection with a lingual to labial bevel for surgical access and visibility and root-end preparation using a round bur [24]. In recent years, a technique ("modern technique") that includes the use of magnification and illumination devices was introduced. The modern technique raised the success rate to above 90 % (compared to about 60 % success with the traditional technique) [19, 20, 25, 26] while allowing a more conservative and precise procedure with significantly less tissue damage [19, 20, 25, 26]. Since the modern technique results in less tissue damage during the surgery [9, 20, 26–28], a lower incidence and milder severity of postoperative pain and swelling following modern technique surgery versus the traditional technique is expected [8, 9, 29]. However, even with the modern technique, pain and swelling may occur [6–9].

Kvist and Reit [6] reported that on the evening after traditional endodontic surgery, almost all patients experienced pain, with 67 % requiring analgesics. Swelling was reported in all patients and reached the maximum on postoperative day 1 [6, 9]. Tsesis et al. [9] compared postoperative quality of life of patient receiving modern versus traditional surgical endodontic treatment and reported a high incidence of symptoms in both groups. It was also reported that patients treated by the modern technique had significantly less postoperative pain but reported more difficulty in mouth opening, mastication, and ability to speak during the immediate postoperative period [9].

Personal Habits

The patient's personal habits, such as the level of oral hygiene, and smoking habits may affect the risk and intensity of postoperative pain. Patients with poor oral hygiene may have higher maximum pain [1]. The same was reported for surgery of impacted third molars [1], and patients who smoke are those who perceived greater pain [1].

García et al. [21] reported that modern endodontic surgery caused little pain and moderate swelling during the first 2 days after the intervention, and these findings were more distinct in patients with poor oral hygiene and in smokers [21], and they recommended that by maintaining good oral hygiene and by avoiding smoking both before and after the surgery, it is possible to minimize the postoperative symptoms [21].

Local Anesthetic, Root-End Filling, and Patient's Age and Gender

The effect of the local anesthesia type, the root-end filling material, and the patients' age or gender on the risk for postoperative symptoms seems to be insignificant. Meechan and Blair [22] compared postoperative pain experience after endodontic surgery using local anesthesia with lignocaine or etidocaine (long-acting local anesthetic) and found no differences in pain experience between the groups despite the much longer anesthesia for long-acting etidocaine [22]. Chong and Pitt Ford [23] evaluated pain experience following root-end resection and filling with MTA or IRM and found that there was no significant difference in the pain experienced by both treatment groups. The age and gender of the patient had no statistically significant effect on any of the postoperative symptoms in endodontic surgery [1, 21]; however, some studies indicate that pain is more acute in females or in males following the extraction of impacted third molars [1].

In conclusion, it seems that the surgical technique characteristics directly affecting the amount of tissue injury during surgery are the most significant confounders for the risk of postoperative symptom development.

Prevention of Postoperative Pain and Swelling

Transmission of pain signals evoked by tissue damage leads to sensitization of the peripheral and central pain pathways [30]. Inadequate pain control during the early postoperative period may contribute to the development of hyperalgesia and likelihood of stronger pain levels later. Thus, because it is easier to prevent than to eliminate pain, the concept of "pre-emptive analgesia" is to treat postoperative pain by preventing the establishment of central sensitization [30, 31].

Pre-emptive analgesia may be defined as "a treatment that is initiated before the surgical procedure in order to reduce central sensitization and ensuing excessive pain" [30]. Thus, due to a "defensive" effect on the nociceptive system, pre-emptive analgesia has the potential to be more effective than a similar analgesic treatment initiated after surgery [30].

Pre-emptive analgesia includes the administration of a drug that blocks painful (nociceptive) input from entering the central nervous system before a surgical procedure in order to attenuate the development of changes that manifest as increased pain at later time points [30]. Clinically, this strategy not only forecasts less pain during the initial postoperative period but also lowers the intensity of pain during the days after the procedure [32].

Studies have been published in which corticosteroids or "nonsteroidal anti-inflammatory drugs" (NSAIDs) have been used before and after surgery to control pain and swelling during the postoperative period [8, 33]. Tsesis et al. [8] in a case series of 82 patients treated using a modern surgical technique, premedicated all patients with a single dose of oral dexamethasone (8 mg) preoperatively and two single doses (4 mg) 1 and 2 days postoperatively. One day postoperatively, 76.4 % of the patients were completely pain free, less than 4 % had moderate pain, and 64.7 % did not report any swelling [8]. In addition, patients with preoperative pain were more likely to have postoperative pain [8].

Lin et al. [33], in a double-blind study of 90 modern endodontic surgery patients, that were randomly premedicated with placebo or with either protocols: a single dose of oral dexamethasone, 8 mg, preoperatively and 2 single doses, of 4 mg, 1 and 2 days postoperatively; or a single dose of etodolac, 600 mg, and 2 single doses, of 600 mg, 1 and 2 days postoperatively. They reported that 1 day postoperatively, 41.8 % of the patients reported no or very mild pain, whereas after 7 days, 87.9 % reported no or very mild pain and that both etodolac and dexamethasone had a significant effect on reducing postoperative pain compared with placebo [33].

Surgical wounds may heal by primary intention (when the wound edges are brought together and detained in place, with minimal scar formation) or by secondary intention (in the presence of infection, when there is no proper approximation of the flap, and flap tension). Thus, the surgical procedure itself may affect the risk of postoperative pain, and a correct surgical technique may prevent postoperative excessive symptoms [34, 35]. It was reported that the type of incision for flap elevation may influence the risk for postoperative pain: 40 patients were randomly assigned to two groups. In one group a sulcular incision (SI) with complete papilla mobilization was made, and in the other group a papilla-base incision (PBI) was used. The papilla-base incision technique was better in reduction of pain levels [34].

In order to minimize postoperative pain and discomfort, the surgical procedure should be as atraumatic as possible [35], and when performing flap elevation, precautions must be taken to avoid perforation or tearing of the flap, and a tension-free primary flap closure is essential; in addition, during osteotomy the bone should be kept moist [35].

Management of Postoperative Pain and Swelling

The pain experienced by patients is mostly limited to the first few days after surgery, and pain and swelling are usually the chief postoperative sequelae [6, 8, 9, 35]. The patient's attitude to development of postoperative symptoms is subjective, and patients may be forced to seek treatment only when the actual pain they are experiencing is greater than their anxiety about the expected pain [31]. Thus, it is important to inform the patients of possible postoperative symptoms [35].

Different therapeutic approaches, both noninvasive and invasive surgical techniques, aimed toward reduction of postoperative inflammatory response following oral surgery have been reported in the literature, such as the use of drugs, cryotherapy (application of ice), low-power laser [36], and incorporation of drains [36, 37].

Analgesics

Postoperative dental pain is usually moderate and of short duration, and analgesics are often required only for the first 1–2 days. The drugs commonly used to minimize the postoperative pain and swelling are analgesics and corticosteroids. The commonly used analgesics following oral surgical procedures are the NSAIDs, due to their anti-inflammatory properties and are therefore able to reduce the inflammatory-related pain and swelling [1, 30–32, 36].

Corticosteroids have been reported to control pain and swelling following endodontic surgery, and the two most widely used are dexamethasone and methylprednisolone [1, 30, 32, 33, 36]. Steroids act on the inflammatory response by inhibiting phospholipase A2 activity. Subsequently, the cyclooxygenase pathways are inhibited, reducing prostaglandin synthesis. This affects the early stages of inflammation by inhibiting vasodilatation, capillary permeability, and leukocyte migration [8]. Therefore, corticosteroids should be administered preoperatively, to allow absorption and distribution of the medication before initial tissue trauma and the subsequent inflammatory response [8, 30]. However, it should be noted that long-term high-dose use of corticosteroids may pose potential side effects, such as adrenal suppression, delayed wound healing, and risk of postoperative infections [36].

Cryotherapy

Cryotherapy ("cold therapy") is the application of cold for therapeutic purposes, and local application of ice has been reported to control postsurgical inflammation, pain, and swelling [35, 36]. Cryotherapy is probably the simplest and oldest therapeutic modality in the treatment of acute tissue injuries. It is proposed that by decreasing tissue temperature, ice can decrease inflammation, inhibit swelling (edema), reduce blood supply (vasoconstriction), decrease hemorrhage, inhibit temperature elevation, reduce metabolic alterations (cold decreases the metabolic rate, thereby lessening secondary injuries due to lack of oxygen), and reduce pain, thereby aiding recovery after tissue trauma [10, 38]. While application of cold can reduce the affected tissue temperature, the effect depends on the method and duration of application, the initial temperature of the ice, and the depth of subcutaneous fat [39]. It was found that after ice application to the cheek, the mucosal temperature was related inversely to cheek thickness. In addition, when an ice bag was wrapped in a towel and applied to the cheek for 30 min, the alveolar mucosa's temperature only decreased an average of 1 °C [40], and even when the ice was directly applied to the cheek, it hardly changed the temperature of the intraoral alveolar mucosa [41]. On the other hand, the placebo effect provided by cold therapy may alter the patient's pain perception, thus providing both psychological and physiological benefits [42].

The current recommendations on the clinical use of topical ice application are variable and range from 10- to 60-min application two to four times per day to application every 10 min [38]. In addition, ice is commonly combined with physical compression, making it difficult to determine the value of the cryotherapy alone [43]. Cryotherapy may also cause side effects such as skin burns and should be used cautiously [38]. In conclusion, using repeated, rather than continuous ice application, ice applications helps sustain reduced temperature without compromising the skin and allows the superficial skin temperature to return to normal while deeper temperature remains low. The ice should be applied in repeated application of 10 min to be most effective, to avoid side effects, and to prevent possible further injury [39].

Low-Power Laser

The use of laser in oral surgery is a new painless, noninvasive technique and was suggested as an adjunct to reduce postsurgical discomfort [36]. It is proclaimed that the laser irradiation induces an increase in the number and width of lymph vessels, decreases blood vessel permeability, increases protein absorption by macrophages, modifies hydrostatic and capillary pressure, and induces the absorption of interstitial fluids [36].

Wound Closure and Drains

The closure technique is an operative factor that has been linked to the intensity of postoperative pain and swelling [36, 37]. Primary closure is the full repositioning of the surgical flap post surgery using sutures such that healing is by primary intention, while in secondary closure the bone remains in communication with the oral cavity and healing is by secondary intention [36, 37]. In third molar surgery, some authors favor secondary closure technique because it is believed to result in less postoperative pain and swelling [36, 37]. In endodontic surgery, the primary goal is to achieve primary flap closure so that healing would be by primary intention. However, in case of severe postoperative pain and swelling, achieving secondary closure may be considered by several alternative techniques such as incorporation of drains [36, 37].

Surgical Site Infection

The introduction of infection to the surgical site may complicate the postoperative sequel [13–15]. Surgical wound classification, introduced by the "National Academy of Sciences" in 1964, has been the foundation for infection risk assessment, operative protocol development, and surgical decision-making [13–15]. A new definition of "surgical site infection" (SSI) was proposed to prevent confusion between the infection of a surgical incision and the infection of a traumatic wound [14].

Surgical site infection was defined by the "Centers for Disease Control and Prevention (CDC)" as:

1. Purulent drainage with or without laboratory confirmation, from the superficial incision.
2. Organisms isolated from an aseptically obtained culture of fluid or tissue from the superficial incision.
3. At least one of the following signs or symptoms of infection – pain or tenderness, localized swelling, redness, or heat – and a superficial incision is deliberately opened by a surgeon, unless incision is culture negative.
4. Diagnosis of superficial incisional SSI made by a surgeon or attending physician [13–15].

Since the oral mucosa is normally colonized by a range of microorganisms that could cause infection, defining an SSI following endodontic surgery requires evidence of clinical signs and symptoms of infection rather than microbiological evidence alone [13]. The majority of SSIs become apparent most often between the 5th and 10th postoperative days and usually up to 30 days of an operative procedure [13].

Surgical Site Infection Risk Factors

Different surgical sites may contribute to the risk of developing infection, and the surgical procedures may be classified into four categories based on the initial surgical site bacterial load [14]: *clean* (when the operative procedure does not enter into a normally colonized viscus or lumen of the body), *clean/contaminated* (when the operative procedure enters into a colonized viscus or cavity of the body, but under elective and controlled circumstances), *contaminated* (when gross contamination is present at the surgical site in the absence of obvious infection), and *dirty/infected* (when active infection is already present) [44].

During endodontic surgery, contamination of the surgical site may occur by a contact with contaminated objects; contact with infected nasal, sinus, or oral mucosa; and also through the dissemination of the infected root dentin. Thus, apical surgery usually starts with "clean/contaminated" status, and when the root apex is reached and surgically manipulated, the bacteria from the infected root canal contaminate the surgical site, and the wound area becomes "contaminated" [14, 45].

The risk of infection is also influenced by various factors such as the type, the location, and the duration of the surgical procedure; the surgeon's skills; the methods of intraoperative management; and by patient-related factors, including the general medical status of the patient [45, 46].

It has been reported that a long-duration surgical procedure may adversely affect the risk for infection. Surgical operations lasting less than 1 h have been shown to be significantly less associated with infection than those lasting more than 3 h with the rate of infection doubling with every hour of the procedure [47].

In any surgical procedure, the skill and experience of the operator are important. It has been demonstrated in implant dentistry to influence the postoperative infection and implant failures [46]. The experience of the operator has been attributed to endodontic surgery and possibly plays a major role both in the long-term outcome and immediate postoperative complications [9].

Prevention and Management of Surgical Site Infection

Prophylactic Antibiotic Use

The main goal of prophylactic antibiotic use is to prevent infection from the surgical wound site, thus decreasing the chance of postoperative complications. The rationale for the use of antibiotics is based on the concept that the primary cause of the periradicular lesion is bacterial infection and that surgical intervention may result in a superimposed bacterial infection in the surgical site [48]. On the other hand, the unwarranted use of antibiotics may contribute to the development of resistant bacteria, adverse reactions, and allergies [48].

While there is a well-established protocol for SBE antibiotic prophylaxis for immunocompromised patients, no consensus exists regarding the use of antibiotics in endodontic surgery, and many practitioners prescribe antibiotics routinely for endodontic surgeries [48, 49].

In a randomized controlled study, Lindeboom et al. found no significant difference between clindamycin prophylaxis and placebo with regard to the prevention of postoperative infection in endodontic surgical procedures [48]. In that study, they found a low infection rate of (2.3 %) indicating that antibiotic prophylaxis did not contribute to the prevention of postoperative infection [48].

Thus, the use of prophylactic antibiotics is not supported by any scientific studies [48], and the prevention of the surgical site infection is best managed by maintenance of good oral hygiene measures and the use of chlorhexidine mouthwashes immediately preoperatively and postoperatively [48, 49].

Postoperative Antibiotics Administration

Antimicrobials should be prescribed where signs of systemic involvement are present such as regional lymphadenopathy, and in combination with surgical drainage if appropriate. A surgical reentry might be indicated to debride the apical tissues [48, 49].

The proper dose and duration of an antibiotic should allow the patient's host defenses to gain control of the infection, and when the infection is resolving, the drug should be terminated [49].

References

1. Garcia B, Larrazabal C, Penarrocha M. Pain and swelling in periapical surgery. A literature update. Med Oral Patol Oral Cir Bucal. 2008;13(11):E726–9.
2. Garcia Garcia A, Gude Sampedro F, Gallas Torrella M, Gandara Vila P, Madrinan-Grana P, Gandara-Rey JM. Trismus and pain after removal of a lower third molar. Effects of raising a mucoperiosteal flap. Med Oral. 2001;6(5):391–6.
3. Gonzalez-Santana H, Penarrocha-Diago M, Guarinos-Carbo J, Balaguer-Martinez J. Pain and inflammation in 41 patients following the placement of 131 dental implants. Med Oral Patol Oral Cir Bucal. 2005;10(3):258–63.
4. Olmedo-Gaya MV, Vallecillo-Capilla M, Galvez-Mateos R. Relation of patient and surgical variables to postoperative pain and inflammation in the extraction of third molars. Med Oral. 2002;7(5):360–9.
5. Penarrocha M, Sanchis JM, Saez U, Gay C, Bagan JV. Oral hygiene and postoperative pain after mandibular third molar surgery. Oral Surg Oral Med Oral Pathol Oral Radiol Endod. 2001;92(3):260–4.
6. Kvist T, Reit C. Postoperative discomfort associated with surgical and nonsurgical endodontic retreatment. Endod Dent Traumatol. 2000;16(2):71–4.
7. Seymour RA, Meechan JG, Blair GS. Postoperative pain after apicoectomy. A clinical investigation. Int Endod J. 1986;19(5):242–7.
8. Tsesis I, Fuss Z, Lin S, Tilinger G, Peled M. Analysis of postoperative symptoms following surgical endodontic treatment. Quintessence Int. 2003;34(10):756–60.
9. Tsesis I, Shoshani Y, Givol N, Yahalom R, Fuss Z, Taicher S. Comparison of quality of life after surgical endodontic treatment using two techniques: a prospective study. Oral Surg Oral Med Oral Pathol Oral Radiol Endod. 2005;99(3):367–71.
10. Greenstein G. Therapeutic efficacy of cold therapy after intraoral surgical procedures: a literature review. J Periodontol. 2007;78(5):790–800.
11. American Association of Endodontics. Glossary of endodontic terms. 8th ed. 2012.
12. Rather LJ. Disturbance of function (functio laesa): the legendary fifth cardinal sign of inflammation, added by Galen to the four cardinal signs of Celsus. Bull N Y Acad Med. 1971;47(3):303–22.
13. NICE Clinical Guidelines. Surgical site infection: prevention and treatment of surgical site infection. National Collaborating Centre for Women's and Children's Health (UK). London: RCOG Press; 2008.
14. Horan TC, Gaynes RP, Martone WJ, Jarvis WR, Emori TG. CDC definitions of nosocomial surgical site infections, 1992: a modification of CDC definitions of surgical wound infections. Infect Control Hosp Epidemiol. 1992;13(10):606–8.
15. Royal Australasian College of Surgeons; Surgical Site Infection (CDC Definition); ANZ Journal of Surgery.

Wiley-Blackwell, 2013. Available at http://www.anzjsurg.com/view/0/surgicalSiteInfectionCDCDef.html. Accessed in Oct 2013.
16. Merskey H, Bogduk N, International Association for the Study of Pain, IASP Task Force on Taxonomy. Classification of chronic pain. 2nd ed. Seattle: IASP Pres; 1994.
17. Bender IB. Pulpal pain diagnosis–a review. J Endod. 2000;26(3):175–9.
18. Tsesis I, Faivishevsky V, Fuss Z, Zukerman O. Flare-ups after endodontic treatment: a meta-analysis of literature. J Endod. 2008;34(10):1177–81.
19. Al-Negrish AR, Habahbeh R. Flare up rate related to root canal treatment of asymptomatic pulpally necrotic central incisor teeth in patients attending a military hospital. J Dent. 2006;34(9):635–40.
20. Tsesis I, Rosen E, Schwartz-Arad D, Fuss Z. Retrospective evaluation of surgical endodontic treatment: traditional versus modern technique. J Endod. 2006;32(5):412–6.
21. Garcia B, Penarrocha M, Marti E, Gay-Escodad C, von Arx T. Pain and swelling after periapical surgery related to oral hygiene and smoking. Oral Surg Oral Med Oral Pathol Oral Radiol Endod. 2007;104(2):271–6.
22. Meechan JG, Blair GS. The effect of two different local anaesthetic solutions on pain experience following apicectomy. Br Dent J. 1993;175(11–12):410–3.
23. Chong BS, Pitt Ford TR. Postoperative pain after root-end resection and filling. Oral Surg Oral Med Oral Pathol Oral Radiol Endod. 2005;100(6):762–6.
24. Gutmann JL, Harrison JW. Surgical endodontics. Boston: Blackwell Scientific Publications; 1991.
25. Tsesis I, Faivishevsky V, Kfir A, Rosen E. Outcome of surgical endodontic treatment performed by a modern technique: a meta-analysis of literature. J Endod. 2009;35(11):1505–11.
26. Tsesis I, Rosen E, Taschieri S, Telishevsky Strauss Y, Ceresoli V, Del Fabbro M. Outcomes of surgical endodontic treatment performed by a modern technique: an updated meta-analysis of the literature. J Endod. 2013;39(3):332–9.
27. Kim S, Kratchman S. Modern endodontic surgery concepts and practice: a review. J Endod. 2006; 32(7):601–23.
28. Setzer FC, Shah SB, Kohli MR, Karabucak B, Kim S. Outcome of endodontic surgery: a meta-analysis of the literature–part 1: comparison of traditional root-end surgery and endodontic microsurgery. J Endod. 2010;36(11):1757–65.
29. Pecora G, Andreana S. Use of dental operating microscope in endodontic surgery. Oral Surg Oral Med Oral Pathol. 1993;75(6):751–8.
30. Dahl JB, Moiniche S. Pre-emptive analgesia. Br Med Bull. 2004;71:13–27.
31. Khan AA, Dionne RA. COX-2 inhibitors for endodontic pain. Endod Top. 2002;3:31–40.
32. Dionne R. Preemptive vs preventive analgesia: which approach improves clinical outcomes? Compend Contin Educ Dent. 2000;21(1):48, 51–4, 6.
33. Lin S, Levin L, Emodi O, Abu El-Naaj I, Peled M. Etodolac versus dexamethasone effect in reduction of postoperative symptoms following surgical endodontic treatment: a double-blind study. Oral Surg Oral Med Oral Pathol Oral Radiol Endod. 2006;101(6):814–7.
34. Del Fabbro M, Taschieri S, Weinstein R. Quality of life after microscopic periradicular surgery using two different incision techniques: a randomized clinical study. Int Endod J. 2009;42(4):360–7.
35. Lindhe J, Lang NP, Karring T. Clinical periodontology and implant dentistry. 5th ed. Oxford: Blackwell Publishing Ltd; 2008.
36. Osunde OD, Adebola RA, Omeje UK. Management of inflammatory complications in third molar surgery: a review of the literature. Afr Health Sci. 2011;11(3): 530–7.
37. Danda AK, Krishna Tatiparthi M, Narayanan V, Siddareddi A. Influence of primary and secondary closure of surgical wound after impacted mandibular third molar removal on postoperative pain and swelling–a comparative and split mouth study. J Oral Maxillofac Surg. 2010;68(2):309–12.
38. Bleakley C, McDonough S, MacAuley D. The use of ice in the treatment of acute soft-tissue injury: a systematic review of randomized controlled trials. Am J Sports Med. 2004;32(1):251–61.
39. Mac Auley DC. Ice therapy: how good is the evidence? Int J Sports Med. 2001;22(5):379–84.
40. Possoff A. External thermal applications in postextraction therapy. J Am Dent Assoc. 1955;50(2):147–56.
41. van der Westhuijzen AJ, Becker PJ, Morkel J, Roelse JA. A randomized observer blind comparison of bilateral facial ice pack therapy with no ice therapy following third molar surgery. Int J Oral Maxillofac Surg. 2005;34(3):281–6.
42. Staats PS, Staats A, Hekmat H. The additive impact of anxiety and a placebo on pain. Pain Med. 2001;2(4): 267–79.
43. Thorsson O. Cold therapy of athletic injuries. Current literature review. Lakartidningen. 2001;98(13):1512–3.
44. Walter CJ, Dumville JC, Sharp CA, Page T. Systematic review and meta-analysis of wound dressings in the prevention of surgical-site infections in surgical wounds healing by primary intention. Br J Surg. 2012;99(9):1185–94.
45. Haley RW, Culver DH, Morgan WM, White JW, Emori TG, Hooton TM. Identifying patients at high risk of surgical wound infection. A simple multivariate index of patient susceptibility and wound contamination. Am J Epidemiol. 1985;121(2):206–15.
46. Resnik RR, Misch C. Prophylactic antibiotic regimens in oral implantology: rationale and protocol. Implant Dent. 2008;17(2):142–50.
47. Cruse PJ, Foord R. The epidemiology of wound infection. A 10-year prospective study of 62,939 wounds. Surg Clin North Am. 1980;60(1):27–40.
48. Lindeboom JA, Frenken JW, Valkenburg P, van den Akker HP. The role of preoperative prophylactic antibiotic administration in periapical endodontic surgery: a randomized, prospective double-blind placebo-controlled study. Int Endod J. 2005;38(12):877–81.
49. Yingling NM, Byrne BE, Hartwell GR. Antibiotic use by members of the American Association of Endodontists in the year 2000: report of a national survey. J Endod. 2002;28(5):396–404.

Nerve Injury During Endodontic Surgical Procedures

13

Eyal Rosen

Abstract

Nerve injuries with altered sensations following endodontic surgical procedures represent a rare but serious complication, and the classification of those injuries is based on their time course and on the potential sensory recovery following the injury.

Direct trauma to the nerve bundle during surgery is the most frequent cause of nerve injury and may lead to long-term disability and to significant negative effects on the patient's quality of life.

Active preventive measures and a timely mannered clinical approach when a nerve injury is suspected are the most efficient measures to minimize the risk for nerve injuries during surgical procedures as well as to prevent permanent damage and enable better clinical and medicolegal outcomes when such injuries do occur.

This chapter is aimed to provide the practitioner with both knowledge and practical tools to prevent and to manage a nerve injury when performing endodontic surgical procedures, thus to enable a safer procedure and a more predictable clinical outcome.

Introduction

Altered sensation due to a nerve injury represents a rare but serious complication of endodontic treatment [1, 2]. Endodontic surgical procedures that are performed in the vicinity of major nerves may also cause an adverse nerve injury [3]. Trauma, tumors, connective tissue diseases, infectious diseases, demineralization, or idiopathic diseases have also been reported as possible causes of altered sensation of maxillofacial nerves [4] and should be considered as a differential diagnosis for altered sensation during or following endodontic treatments [4–7].

Most cases of inferior alveolar nerve (IAN) injuries have been reported in second mandibular molars but also in 1st molars and in premolars [6]. Garisto et al. [8] evaluated the occurrence of altered sensation following dental local anesthetic administration in the United States. They reported 248 cases of altered sensation, of which 13 cases (5 %) included an endodontic treatment.

E. Rosen, DMD
Department of Endodontology, Maurice and Gabriela Goldschleger School of Dental Medicine, Tel Aviv University, Tel Aviv, Israel
e-mail: dr.eyalrosen@gmail.com

I. Tsesis (ed.), *Complications in Endodontic Surgery*,
DOI 10.1007/978-3-642-54218-3_13, © Springer-Verlag Berlin Heidelberg 2014

The risk of nerve injury during surgical endodontic procedures is a matter of great concern, and several diagnostic [9–13] and surgical [14, 15] methods have been developed in order to prevent nerve injury during endodontic surgical procedures [14]. However, the available literature assessing the prevalence and the clinical manifestation of endodontic surgery-related nerve injuries is scarce; thus, our understanding of its clinical and medicolegal aspects is insufficient [5, 6, 14].

This chapter will review the classification, etiology, preventive measures, diagnosis, and management of endodontic surgery-related nerve injuries and is aimed to provide the practitioner with both knowledge and practical tools to prevent and to manage a nerve injury when performing endodontic surgical procedures, thus to enable a safer procedure and a more predictable clinical outcome.

Classification

Back in 1942, Seddon [16, 17] presented a classification of mechanical nerve injuries ("Seddon's classification": neuropraxia, axonotmesis, and neurotmesis) [16, 17] that remained relevant till today and may also be used to describe trigeminal nerve injuries during endodontic surgery based on the time course and the potential sensory recovery [16, 17]:

Neuropraxia (meaning "nonaction") is used to describe cases in which there is a short-lived altered sensation, so short that recovery could not possibly be explained in terms of true regeneration. Neuropraxia may result from nerve trunk traction, manipulation, or compression, without degeneration of the axon, and is characterized by a conduction block, followed by a complete and fast return of sensation or function. The trauma may injure the endoneurial capillaries, resulting in intrafascicular edema and ensuing a conduction block. Normal sensation or function usually returns following the resolution of the intrafascicular edema, generally within a few days following the nerve injury. If the pressure resulted in segmental demyelination or mechanical disruption of the myelin sheaths, sensory and functional recoveries are complete within 1–2 months. The common clinical manifestation of this type of injury is paresthesia [16, 17].

Axonotmesis is described as a damage to the nerve fibers which is severe enough to cause complete peripheral degeneration; however, the sheath and the more intimate supporting structures of the nerve have not been completely divided, which means that the nerve tissues are still in continuity. Axonotmesis may be followed by subsequent regeneration or degeneration of the nerve. Nerve compression and traction may cause intrafascicular edema, severe ischemia, or demyelination. Although there is damage to the axons, there is no disruption of the endoneurial sheath, perineurium, or epineurium. Complete recovery may occur in 2–4 months, but sometimes the improvement process leading to complete recovery may last up to 12 months. The clinical manifestation of axonotmesis is an initial anesthesia followed by paresthesia as recovery begins [16, 17].

Neurotmesis (meaning "cutting") is described as a nerve that has been completely cut. Neurotmesis may result from severe trauma, such as nerve traction, compression, injection injury, or chemical injury, and is characterized by severe disruption of all components of the nerve trunk. The clinical manifestation of these injuries is an immediate anesthesia. It will then be followed by paresthesia or possibly other neurosensory responses such as allodynia, hyperalgesia, or chronic pain. This type of nerve injury has a poor prognosis for recovery – sensory and functional recovery is never complete and there is a high probability of developing a central neuroma [16, 17].

The clinical manifestations of endodontic surgery-related nerve injuries are complex and include a combination of both objective neurological signs and subjective complaints of the patients. However, for simplicity, most cases of altered sensation following endodontic surgery may be classified as follows: *anesthesia*, insensitivity to all forms of stimulation; *paresthesia*, a sensation,

Table 13.1 Nerve injury classification

Classification	Mechanism of injury	Clinical manifestation	Prognosis
Neurapraxia (Transient block)	Mild injury to the nerve; no loss of continuity of the nerve	Paresthesia[a]	Good prognosis; recovery usually within days or up to 1–2 months
Axonotmesis (Lesion in continuity)	Moderate injury to the nerve; nerve is damaged but not completely severed	Initial anesthesia[b] followed by paresthesia[a] as recovery begins	Moderate prognosis; recovery may occur in 2–4 months, but improvement leading to recovery may last up as 12 months
Neurotmesis (Nerve cut)	Severe injury to the nerve; severed nerve	Initial anesthesia[b], which may be followed by paresthesia[a], or other neurosensory responses such as allodynia[c], hyperalgesia[d], or chronic pain	Poor prognosis; sensory recovery is never complete

Classification of nerve injuries based on Seddon [17] and Juodzbalys et al. [16]
[a]Paresthesia: a sensation, such as burning, prickling, or partial numbness
[b]Anesthesia: insensitivity to all forms of stimulation
[c]Allodynia: pain due to a stimulus that does not normally provoke pain
[d]Hyperalgesia: increased response to a stimulus that is normally painful

such as burning, prickling, or partial numbness; or *hyperesthesia*, increased sensitivity to all forms of stimulation, all affecting the teeth, lips, tongue, or the surrounding skin and mucosa [18]. Additional possible neurosensory impairment deficits may be classified by the response to stimuli as follows: *allodynia*, pain due to a stimulus that does not normally provoke pain; *hypoalgesia*, decreased response to a stimulus that is normally painful; and *hyperalgesia*, increased response to a stimulus that is normally painful [16].

It is important to recognize that the pathological process following the initial nerve injury is a dynamic process. Consequently, the altered sensation clinical presentation may often change a long time after the initial injury [1, 4–6, 8, 17].

Table 13.1 presents a classification of nerve injuries following endodontic surgery.

Etiology

The most routine surgical endodontic procedures, such as anesthetic procedures [8], flap procedures, osteotomy, and apicectomy, may lead to nerve injury during surgical endodontic treatments [14, 15].

The possible causes of nerve injury include both preoperative factors, such as poor flap design, and intraoperative factors, such as traumatic flap reflection, accidental intraneural injection, traction of the mental nerve during flap elevation, penetration of the osteotomy preparation into the nerve canal, and more [19]. In addition, nerve injuries may be caused indirectly by postsurgical complications such as the development of intra-alveolar hematoma or edema inside the mandibular canal applying temporary pressure increase on the nerve bundle or neuritis with prolonged pressure increase that may lead to permanent degeneration of the affected nerve [20].

Nevertheless, direct trauma to the nerve bundle during surgery is the most frequent cause of nerve injury and may occur through several mechanisms such as nerve compression, stretching, cutting, overheating, and accidental puncture [2, 4, 5, 16, 21].

Prevention

Prevention is the most efficient clinical approach to minimize the risk of nerve injuries during endodontic surgical procedures and ensuing medical and medicolegal consequences. For medicolegal reasons, it is important to include nerve injury as an item in the informed consent document [5, 22–25]. The medicolegal aspects of altered sensation following endodontic surgical procedures are presented in a separate chapter of this book.

Nerve injury preventive measures should be implemented preoperatively, intraoperatively, and postoperatively, as described below.

Preoperative Preventive Measures

"Primum non nocere" (a Latin phrase that means "first, do no harm") is a fundamental principle that should be implemented in the planning of any treatment procedure. Thus, the practitioner should take into account all possible complications and preventive measures prior to treatment, i.e., during the evaluation and treatment planning phase. In order to apply this principle in endodontic surgery, the practitioner is obligated to perform a thorough clinical and radiographic evaluation, to be aware of possible risk factors, to recognize all necessary anatomical considerations in advance, to plan the treatment adequately, and to verify that the procedure is within his/her skills [5–7, 9, 11, 12, 14, 15].

Table 13.2 presents preventive measures for altered sensation in endodontic surgery.

Thorough medical history and clinical examination and good-quality radiographs are essential for preoperative diagnosis of teeth scheduled to undergo apical surgery [9, 11, 12, 14, 15]. Periapical (PA) radiography is the principal radiographic modality used for diagnosis and treatment planning prior to endodontic surgery. However, in certain cases, PA radiography alone may be clinically limited by the fact that the information is rendered in only two dimensions [9, 11, 12, 14, 15]. The use of computed tomography (CT) scans and more recently cone-beam CT (CBCT) enables the visualization of the dentition, the maxillofacial skeleton, and the surrounding anatomical structures in three dimensions [26]. In endodontic surgery, CBCT facilitates the evaluation of the true extent of PA lesions and of the relationships between the PA lesions/root apices and anatomical landmarks such as neurosensory structures. Thus, the CBCT enables the planning of a more predictable surgical approach [9, 10, 13, 26–29]. However, the decision whether to use CBCT scan or not must be based on the patient's history, clinical examination, and an initial PA radiographic evaluation and should be justified on an individual basis [9, 27]. Figure 13.1 presents a case selection algorithm for performing a CBCT scan, aimed at either prevention or management of nerve injuries related to endodontic surgical treatments [27].

Several possible risk factors for nerve injury related to endodontic treatments have been reported, including the patient's gender [22, 24, 25] and the tooth location [7]; some may be relevant specifically to endodontic surgical procedures. Knowing the possible risk factors for nerve injury may be useful for prevention, screening, and diagnosis of such injuries.

A female predominance was described in several nerve injury studies, such as nerve injury related to local anesthesia injection, third molar

Table 13.2 Preventive measures for altered sensation during and following endodontic surgery

Preoperative measures	Thorough clinical and radiographic evaluation (computed tomography when indicated)
	Risk factors evaluation
	Anatomical considerations
	Adequate treatment planning
	The procedure is within the practitioners skills
	Medicolegal precautions (informed consent)
Intraoperative measures	Anatomical considerations
	Magnification and conservative microsurgical techniques
	Adequate surgical procedures (injection, flap design and management, osteotomy, suturing)
	Case-specific surgical adjustments
	Consideration of early intervention in case a possible nerve injury is suspected
Postoperative measures	Postoperative anti-inflammatory adjuncts consideration
	Follow-up
	Timely mannered and adequate clinical and medicolegal response in case a nerve injury is suspected

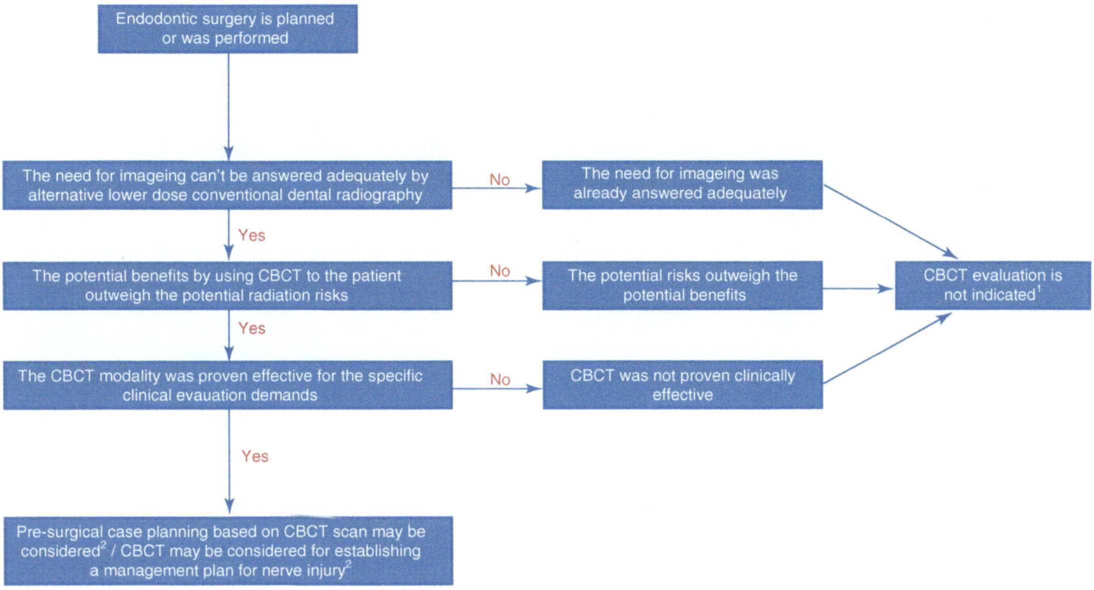

Fig. 13.1 Case selection algorithm for CBCT scan aimed for the prevention or management of nerve injuries related to endodontic surgical treatments. (*1*) Unless, CBCT evaluation may be indicated for clinical demands other than the prevention or management of nerve injuries. (*2*) Specific indications for CBCT evaluation in order to prevent or manage nerve injuries related to endodontic surgery: determine the exact location of root apex/apices and/or periapical lesion and their anatomical relation to adjacent neurosensory structures; suspected complex tooth morphology or surrounding anatomical structures or anatomical superimposition of roots or areas of the maxillofacial skeleton that might contribute to an increased risk of nerve injury during surgery; patients with nonspecific clinical signs and symptoms that may be related to a nerve injury; and assessment of endodontic treatment complications related to potential nerve injury [27]

surgery, lingual nerve repair, and nerve injury caused by dental treatment and traumatic injuries [18, 22, 24, 25]. The reason for this gender discrepancy may be explained by the fact that relatively more female patients are seeking dental treatment [24, 30]. Gender anatomical variation may be another possible explanation – females have significantly shorter vertical distances from the IAN to the root apices of mandibular molar teeth, which may potentially pose an increased risk of nerve injury during mandibular molar endodontic surgery in female patients compared to male patients [13].

A relative predominance of nerve injuries related to endodontic treatments of the second mandibular molars has been reported (example in Fig. 13.2) [5]. The anatomical structure of the IAN and its relations to the surrounding anatomical structures may have a significant role in this finding: The trabecular pattern of the cancellous bone in the mandibular molar region is characterized by a consistently loose appearance, numerous vacuoles and often without any cortical bone protecting the pedicle [5–7]. In the second mandibular molar, the distance between the apices and the pedicle of the IAN is often less than 1 mm, compared to a more variable distance observed in the first molar teeth (1–4 mm) [7]. The artery usually follows the IAN, running along the superomedial side from the mandibular foramen to the 1st molar and then becoming lateral, up to the mental foramen (Fig. 13.3) [7].

The nerve supply of the maxillary sinus membrane is provided by the three superior alveolar nerves, the anterior palatine nerve, and the infraorbital nerve [31]. These nerves pass enclosed within the wall of the sinus and innervate also the related maxillary teeth. Thus, endodontic surgery of maxillary teeth may involve these nerves and induce nerve injuries [31].

Damage to the mental nerve is also a major concern during endodontic surgical procedures

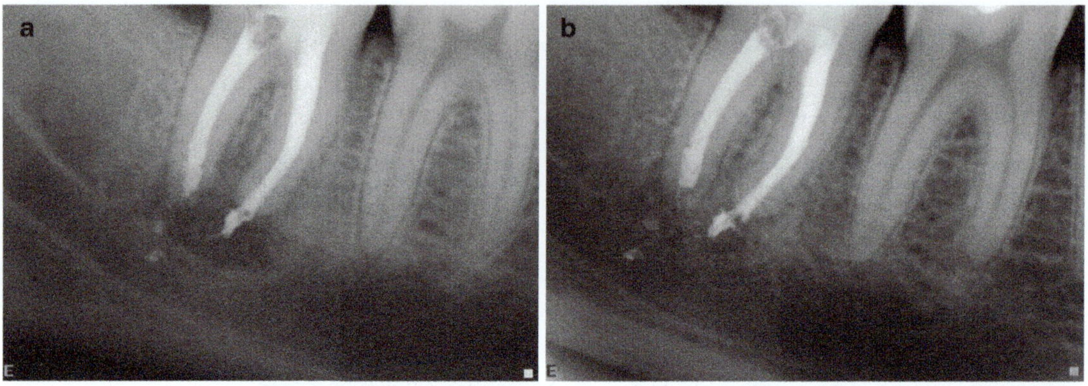

Fig. 13.2 Nerve injury following an endodontic treatment of mandibular second molar. (**a**) Nonsurgical endodontic treatment in the mandibular second molar. Radiographic evidence of overfilling of the endodontic filling material in the vicinity of the IAN. The patient presented with IAN paresthesia following the treatment, and was treated by corticosteroids for 1 week and then was followed up for several months. (**b**) At 6 months follow-up, healing process of the periapical lesion was demonstrated. A gradual resolution of the paresthesia symptoms was demonstrated in the months following the endodontic treatment, with return to normal neural function 3 months following the treatment

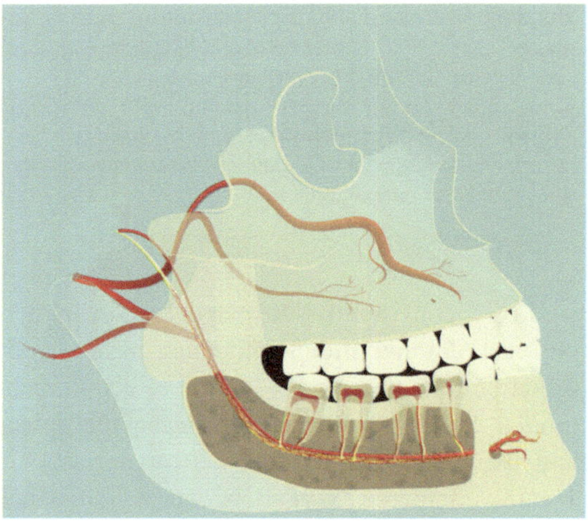

Fig. 13.3 The inferior alveolar nerve (IAN) anatomy. The artery (in *red*) usually follows the IAN (in *yellow*)

of mandibular posterior teeth [5, 7, 14, 15, 32, 33]. The mental nerve exits the body of the mandible through the mental foramen (MF, Fig. 13.3) and innervates the skin of the chin and the skin and mucous membrane of the lower lip [32, 33]. The common location of the MF is inferior to the second premolar, but the MF location may be variable [32, 33]. In addition, small accessory foramina (accessory mental foramina (AMF)) may also exist in the surrounding area of the MF, usually located in the apical area of the first molar and in the posterior or inferior areas of the mental foramen [32, 33]. It is important to know in advance the location of the MF and the innervation map of the mental nerve, in order to avoid damage to the neurovascular bundle during endodontic surgical procedures in this region [14, 15] as well as for an accurate and specific diagnosis of such damage in case it occurs following the procedure.

The clinical and surgical competence of the practitioner to perform the surgical procedure is an important prerequisite to performing surgical procedures. This competence exists when the practitioner has sufficient knowledge and skills such that the procedure can be performed to obtain the intended outcomes with minimal risks of harm to the patient [34, 35]. A practitioner's clinical competence is a combination of several components, including the following: knowledge, clinical decision-making capability, good judgment, technical skills, clinical attitudes, professional habits, and interpersonal skills. Each of these must be mastered by the practitioner, using a variety of sources of information and skill acquisition prior to performing any surgical procedure, in order to achieve predictable clinical results while minimizing the risk for potential complications, including nerve injuries [5, 24, 34, 35].

Therefore, practitioners should consider whether the procedure is relevant to their practice, recognize the expected outcomes, be familiar with potential risks and complications, and practice self-evaluation [34, 35]. It is prudent to verify that the procedure is within the practitioner's clinical skills and also that the practitioner is capable to prevent, diagnose, and manage possible complications such as nerve injuries.

Intraoperative Preventive Measures

All surgical procedures should be performed while balancing between two parallel aims: to provide the most favorable conditions for success and to take all measures to prevent potential complications. The preventive measures include the following: implementation of relevant anatomical considerations, the use of magnification and conservative microsurgical techniques, practicing adequate surgical procedures (such as proper and careful injection techniques, adequate flap design and management, cautious osteotomy, and careful suturing), implementation of case-specific surgical adjustments, and considering early intervention in case a possible nerve injury is suspected (Table 13.2) [5–7, 9, 11, 12, 14, 15].

It is prudent to balance between the two aforementioned aims of providing the most favorable conditions for success while preventing possible nerve injury, and it requires knowledge, experience, and awareness from the practitioner. For example, the osteotomy is aimed to provide an adequate surgical approach for proper management of the apical part of the root, thus providing the optimal conditions for success [14], but on the other hand, an excessive osteotomy may cause damage to adjacent anatomical structures such as nerve bundles [7, 14–16, 36]. Thus, the practitioner is required to achieve a complex equilibrium between the clinical demands required for a successful procedure and measures required for preventing damage.

During surgery of mandibular posterior teeth, damage to the mental nerve may occur by direct cutting of the nerve bundle or by stretching or crushing the neurovascular bundle with the retractor [14, 15]. Cutting and stretching may be avoided by an adequate flap design; crush injuries are often caused by impinging the retractor against the base of the flap in which the mental nerve is contained [14, 15]. Kim and Kratchman [14] suggested to first identify the mental foramen, then to carefully cover it with the retractor, and then to make a 15-mm long horizontal groove in the bone just above it and beyond the apex, to allow space for the osteotomy and subsequent apicoectomy. Once the retractor is in position within the groove, there should be no movement or slippage [14]. While it sometimes may be necessary to make such a groove, generally it is desirable to avoid unnecessary manipulations in the vicinity of nerve bundles. It is also advised to be aware of the risk of injury to the nerve when performing surgery of mandibular posterior teeth.

Endodontic surgery of mandibular molars poses even greater technical challenges, attributed to factors as the close proximity of the apices to the mandibular canal [12], the difficult access to the roots as a result of the posterior location [11, 14], and the thickness of the buccal cortical bone plate [9, 14]. This challenging anatomical situation may increase the risk of nerve injury during the endodontic surgical procedure [9, 36].

Therefore, case-specific anatomical challenges may require specific treatment planning and specific surgical adjustments, in order to achieve predictable clinical results safely.

In modern endodontics, the use of magnification and illumination devices has been implemented, enabling the practitioners to magnify the treatment field [37], with the aim of improving the accuracy and quality of treatment [38, 39]. The basic principle of microsurgery is that the surgeon's hands can execute remarkable micromanipulations as long as the surgeon's eyes can see a magnified operation field [37, 40]. Therefore, the application of magnification and illumination in surgical endodontic treatments, which allows easier and more precise identification of anatomical and pathological structures [41–45], may facilitate all phases of the surgical treatment to be done with greater accuracy and safety [38]. In this sense, it may allow a more conservative surgical treatment, especially when it is performed in the vicinity of neurovascular bundles, and therefore may reduce nerve injury risks.

Additional intraoperative surgical procedures that may be related to potential nerve injury, such as anesthetic injections, are discussed in other chapters of this book.

Postoperative Preventive Measures

Endodontic surgical procedures are usually performed under local anesthesia. Thus, the clinical symptoms of surgery-related nerve injuries will usually be evident only after the surgical procedure, when the local anesthesia wears out. On the other hand, in many cases, when a nerve injury did occur during the procedure, early intervention is of utmost importance. Thus, following the surgical procedure the practitioner, with the cooperation of the patient, needs to be alert to detect any possible sign of altered sensation [5, 6, 16, 24].

Early symptoms that may suggest a possible nerve injury include acute pain during or after the surgical procedure or neurosensory alterations, such as paresthesia, anesthesia, or hyperesthesia [46].

If a nerve injury is suspected, the clinician should perform a basic neurosensory evaluation, to ascertain whether the patient indeed experiences altered sensation signs, and document the findings [5, 6, 16, 24]. Then, a rigorous follow-up protocol should be followed.

In the absence of a definitive nerve injury diagnosis, a preventive approach of early intervention may be considered [5, 6, 16, 24], consisting the use of corticosteroids and nonsteroidal anti-inflammatory drugs (NSAIDs). The use of corticosteroids, if administered within a few days of the nerve injury, may minimize neuropathy, inhibit axon sprouting, and prevent neuroma formation [5, 6, 16, 24, 47, 48].

Diagnosis

Prevention is the most efficient way to address a nerve injury. However, when this serious complication occurs, a correct and timely mannered diagnosis is of outmost importance for preventing further damage, enabling appropriate management, and improving the healing prospect [2–4, 6, 8, 23–25, 49, 50].

Neurosensory impairment represents a complex clinical scenario with various clinical and psychological manifestations. Thus, sometimes the clinical manifestation of the nerve injury, such as persistent pain, may be confused with other postoperative symptoms [4, 16, 51–56]. Polycarpou et al. [55] evaluated cases of persistent pain after apparently successful nonsurgical and surgical endodontic treatments and reported the following risk factors: presence of preoperative pain from the tooth site lasting at least 3 months, history of previous chronic pain experience or painful treatment in the orofacial region, and female gender [55]. Nevertheless, it is conceivable to assume that at least in some of the cases, the persistent pain reported by the patients after the procedure was related to altered sensation.

Campbell et al. [51] evaluated 118 patients who underwent a nonsurgical endodontic treatment followed by a surgical endodontic treatment and found that 6 of the patients had continuous pain after the surgery for an average of 21 months [51]. Three of these patients had radiographic evidence of success and were suspected of having a nerve injury, and the other 3 patients were suspected of experiencing phantom tooth pain [51].

Thus, the clinician is obligated to extend his attention to this etiologic alternative, especially in cases with persistent symptoms following apparently successful surgical endodontic treatments [4, 16, 51–56].

When nerve injury is suspected, a timely mannered clinical approach is advised aimed to determine the sensory disturbance, quantify the sensory disturbance, determine treatment needs, and monitor recovery [2, 3, 6, 16, 17, 49, 50].

Figure 13.4 presents an algorithm for the diagnosis and management process of suspected nerve injury following an endodontic surgery.

The methods used for neurosensory function evaluation vary significantly, ranging between simple patient questioning and complicated technological examination modalities [3, 6, 16, 57, 58].

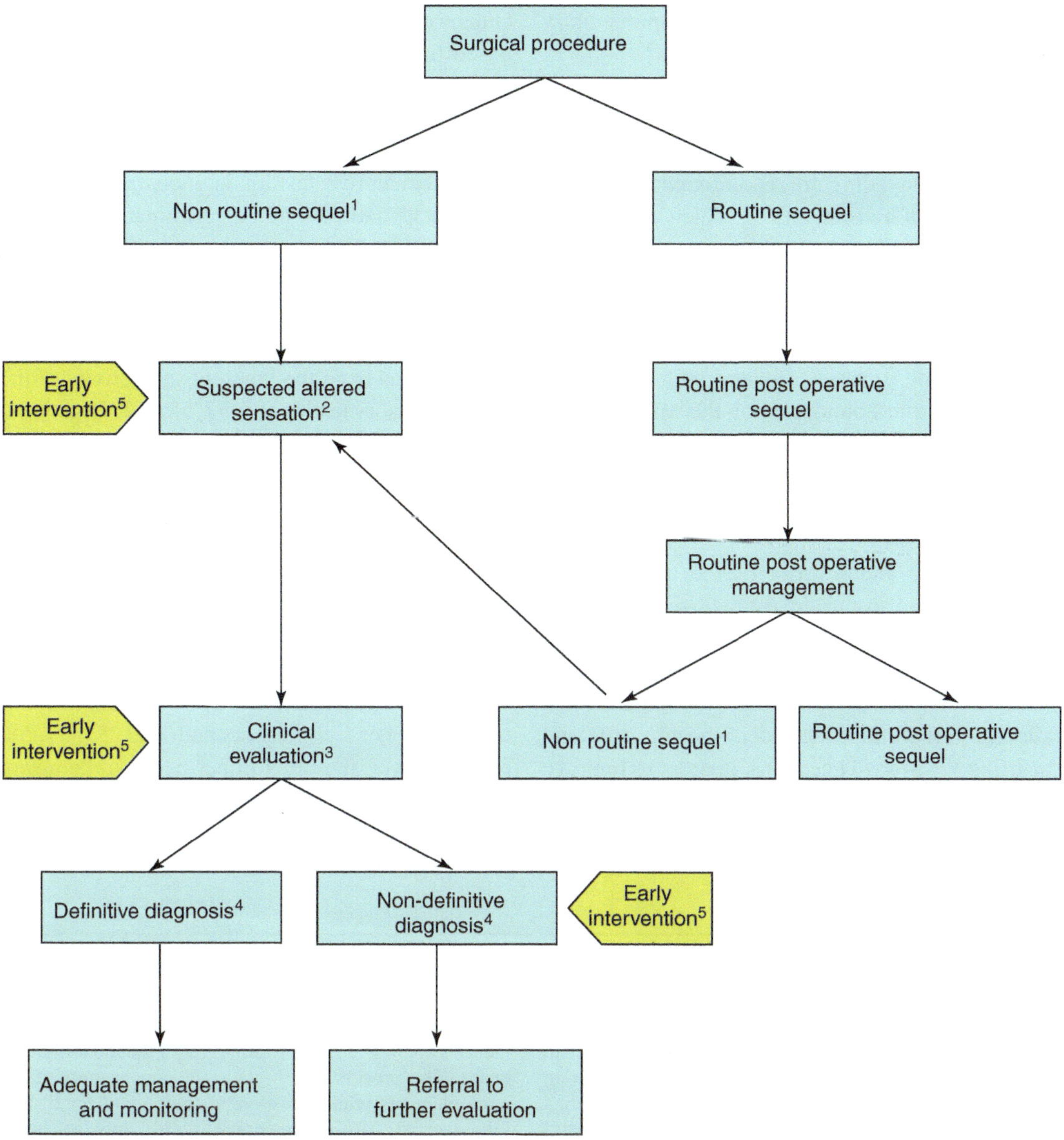

Fig. 13.4 Diagnosis and management of a nerve injury following endodontic surgery. (*1*) Nonroutine sequel: any event that is not part of the routine and/or expected sequel during or following the surgical procedure. (*2*) Suspected altered sensation: any event that occurred during or following the surgical procedure, was reported by the patient, or is suspected based on clinical and/or radiographic evaluation, which may suggest the presence of altered sensation following the surgical procedure. (*3*) Clinical evaluation: evaluation performed to determine the presence, nature, and extent of the sensory disturbance. (*4*) Definitive/non-definitive diagnosis: the practitioner is able/unable (respectively) to determine the presence, nature, and extent of the suspected altered sensation; OR is able/unable (respectively) to determine the required treatment and/or to monitor recovery. (*5*) Early intervention: an intervention performed even prior to a definitive diagnosis, aimed at preventing permanent nerve damage and enabling a better clinical and medicolegal response

However, the basic indicator of a sensory abnormality is the patient's own subjective report [3, 6, 16, 57, 58]. Currently there is no consensus as to the optimal method to be applied to measure nerve injury following endodontic surgery. Nevertheless, the diagnosis should be based on clinical sensory testing and complementary objective sensory tests [3, 6, 16, 56–58].

Unique clinical tests such as the "light touch" test performed with specially designed evaluation equipment such as the "Semmes-Weinstein monofilaments" for grading are recommended. In addition, the use of a visual analog scale (VAS)-based questionnaire rather than arbitrary questions may improve the objectivity of the evaluation [56].

The clinical sensory tests are aimed to better specify the sensory disturbance and to improve the diagnostic process [16] and should start by determining the boundaries of the affected area of altered sensation [54]. Once the affected area boundaries are determined, the next goal is to define the nature and severity of the neurosensory impairment [54].

The nature and severity of the neurosensory impairment are evaluated using a set of clinical tests, each of them aimed to evaluate specific neural receptors [59]. All tests should be performed with the patient's eyes closed, by comparing the affected side to the contralateral healthy side and by using VAS-based questions, in order to improve the objectivity of the tests [54, 56, 59].

The clinical neurosensory testing with cutaneous contact may grossly be divided into two categories: mechanoceptive and nociceptive, based on the specific stimulated receptors being evaluated [16, 59]. Mechanoceptive testing includes tests such as "two-point discrimination," "static light touch," and "brush directional stroke" [59]. Nociceptive testing includes tests such as "pin prick" and "thermal discrimination" [59].

Figure 13.5 presents several clinical evaluation methods of a suspected nerve injury following an endodontic surgical treatment.

Objective sensory tests are aimed to bypass a possible bias from the inherent subjectivity of the clinical sensory testing [53, 57, 58, 60]. Trigeminal evoked potentials (TEP) test is an electrophysiologic method of evaluating the trigeminal pathway and is an example of a noninvasive and objective method to quantify peripheral neural function. TEP may serve as an important adjunct in the diagnostic process for nerve injuries related to endodontic surgery [53, 57, 58, 60].

Some of the abovementioned evaluation methods require expertise that may be beyond the dental practitioner's clinical scope [6, 23, 53, 57, 58, 60]. However, the practitioner needs to be aware of the possibility of nerve injury following endodontic surgery and should know its possible risk factors, its major clinical manifestations, and the

Fig. 13.5 Clinical evaluation methods of suspected nerve injury following endodontic surgical treatment [52, 54, 56, 59]. (**a**) Determining the boundaries of the area of suspected altered sensation, is the first clinical test: An explorer is advanced (in a direction marked here with an *arrow*) with multiple gentle contact points starting from a peripheral area with normal sensation, propagating toward the center of the suspected area, until the patient indicates a change or loss of sensation. That specific point is considered as the border of the affected area. The procedure is repeated on multiple spots (indicated here by *dots*) to form the outline of the area of altered sensation. Eventually, the area of altered sensation is outlined and marked. (**b**) Two-point discrimination: tested by contact with sharp tweezers, initially with attached arms, and then followed by succeeding contacts, with increasingly growing distance between the tweezers arms. The distance at which the patient is capable of distinguishing two contact points is considered the baseline two-point discrimination distance. (**c**) Static light touch: a device holding a monofilament (calibrated by the force required to bend the monofilament) is applied to the skin surface until the monofilament bends. The process is repeated with increasingly stiffer monofilaments while questioning the patient for his\her response. (**d**) Brush directional stroke: moving brush strokes of a monofilament (same as previously used for the static light touch test) in different directions (the *arrows* indicate the directions of the strokes that are applied). The patient is asked to confirm the direction of the stroke. (**e**) Pin prick: a needle is applied in a pricking motion. An appropriate response should be a feeling of sharp (not dull) pain. (**f**) Thermal discrimination: a cotton-tipped applicator is sprayed with a topical anesthetic skin refrigerant (such as "ethyl chloride"), or without spray (as control), and then applied to the evaluated area. A normal response is considered correct answer of a cold or normal feeling

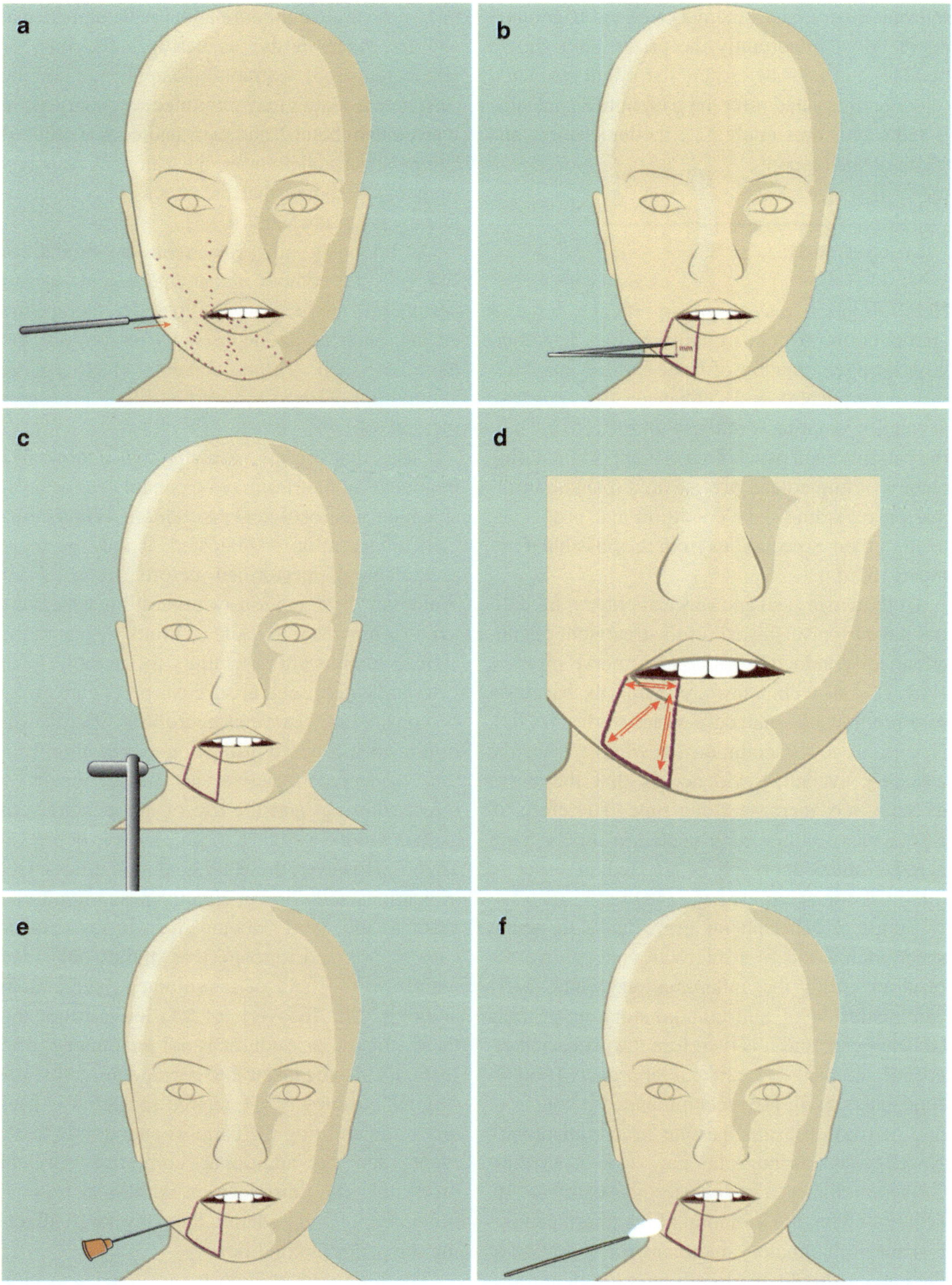
a
b
mm
c
d
e
f

relevant anatomical landmarks of the trigeminal nerve. Most importantly the practitioner should be able to at least determine the initial suspicion of nerve injury and refer the patient to a specialist if indicated, thus enabling a better clinical and medicolegal response.

Management

Nerve injuries may have significant negative effects on the patient's quality of life. The common iatrogenic nature of these injuries may further complicate and enhance the negative psychological effects of these injuries [61]. Thus, the patients need psychological support including receipt of immediate, precise, and realistic information regarding their condition and prognosis, to align their expectations from the possible treatments [5, 61].

Both nonsurgical and surgical clinical modalities have been suggested for the treatment of endodontically induced symptomatic nerve injuries. However, all techniques are primarily based on case reports and small case-series studies [6, 62]. Nevertheless, the common knowledge from the currently available evidence is that the nerve damage may increase along time. Therefore, in case a nerve injury is suspected, a timely mannered clinical approach is advised in order to minimize long-term damage [49].

Injury of a peripheral nerve leads to neural sheet edema and to a microcirculatory disorder resulting from the inflammation. Thus, early administration of anti-inflammatory drugs may be beneficial, and it is therefore the primary therapeutic noninvasive clinical approach [6, 46]. Juodzbalys et al. [16] recommended a course of oral steroids (dexamethasone or prednisolone). NSAIDs such as ibuprofen may serve as an alternative or adjunct to an oral steroid treatment [16, 46]. Following the initiation of the pharmacological anti-inflammatory treatment, the condition of the patient should be closely monitored, and if it improves, another course of anti-inflammatory drugs may be considered [16].

Cryotherapy ("cold therapy") is the application of cold for therapeutic purposes, such as to minimize postsurgical inflammation, pain, and edema, and has been in use as early as the time of Hippocrates [63]. Extraoral ice application on the para-neural tissues may minimize secondary nerve injury from the inflammation and edema-induced compression and improve postsurgical recovery. It should be noted that the exact effect of cryotherapy is yet unclear [16, 63].

Additional noninvasive treatment modalities suggested for complicated and persistent cases of peripheral nerve injuries include therapeutic agents, such as antidepressants, or physiologic therapies, such as transcutaneous electric nerve stimulation (TENS) [64, 65] and low-level laser therapy [66].

Cases that are not responsive to noninvasive treatment modalities may be candidates for invasive microneurosurgical procedures. When a surgical intervention is indicated, it may be more predictable if performed before the setup of Wallerian degeneration (a process in which the axon stump distal to a site of injury degenerates) about 3 months after the injury [6, 16, 66].

If indicated, several surgical procedures may be considered: "external neurolysis," flap elevation for direct nerve inspection and freeing from the adjacent constrictive scar tissue; repair by direct suturing; and the use of autogenous vein graft or Gore-Tex tube to bridge a nerve defect [6, 16, 66]. However, these surgical modalities exact indications and clinical effectiveness seem to be variable and poorly documented, in low-quality case reports and retrospective studies published mainly in the field of maxillofacial surgery. In addition, full recovery of sensation following these surgical procedures is not guaranteed [66]. It should also be taken into consideration that the original etiology of the altered sensation is usually trauma during the surgical endodontic treatment, and an additional corrective surgical procedure may introduce an additional trauma, inflammation, and edema, thus adversely affecting the patient's condition.

The long-term prognosis of altered sensation following endodontic surgery is yet unknown, but it is believed to be related to the type and extent of injury (Table 13.1), to the timing of a corrective intervention, and to the selected treatment protocol [6, 16, 17, 61, 66]. From the currently available literature, it seems that most patients, especially those with a relatively low extent of injury and who received an appropriate early intervention treatment, did tend to improve with time, sometimes using several different coping mechanisms [61]. However, unknown portion of the patients may suffer from long-term or permanent disability, with significant medical and medicolegal consequences and a destructive effect on their quality of life [6, 16, 17, 61, 66]. Pogrel et al. [61] reported that among 145 patients who were evaluated at least 3 years since their initial consultation regarding dental treatment related injury to the trigeminal nerve, a considerable portion reported significant effects on their quality of life, manifesting as eating disorders (43 %), speech problems (38 %), depression (37 %), relationship changes (14 %), and adverse effects on employment (13 %) [61]. Among this cohort of patients, it was also found that patients over 40 years old reported more long-term pain than younger patients, that males reported on a greater decrease in symptoms than females, and that symptoms of lingual nerve injury improved more than symptoms of the inferior alveolar nerve [61].

In conclusion, active preventive measures based on a thorough clinical evaluation, adequate treatment planning, and case-specific adjustments during and following the surgical procedure are the most efficient measures to minimize the risk of nerve injuries during endodontic surgical procedures. However, when a nerve injury is suspected, a timely mannered clinical approach is of outmost importance, aimed at preventing permanent damage and enabling a better clinical and medicolegal response.

References

1. Escoda-Francoli J, Canalda-Sahli C, Soler A, Figueiredo R, Gay-Escoda C. Inferior alveolar nerve damage because of overextended endodontic material: a problem of sealer cement biocompatibility? J Endod. 2007;33(12):1484–9.
2. Grotz KA, Al-Nawas B, de Aguiar EG, Schulz A, Wagner W. Treatment of injuries to the inferior alveolar nerve after endodontic procedures. Clin Oral Investig. 1998;2(2):73–6.
3. Yatsuhashi T, Nakagawa K, Matsumoto M, Kasahara M, Igarashi T, Ichinohe T, et al. Inferior alveolar nerve paresthesia relieved by microscopic endodontic treatment. Bull Tokyo Dent Coll. 2003;44(4):209–12.
4. Gallas-Torreira MM, Reboiras-Lopez MD, Garcia-Garcia A, Gandara-Rey J. Mandibular nerve paresthesia caused by endodontic treatment. Med Oral. 2003;8(4):299–303.
5. Givol N, Rosen E, Bjorndal L, Taschieri S, Ofec R, Tsesis I. Medico-legal aspects of altered sensation following endodontic treatment: a retrospective case series. Oral Surg Oral Med Oral Pathol Oral Radiol Endod. 2011;112(1):126–31.
6. Pogrel MA. Damage to the inferior alveolar nerve as the result of root canal therapy. J Am Dent Assoc. 2007;138(1):65–9.
7. Tilotta-Yasukawa F, Millot S, El Haddioui A, Bravetti P, Gaudy JF. Labiomandibular paresthesia caused by endodontic treatment: an anatomic and clinical study. Oral Surg Oral Med Oral Pathol Oral Radiol Endod. 2006;102(4):e47–59.
8. Garisto GA, Gaffen AS, Lawrence HP, Tenenbaum HC, Haas DA. Occurrence of paresthesia after dental local anesthetic administration in the United States. J Am Dent Assoc. 2010;141(7):836–44.
9. Bornstein MM, Lauber R, Sendi P, von Arx T. Comparison of periapical radiography and limited cone-beam computed tomography in mandibular molars for analysis of anatomical landmarks before apical surgery. J Endod. 2011;37(2):151–7.
10. Kamburoglu K, Kilic C, Ozen T, Yuksel SP. Measurements of mandibular canal region obtained by cone-beam computed tomography: a cadaveric study. Oral Surg Oral Med Oral Pathol Oral Radiol Endod. 2009;107(2):e34–42.
11. Kim TS, Caruso JM, Christensen H, Torabinejad M. A comparison of cone-beam computed tomography and direct measurement in the examination of the mandibular canal and adjacent structures. J Endod. 2010;36(7):1191–4.
12. Kovisto T, Ahmad M, Bowles WR. Proximity of the mandibular canal to the tooth apex. J Endod. 2011;37(3):311–5.
13. Simonton JD, Azevedo B, Schindler WG, Hargreaves KM. Age- and gender-related differences in the position of the inferior alveolar nerve by using cone beam computed tomography. J Endod. 2009;35(7):944–9.
14. Kim S, Kratchman S. Modern endodontic surgery concepts and practice: a review. J Endod. 2006;32(7):601–23.
15. Moiseiwitsch JR. Avoiding the mental foramen during periapical surgery. J Endod. 1995;21(6):340–2.
16. Juodzbalys G, Wang H, Sabalys G. Injury of the inferior alveolar nerve during implant placement: a literature review. J Oral Maxillofac Res. 2011;2(1):e1.
17. Seddon HJ. A classification of nerve injuries. Br Med J. 1942;2(4260):237–9.

18. Hillerup S, Jensen R. Nerve injury caused by mandibular block analgesia. Int J Oral Maxillofac Surg. 2006;35(5):437–43.
19. Misch K, Wang HL. Implant surgery complications: etiology and treatment. Implant Dent. 2008;17(2):159–68.
20. Park SH, Wang HL. Implant reversible complications: classification and treatments. Implant Dent. 2005;14(3):211–20.
21. Annibali S, Ripari M, La Monaca G, Tonoli F, Cristalli MP. Local accidents in dental implant surgery: prevention and treatment. Int J Periodontics Restorative Dent. 2009;29(3):325–31.
22. Bjorndal L, Reit C. Endodontic malpractice claims in Denmark 1995–2004. Int Endod J. 2008;41(12):1059–65.
23. Chaushu G, Taicher S, Halamish-Shani T, Givol N. Medicolegal aspects of altered sensation following implant placement in the mandible. Int J Oral Maxillofac Implants. 2002;17(3):413–5.
24. Givol N, Rosen E, Taicher S, Tsesis I. Risk management in endodontics. J Endod. 2010;36(6):982–4.
25. Givol N, Taicher S, Halamish-Shani T, Chaushu G. Risk management aspects of implant dentistry. Int J Oral Maxillofac Implants. 2002;17(2):258–62.
26. Patel S. New dimensions in endodontic imaging: part 2. Cone beam computed tomography. Int Endod J. 2009;42(6):463–75.
27. American Association of Endodontics, American Academy of Oral and Maxillofacial Radiology. AAE and AAOMR joint position statement – use of cone-beam-computed tomography in endodontics. Chicago. 2010.
28. de Paula-Silva FW, Wu MK, Leonardo MR, da Silva LA, Wesselink PR. Accuracy of periapical radiography and cone-beam computed tomography scans in diagnosing apical periodontitis using histopathological findings as a gold standard. J Endod. 2009;35(7):1009–12.
29. Pinsky HM, Dyda S, Pinsky RW, Misch KA, Sarment DP. Accuracy of three-dimensional measurements using cone-beam CT. Dentomaxillofac Radiol. 2006;35(6):410–6.
30. Manski RJ, Moeller JF, Maas WR. Dental services. An analysis of utilization over 20 years. J Am Dent Assoc. 2001;132(5):655–64.
31. Wallace JA. Transantral endodontic surgery. Oral Surg Oral Med Oral Pathol Oral Radiol Endod. 1996;82(1):80–3.
32. Concepcion M, Rankow HJ. Accessory branch of the mental nerve. J Endod. 2000;26(10):619–20.
33. Katakami K, Mishima A, Shiozaki K, Shimoda S, Hamada Y, Kobayashi K. Characteristics of accessory mental foramina observed on limited cone-beam computed tomography images. J Endod. 2008;34(12):1441–5.
34. Czarnowski C, Ponka D, Rughani R, Geoffrion P. See one. Do one. Teach one: office-based minor surgical procedures. Can Fam Physician. 2008;54(6):893.
35. Miller MD. Office procedures. Education, training, and proficiency of procedural skills. Prim Care. 1997;24(2):231–40.
36. Wesson CM, Gale TM. Molar apicectomy with amalgam root-end filling: results of a prospective study in two district general hospitals. Br Dent J. 2003;195(12):707–14; discussion 698.
37. Bahcall JK. Visual enhancement. In: Ingle JI, Bakland LK, Baumgartner JC, editors. Ingle's endodontics. Hamilton: BC Decker Inc; 2008. p. 870–6.
38. Del Fabbro M, Taschieri S. Endodontic therapy using magnification devices: a systematic review. J Dent. 2010;38(4):269–75.
39. Del Fabbro M, Taschieri S, Lodi G, Banfi G, Weinstein RL. Magnification devices for endodontic therapy. Cochrane Database Syst Rev. 2009;(3):CD005969.
40. Taschieri S, Del Fabbro M, Weinstein T, Rosen E, Tsesis I. Magnification in modern endodontic practice. Refuat Hapeh Vehashinayim. 2010;27(3):18–22, 61.
41. Baldassari-Cruz LA, Lilly JP, Rivera EM. The influence of dental operating microscope in locating the mesiolingual canal orifice. Oral Surg Oral Med Oral Pathol Oral Radiol Endod. 2002;93(2):190–4.
42. de Carvalho MC, Zuolo ML. Orifice locating with a microscope. J Endod. 2000;26(9):532–4.
43. Gorduysus MO, Gorduysus M, Friedman S. Operating microscope improves negotiation of second mesiobuccal canals in maxillary molars. J Endod. 2001;27(11):683–6.
44. Slaton CC, Loushine RJ, Weller RN, Parker MH, Kimbrough WF, Pashley DH. Identification of resected root-end dentinal cracks: a comparative study of visual magnification. J Endod. 2003;29(8):519–22.
45. Zaugg B, Stassinakis A, Hotz P. Influence of magnification tools on the recognition of simulated preparation and filling errors. Schweiz Monatsschr Zahnmed. 2004;114(9):890–6.
46. Froes FG, Miranda AM, Abad Eda C, Riche FN, Pires FR. Non-surgical management of paraesthesia and pain associated with endodontic sealer extrusion into the mandibular canal. Aust Endod J. 2009;35(3):183–6.
47. Han SR, Yeo SP, Lee MK, Bae YC, Ahn DK. Early dexamethasone relieves trigeminal neuropathic pain. J Dent Res. 2010;89(9):915–20.
48. Seo K, Tanaka Y, Terumitsu M, Someya G. Efficacy of steroid treatment for sensory impairment after orthognathic surgery. J Oral Maxillofac Surg. 2004;62(10):1193–7.
49. Scolozzi P, Lombardi T, Jaques B. Successful inferior alveolar nerve decompression for dysesthesia following endodontic treatment: report of 4 cases treated by mandibular sagittal osteotomy. Oral Surg Oral Med Oral Pathol Oral Radiol Endod. 2004;97(5):625–31.
50. Seddon HJ, Medawar PB, Smith H. Rate of regeneration of peripheral nerves in man. J Physiol. 1943;102(2):191–215.
51. Campbell RL, Parks KW, Dodds RN. Chronic facial pain associated with endodontic therapy. Oral Surg Oral Med Oral Pathol. 1990;69(3):287–90.
52. Cruccu G, Sommer C, Anand P, Attal N, Baron R, Garcia-Larrea L, et al. EFNS guidelines on neuropathic pain assessment: revised 2009. Eur J Neurol. 2010;17(8):1010–8.

53. Fagade OO, Wastell DG. Trigeminal somatosensory evoked potentials: technical parameters, reliability and potential in clinical dentistry. J Dent. 1990;18(3):137–41.
54. Meyer RA, Bagheri SC. Clinical evaluation of peripheral trigeminal nerve injuries. Atlas Oral Maxillofac Surg Clin North Am. 2011;19(1):15–33.
55. Polycarpou N, Ng YL, Canavan D, Moles DR, Gulabivala K. Prevalence of persistent pain after endodontic treatment and factors affecting its occurrence in cases with complete radiographic healing. Int Endod J. 2005;38(3):169–78.
56. Poort LJ, van Neck JW, van der Wal KG. Sensory testing of inferior alveolar nerve injuries: a review of methods used in prospective studies. J Oral Maxillofac Surg. 2009;67(2):292–300.
57. Bennett AJ, Wastell DG, Barker GR, Blackburn CW, Rood JP. Trigeminal somatosensory evoked potentials. A review of the literature as applicable to oral dysaesthesias. Int J Oral Maxillofac Surg. 1987;16(4): 408–15.
58. Bennett MH, Jannetta PJ. Trigeminal evoked potentials in humans. Electroencephalogr Clin Neurophysiol. 1980;48(5):517–26.
59. Ghali GE, Epker BN. Clinical neurosensory testing: practical applications. J Oral Maxillofac Surg. 1989;47(10):1074–8.
60. Barker GR, Bennett AJ, Wastell DG. Applications of trigeminal somatosensory evoked potentials (TSEPs) in oral and maxillofacial surgery. Br J Oral Maxillofac Surg. 1987;25(4):308–13.
61. Pogrel MA, Jergensen R, Burgon E, Hulme D. Long-term outcome of trigeminal nerve injuries related to dental treatment. J Oral Maxillofac Surg. 2011;69(9):2284–8.
62. Graff-Radford SB, Evans RW. Lingual nerve injury. Headache. 2003;43(9):975–83.
63. Osunde OD, Adebola RA, Omeje UK. Management of inflammatory complications in third molar surgery: a review of the literature. Afr Health Sci. 2011;11(3): 530–7.
64. Cotter DJ. Overview of transcutaneous electrical nerve stimulation for treatment of acute postoperative pain. Med Instrum. 1983;17(4):289–92.
65. Singla S, Prabhakar V, Singla RK. Role of transcutaneous electric nerve stimulation in the management of trigeminal neuralgia. J Neurosci Rural Pract. 2011;2(2):150–2.
66. Leung YY, Fung PP, Cheung LK. Treatment modali ties of neurosensory deficit after lower third molar surgery: a systematic review. J Oral Maxillofac Surg. 2012;70(4):768–78.

Bisphosphonate-Related Osteonecrosis of the Jaw (BRONJ) 14

Samantha Pozzi, Alexandre Anesi, Luigi Generali, Alessia Bari, Ugo Consolo, and Luigi Chiarini

Abstract

Osteonecrosis of the jaw (ONJ) is a rare condition that has been mainly related to the treatment with i.v. bisphosphonates in patients affected by cancer bone disease. The ethiopathology is still unknown and the frequency is between 0.8 and 12 %. It can appear in edentulous patients, but invasive procedures have been demonstrated to increase the risk of developing this complication. Few cases have been described in the endodontic literature. In the next chapter, we will describe ONJ, will analyze the data from literature, and will report expert opinions and guidelines about the best clinical practice in the endodontic field. Finally, since data in this field are limited, we would like to underline that the best treatment plan for cancer patients receiving bisphosphonates and requiring dental procedures is a multidisciplinary, case-by-case approach.

Introduction

Ischemic osteonecrosis refers to avascular necrosis that can affect any bone of the skeleton. It was first described in the eighteenth century in the femoral head [1]. Since 2003, however, osteonecrosis

S. Pozzi, MD (✉) • A. Bari, MD
Program of Innovative Therapy in Oncology and Hematology, University of Modena and Reggio Emilia, Modena, Italy

Dipartimento di Medicina Diagnostica, Clinica e di Sanità Pubblica,
Centro Oncologico Modenese, Policlinico di Modena, Università di Modena e Reggio Emilia,
Largo del Pozzo 71, stanza #4.20, Modena 41122, Italy
e-mail: samantha.pozzi@unimore.it; alessia.bari@unimore.it

A. Anesi, MD • L. Chiarini, MD
Unit of Cranio-Maxillofacial Surgery, University of Modena and Reggio Emilia, Modena, Italy

Dipartimento di Scienze Mediche e Chirurgiche Materno-Infantili e dell'Adulto, Chirurgia Maxillofacciale, Policlinico di Modena,
Largo del Pozzo 71, Modena 41122, Italy
e-mail: alexandre.anesi@unimore.it; luigi.generali@unimore.it

L. Generali, MD • U. Consolo, MD
Unit of Dentistry and Oral-Maxillofacial Surgery, University of Modena and Reggio Emilia, Modena, Italy

Dipartimento Chirurgico, Medico, Odontoiatrico e di Scienze Morfologiche con interesse Trapiantologico, Oncologico e di Medicina Rigenerativa, Odontoiatria, Policlinico di Modena,
Università di Modena e Reggio Emilia,
Largo del Pozzo 71, Modena 41122, Italy
e-mail: luigi.chiarini@unimore.it; ugo.consolo@unimore.it

I. Tsesis (ed.), *Complications in Endodontic Surgery*,
DOI 10.1007/978-3-642-54218-3_14, © Springer-Verlag Berlin Heidelberg 2014

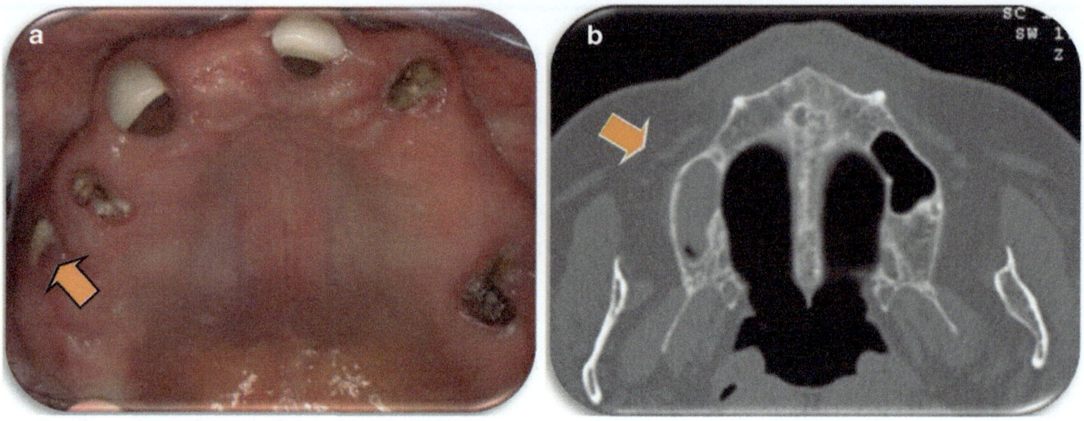

Fig. 14.1 (**a**) Patient affected by metastatic breast cancer treated with i.v. zoledronic acid for 16 months. The *arrow* shows the presence of exposed bone in the posterior right maxilla after a tooth extraction. (**b**) Multislice CT scan with bone algorithm. Cortical osteosclerosis with maxilla sinus inflammation is detectable

of the jaw (ONJ) was an extremely rare condition, secondary to local and systemic factors, from rheumatological to thrombophilic disorders [1]. In the oncological setting, it was mainly consequent to radiation therapy of head and neck and it was defined osteoradionecrosis [2]. In 2003, Marx and colleagues described an increasing number of cases of ONJ in patients affected by cancers, mainly multiple myeloma and breast cancer, not undergoing radiation therapy [3]. All the 36 cases described by Marx received treatment with i.v. bisphosphonates (BP), mainly pamidronate and zoledronic acid. Soon after Marx, other authors [4–11] confirmed the observation in retrospective epidemiologic surveys in dental clinics and cancer centers worldwide confirming the association between ONJ and BP administration (Fig. 14.1a, b). Despite that the causality and the pathogenesis have not been clarified, the almost constant association with BP named this new condition bisphosphonate-related osteonecrosis of the jaw (BRONJ) [12].

BP belong to the category of bone antiresorptive agents, prescribed to patients with altered bone turnover, mainly osteoporosis, Paget's disease, bone metastasis, and multiple myeloma [13]. BP inhibit the mevalonate pathway and consequently osteoclastogenesis and bone resorption [14]. However, in the past few years, a growing amount of data supports the theory that there might be new target cells and BP might have a more pleiotropic effect [15]. Based on the chemical structures, BP are divided into two main categories: nitrogen- and not-nitrogen-containing BP (Table. 14.1). The nitrogen-containing BP are more potent, and comprehend pamidronate and zoledronic acid, the two main drugs prescribed in oncological patients. Pamidronate was approved by FDA in 2001 and zoledronic acid in 2002 [16] and they are the BP more often related to ONJ, compared with not-nitrogen-containing BP. Not-nitrogen-containing BP are prescribed in patients with osteoporosis; they are usually orally available and are less potent BP.

Criteria for the definition of BRONJ have been established by the American Association of Oral and Maxillofacial Surgeons (AAOMS) in 2007 [17] and take into account three characteristics: current or previous treatment with a BP, identification of exposed bone in the maxillofacial region that has persisted for more than 8 weeks, and no history of radiation therapy to the jaws. Since not all the cases manifest with exposed bone, a revision of the definition has been proposed [18, 19] with the introduction of stage "0" (Table 14.2a).

Despite the extensive ongoing research, the mechanism that induces ONJ is still unclear. Recently several cases of ONJ related to other antiresorptive agents such as denosumab, an anti-RANKL monoclonal antibody, have been described, hypothesizing that ONJ is not related

Table 14.1 Major bisphosphonates, potency, primary indication, and route of administration

Drug name	Potency	Primary indication	Route of administration
Non-N-BP			
Etidronate disodium	1×	Osteoporosis, Paget's disease	Oral and i.v.
Tiludronic acid	10×	Paget's disease, hypercalcemia in malignancy	Oral
Sodium clodronate	10×	Bone pain, bone metastasis, hypercalcemia	Oral
N-BP			
Pamidronate disodium	100×	Paget's disease, bone pain, bone metastasis, hypercalcemia	i.v.
Alendronate	>100–<1,000×	Osteoporosis	Oral and i.v.
Risedronate sodium	>1000–<10,000×	Osteoporosis, Paget's disease	Oral
Ibandronic acid	>1,000–<10,000×	Osteoporosis, bone metastasis, hypercalcemia	Oral and i.v.
Zoledronic acid	>1,000–<10,000×	Bone metastasis, Paget's disease, hypercalcemia	i.v.

Non-N-BP not-nitrogen-containing bisphosphonates, *N-BP* nitrogen-containing bisphosphonates

Table 14.2a ONJ staging system

Stage	Clinical presentation
At risk	No evidence of necrotic bone in patients treated with oral or i.v. BP
Stage 0	No clinical evidence of necrosis, but nonspecific clinical findings and symptoms
Stage 1	Asymptomatic patient with exposed necrotic bone, no evident infection
Stage 2	Symptomatic patient with exposed necrotic bone + infection (pain, erythema ± purulent discharge)
Stage 3	Exposed necrotic bone in symptomatic patient with pain, infection, and one or more of the following:
	Exposed and necrotic bone extending beyond the region of alveolar bone resulting in pathologic fracture
	Extraoral fistula
	Oral-antral or oral-nasal communication
	Osteolysis extending to the inferior border of the mandible or sinus floor

Modified from Ruggiero et al. [16]

to BP, but to a class of drugs with antiresorptive activity, and a new terminology has been proposed: antiresorptive agent-induced osteonecrosis of the jaw (ARONJ) [20, 21]. Moreover, few cases of ONJ have been described in cancer patients treated with anticancer drugs [21] and the terminology might change again in the future. All these observations highlight the complexity of the pathogenesis of ONJ.

In the following chapter, we will try to better define the characteristics, the diagnostic, and the therapeutic approach to ONJ in the context of endodontic surgery. Currently very few cases of ONJ after endodontic surgery have been described in literature and guidelines on this topic are scarce.

In the course of this chapter, we will use the term ONJ as a generic term of necrosis of the jaw and BRONJ when specifically related to bisphosphonates, and we will use the more wide term of ARONJ when the ONJ can be related to both bisphosphonates and other antiresorptive agents.

Epidemiology

BRONJ is a very rare condition, with a highly inhomogeneous distribution based on the chemical structure and the potency of BP, schedule of administration, duration of treatment, and the type of bone disorder (malignant vs. not malignant bone disease). Cases of spontaneous not BP-related ONJ are very rare in the general population [4]. Based on case series, case-controlled studies, and cohort studies, the cumulative incidence of BRONJ is estimated to be between 0.8 and 12 % in patients receiving i.v. BP [22–29]. The incidence is higher in oncological patients, mainly affected by multiple myeloma (3.8 cases per 100 patients), prostate cancer (2.9 per 100 patients), and breast cancer (2.5 per 100 patients) [27]. The incidence is also influenced by dental procedures. In an Australian population-based survey [30], the frequency of BRONJ in cancer patients treated with i.v. BP is as low as 0.88–1.15 %, but it reaches 6.7–9.1 % after dental extraction [31]. BRONJ is even more rare in patients affected by osteoporosis receiving oral BP (0.01–0.04 %) from an Australian survey, with incidence rising to 0.09–0.34 % after dental extraction [31].

The discrepancy of the frequency in cancer population compared with osteoporosis can be partly related to different biology of the bone disease and to the different types of BP administered, the schedule of administration, and the cumulative dose of BP. As far as duration of treatment, the risk in multiple myeloma patients seems to be increased after 2 years of monthly administration of i.v. N-BP [23, 29].

Despite the observation that invasive dental procedures increase the risk of BRONJ, likely as a consequence of bone exposure and the increased risk of infections, cases of spontaneous BRONJ have been described in toothless patients, possibly related to the mucosal trauma from dental prosthesis, but sometimes no preceding factor is observed [32].

In the study by Hsiao that analyzed patients undergoing root canal treatments, the probability of healing after conventional root canal procedures in patients treated with oral BP was not statistically different from patients not receiving BP [33]. In the endodontic literature, very few publications reported cases of BRONJ in patients treated with BP [34–37]. Gallego described one case of BRONJ possibly precipitated by the mucosal damage induced by rubber dam clamp [34]. Goodell reported two cases of BRONJ precipitated by endodontic procedures. One patient was a 72-year-old man affected by prostate cancer and treated with i.v. BP that developed an ulcerated area after endodontic treatment on tooth #18. Tooth #18 also had a porcelain-fuse-to-metal restoration. The second case was a 74-year-old man affected by prostate cancer that has been treated with oral BP followed by i.v. BP. The patient received a nonsurgical endodontic treatment on tooth #15. After the procedure, the patient complained of persistent pain and underwent an apicoectomy without benefit of the symptoms. The patient developed tooth mobility in correspondence of fixed partial denture and exposed bone. The conservative treatment did not obtain any benefit, and he complained of pain and foul odor. After debridement of the maxilla and extraction of tooth #15 followed by antibiotic treatment, the patient improved, and the follow-up at 6 months showed a subjective and clinical amelioration [35]. Two more cases of BRONJ secondary to nonsurgical and surgical root canal treatments have been described by Sarathy et al. [36]. Finally, one case has been described by Katz in a 60-year-old female affected by multiple myeloma and treated with i.v. BP that underwent a bone graft procedure in the area of teeth #2–3. Tooth #3 was also treated with nonsurgical root canal and periradicular surgery. The clinical examination showed an area of exposed bone adjacent to tooth #2–4. The patient received a conservative treatment on #2 with rapid improvement [37].

Risk Factors

Despite the extensive research directed to determine the etiopathology of BRONJ, data that demonstrate the causality of BP in the development of BRONJ are still circumstantial, and hypothesis about the risk factors and the mechanisms involved are even less clear. Due to the low frequency of ONJ compared with the extensive use of BP, it is evident that cofactors should be implicated in the development of this complication.

Several attempts have been addressed to identify risk factors, related to both patient's features and drug characteristics [16, 19, 25, 30, 38]. In the 2009 paper by the American Association of Oral and Maxillofacial Surgeons, the risk factors are categorized in drug-related factors, local, demographic, genetic, and preventive [16]. The drug-related factors evaluate the type of BP, the potency of BP, the schedule of administration, and the duration of the treatment and more recently even their pharmacokinetics and pharmacodynamics [39]. About the potency, pamidronate and zoledronic acid are the types of BP more frequently associated with ONJ. Concerning the exposition to the treatment, several studies observed an increased risk for patients affected by multiple myeloma treated over 2 years, and the updated guidelines for the treatment of patients affected by multiple myeloma suggest a 2-year treatment and to evaluate case by case for longer therapy [40]. For breast cancer patients, the American Society of Clinical Oncology guidelines do not indicate a limit for the use of bone-modifying agents like BP and denosumab but suggest that should be continued based on the patients' performance status [41]. The 2013 American National Osteoporosis Foundation guidelines observe that no treatment should be administered for indefinite time, but due to the lack of evidence in this field, especially for treatments longer than 5 years, they conclude that the duration of treatment should be individualized based on the fracture risk of each patient [42]. About local risk factors, the mandible is interested two times more than the maxilla. In the mandible the region of lingual tori and mylohyoid ridge are more prone to develop the complication, and in the maxilla the palatal tori is more often interested by ONJ [17, 39]. Cancer type should be taken into account as well, since multiple myelomas seem to be more prone to develop this complication [4, 27]. Moreover, the concomitant use of other drugs such as steroids and thalidomide may affect the bone biology as observed in some papers, but not confirmed by others [25]. Despite that lesions can be spontaneous, invasive dental procedure is one of the major risk factors for the development of BRONJ [17].

Etiopathology: Osteonecrosis and/or Osteomyelitis

The three main hypotheses about the etiopathology of BRONJ evaluate the importance of local infections, the damage of the microcirculation (antiangiogenetic effect of BP), and the inhibition of the bone remodeling. It is still unclear if the osteonecrosis is the consequence of an osteomyelitis or if the osteomyelitis is secondary to the necrosis. Antiangiogenetic mechanism has been proposed by Ruggiero based on several research data of BP in vitro and in vivo [4], while other hypothesis are in support of altered bone remodeling and local infection [4]. It is important to note that since the frequency of BRONJ is extremely low (between 0.8 and 12 % in i.v. BP), BP probably act in a multifactorial context leading to avascular necrosis by a multistep pathogenesis.

Clinical Presentation and Staging

The most widely used definition of BRONJ refers to the one given by the American Association of Oral and Maxillofacial Surgeons (AAOMS) in 2007 that refers to "patients with exposed bone of the maxillofacial region for at least 8 weeks (that) are currently on or have taken bisphosphonates and have no history of radiotherapy to the jaw" [17]. Differential diagnosis with similar conditions and delayed healing is necessary [16] as alveolar osteitis, sinusitis, gingivitis, and periodontal disease.

Based on the clinical presentation, BRONJ is classified into four stages (0–III) [16] (Table 14.2a).

Patients can present with asymptomatic exposed bone or can be symptomatic complaining pain, periapical/periodontal fistula, halitosis, tingling, and swollen gum.

An alternative definition and staging has been proposed by Bedogni that redefined BRONJ as follows: "bisphosphonate-related osteonecrosis of the jaw (BRONJ) is an adverse drug reaction described as the progressive destruction and death of bone that affects the mandible or maxilla of patients exposed to the treatment with nitrogen-containing bisphosphonates, in the absence of a previous radiation treatment" [19]. Bedogni proposes a staging on both clinical and radiological findings (Table 14.2b).

Table 14.2b Staging system proposed by Bedogni based on clinical and radiological findings

	Clinical signs and symptoms	CT findings
Stage 1 Focal BRONJ	Bone exposure	Increased bone density limited to the alveolar bone region (trabecular thickening and/or focal osteosclerosis), *with or without the following signs*:
	Sudden dental mobility	Markedly thickened and sclerotic lamina dura
	Nonhealing postextraction socket	Persisting alveolar socket
	Mucosal fistula	Cortical disruption
	Swelling of the gum	1a. Asymptomatic
	Abscess formation	1b. Symptomatic (pain and purulent discharge)
	Trismus	
	Gross mandibular deformity and/or hypoesthesia of the lips	
Stage 2 Diffuse BRONJ	Same signs and symptoms as stage 1	Increased bone density extended to the basal bone (diffuse osteosclerosis), *with or without the following signs*:
		Prominence of the inferior alveolar nerve canal
		Periosteal reaction
		Sinusitis
		Sequestrum formation
		Oral-antral fistula
		2a. Asymptomatic
		2b. Symptomatic (pain and purulent discharge)
Stage 3 Complicated BRONJ	Same signs and symptoms as stages 1 and 2, *with one or more of the following clinical signs and symptoms*:	Osteosclerosis of adjacent bones (zygoma, hard palate), pathologic mandibular fracture, and/or osteolysis extending to the sinus floor
	Extraoral fistula	
	Displaced mandibular stumps	
	Nasal leakage of fluids	

Modified from Bedogni et al. [19]

Prevention of BRONJ

The majority of available guidelines [16, 38] suggests oral examination and removal of unsalvageable teeth: complete all-invasive procedures and complete recovery before the start of BP treatment. It has been demonstrated that the prevention reduces the risk of BRONJ, without completely eliminating the risk. For patients that are already receiving treatment, the approach is not quite clear. Avoiding invasive procedures and adequate prophylaxis should be guaranteed. Still controversial is the utility of suspension of BP for a maximum of 3 months before dental procedures.

Patients receiving BP should be aware of the risk of ONJ and should be educated as to the importance of dental hygiene and to report any pain, swelling, or exposed bone [16].

Management of Patients Receiving Bisphosphonate in Endodontic Therapy and Endodontic Surgery

Dental extractions or invasive surgical procedure is considered one of the precipitating factors for the development of BRONJ [31, 43].

Nonsurgical endodontic treatment is preferred over extraction if pulpal disease is identified or for severely decayed teeth in patients with a history of receiving intravenous bisphosphonates or prolonged use of oral bisphosphonates [4, 33, 36]. In agreement with the position statement of the American Association of Endodontists of 2012, teeth to be extracted may be treated by crown resection, endodontic treatment of the roots, and restoration similar to preparing an overdenture abutment [44]. Moreover, nonsurgical root canal treatment is less traumatic to the oral tissue when compared to the extraction and is associated with ONJ only in 0.8 % of all cases [43].

When nonsurgical root canal treatment has failed, nonsurgical retreatment is considered as the first-choice treatment [45, 46].

Nonsurgical root canal treatment or retreatment has a success rate of up to 74 % for necrotic teeth with apical periodontitis [47]. Currently there are no data in the literature regarding the healing of periradicular lesions in patients taking intravenous bisphosphonates. We find only a short-term retrospective clinical and radiographic study that evaluated the healing of periradicular lesions in patients taking long-term oral bisphosphonates after nonsurgical root canal treatment. The authors conclude that these patients can expect a satisfactory outcome with evidence of periradicular healing [33].

When also nonsurgical root canal retreatment is impractical, surgical canal treatment is considered [45, 48]. The modern endodontic microsurgery is performed by using operating microscope, micro-instruments, ultrasonic tips, and biocompatible root-end filling materials and has a successful outcome in a follow-up of more than 1 year postoperatively in 89.0 % of cases [49, 50].

Currently there are few data about the outcome of surgical endodontic treatment in patients taking bisphosphonates. Sarathy et al. describe a case report where surgical endodontic treatment was a precipitating factor [36].

Surgical endodontic treatment is considered less invasive than tooth extraction, but several authors state that it is not recommended in patients taking bisphosphonates [36, 37, 51–53].

Surgical endodontic treatment should follow the same recommendation of any oral surgical procedures [54] and should be suggested to an assessment of the risk and potential benefits of the treatment for each individual patient [55].

Diagnostic Criteria for BRONJ/ARONJ

The diagnostic criteria for BRONJ developed by the American Association of Oral and Maxillofacial Surgeons include a history of bisphosphonate use, absence of radiotherapy to the head/neck, and presence of exposed bone in the maxilla or mandible persisting for more than 8 weeks. The guidelines were revised in 2009 to include patients with stage 0 disease, characterized as those with no evidence of necrotic bone but with the following: (1) nonspecific symptoms such as pain or odontalgia not explained by odontogenic causes or dull aching bone pain, (2) clinical findings including loosening of teeth not explained by chronic periodontal disease and/or periapical/periodontal fistula not associated with pulpal necrosis due to caries, or (3) radiographic findings including alveolar bone loss not attributable to chronic periodontal disease, trabecular bone alterations including dense woven bone, and persistent unremodeled bone in extraction sites, thickening of the lamina dura, and inferior alveolar canal narrowing [16].

Clinical judgment may underestimate the extent of bone involvement, and ARONJ may extend well beyond the exposed bone in the oral cavity. In addition, clinical judgment may underestimate the amount of bone resection if surgical treatment is planned [56].

A wide spectrum of radiographic features have been reported in ARONJ, with the emergence of typical patterns now readily identifiable in affected patients. These include osteosclerosis, thickened and disorganized medullary trabeculation, cortical disruption, increased thickness of the lamina dura and inferior alveolar nerve canal (IAN) margins, periosteal bone formation, and sequestration. Hutchinson et al. reported that in stage 0 patients with radiographic abnormalities, a consistent finding is the presence of osteosclerosis in clinically symptomatic areas, ranging from distinct focal density of the surrounding alveolar bone to more widespread involvement. In most patients the posterior mandible is involved, and prominence of the IAN canal, increased trabecular density, and lack of differentiation between cortical and medullary bone are common findings. Uniform periradicular radiolucencies are often noted in the mandibular cases, and one-third had evidence of buccal or lingual cortical disruption [57].

Radiological features of advanced clinically apparent ARONJ have been well documented, particularly by CT. Although CT scanning provides a three-dimensional reconstruction of bony architecture, it provides little information about local metabolic or vascular changes and therefore may not be as sensitive in detecting early lesions as is radionuclide imaging. In the study of Ryan and coworkers, 65.7 % of patients showed tracer uptake in areas that subsequently developed BRONJ. This sensitivity in detecting increased metabolic activity in the form of bone turnover is a precise though nonspecific indicator of vascularity and bone metabolism because labeled bisphosphonates depend on increased local osteoblastic activity. It has been speculated that bone turnover in ARONJ is actually greater than normal in response to bacterially mediated bone resorption. Therefore, scintigraphy may have prognostic value. Reports of negative bone scans in patients with known ARONJ indicate that scintigraphy may not detect photopenic foci, so-called cold lesions, possibly because of alterations in microcirculation due to microthrombotic occlusion. Early lesions in the maxilla, especially in avascular areas such as palatal tori, can be more difficult to detect because normal scintigrams frequently show mild uptake in the nasopharynx [58].

Cone beam computed tomography (CBCT) is adequate to investigate the prevalence of typical radiological findings of ARONJ, with the same accuracy of multislice CT. Anyway, during surgical therapy, the exact resection margins are not possible to be determined using any mode of imaging. CBCT imaging and multislice CT of BRONJ offer only the possibility of estimating the extent of the BRONJ lesion and depicting the involvement of important anatomical structures, for example, the mandibular nerve, the maxillary sinus, or the teeth. This information is essential if surgical therapy is considered. However, the substantial advantages of CBCT are its ready availability, the reduced radiation dose, and the lower cost in comparison with multislice CT [59].

The MRI showed two patterns of bone disease in ARONJ. In the first pattern, characteristic of exposed areas of diseased bone, low signal was observed in T1- and T2-weighted images, with a relatively low signal in inversion recovery images, which was suggestive of low water content. The second pattern, typical of unexposed diseased bone, was characterized by T1 hypointensity and T2 and inversion recovery hyperintensity, suggesting high water content. In advanced disease with extensive bone exposure, the two patterns coexist, with the second one being always present in a peripheral distribution [56].

Clinical Care of Patients with Established BRONJ/ARONJ

There are currently many protocols for the treatment strategies of ARONJ. These are recommendations published by manufacturers of drugs, scientific associations, or those based on literature reviews [17, 60–62]. At present, two different approaches can be differentiated: conservative approach including antibiotics, oral rinses, pain control, and limited debridement with the aim of reducing the stage of necrosis and avoiding progression which may be associated with surgery. These guidelines recommend invasive surgery only for large and extended necrosis [63].

When patients develop ARONJ, recommendations for the treatment approach to ARONJ depend on severity. Generally, a conservative approach is recommended with the use of antiseptic mouth rinse (0.12 % chlorhexidine gluconate) and broad-spectrum antibiotics (amoxicillin/clavulanic acid, metronidazole, or clindamycin). A limited surgery, including surface debridement, tooth extraction, necrotic bone sequestrectomy, or aggressive surgeries, such as resection of the affected bone, may be required in patients with more severe stages of ARONJ [52].

When dental treatment is performed on such a patient, the use of antiseptic mouth rinse (0.12 % chlorhexidine gluconate) and broad-spectrum antibiotics (amoxicillin/clavulanic acid, metronidazole, or clindamycin) has been recommended but not yet substantiated [32].

In Table 14.3, modified from Yamashita [52], we report the suggestion for the treatment goals, follow-up, and ONJ management.

Table 14.3 Management of patients with ONJ

Treatment objectives	Eliminate pain
	Control infection
	Reduce the progression or the occurrence of bone necrosis
Management of infections	Oral antimicrobial rinse
	Systemic antibiotic in case of infection
Conservative therapy	Remove sharp bone edges to prevent trauma to adjacent soft tissues
	Remove loose segments of bony sequestra avoiding the exposition of uninvolved bone
	Consider extraction of symptomatic teeth within exposed, necrotic bone
	Segmental jaw resection may be needed in case of symptomatic patients with extensive necrotic bone or pathologic fracture
Follow-up	Every 2–3 weeks
Prosthesis	Prosthesis appliances should be reevaluated for fit and soft denture relines may be recommended
Antiresorptive treatments	No scientific evidence to support discontinuation of antiresorptive agents to promote healing of the necrotic bone in the jaw

Modified from Yamashita and McCauley [52]

In contrast to these general guidelines, others already recommend surgical treatment at earlier stages with the aim of avoiding progression of the necrosis. There is a consensus that cases refractory to conservative management may benefit from investigational therapies [32]. The roles of surgical treatment and hyperbaric oxygen therapy are still under investigation. While a drug holiday for the administration of antiresorptive agents is recommended by several guidelines, there are no studies proving its efficacy. Comparing the results between conservative and surgical treatment, it seems that there is no difference regarding the success of treatment (e.g., 60.5 % vs. 60.4 %). This comparison is biased since, according to some recommendations, surgery is rather performed in cases with extended necrotic bone. However, if the results for acceptable healing and resolution of pain are compared between conservative and surgical treatment, the former shows worse outcomes than the group with surgical treatment. The group receiving surgical treatment has fewer new cases of ARONJ than the group with conservative treatment (e.g., 3.1 % vs. 8.1 %). Both results are related to the fact that surgical treatment is mostly performed in cases with a higher stage of ARONJ than for conservative treatment. It is not known to what extent early surgery might be beneficial for patients at a low stage when compared to conservative treatment. The higher stages are often associated with worse general health conditions that might negatively affect the surgical results. Unfortunately not every study on treatment outcomes revealed information concerning the staging and thereby extension and severity of the necrosis. However, it seems that total healing of ARONJ after conservative treatment is only successful in low stages [64, 65]. We conclude that conservative treatment might only lead to complete healing in stage I patients. The review performed by Kühl et al. [63] shows that surgical procedure in terms of exploration and resection of necrotic bone results in successful healing of 60 % (Fig. 14.2a–c). Although complete healing was not achievable in 20 %, patients showed at least a relief of pain. With regard to these results, almost 80 % of the patients had a direct benefit related to surgical intervention. Only 3 % showed worse outcomes with refractory healing and resolution of pain after surgery and 16.5 % were either lost to follow-up or showed the same stage. Most studies with surgical procedure included patients with high stages of necrosis. With regard to the poor conditions associated with high stages of necrosis in these groups, it might be concluded that surgical therapy in cases with low-grade necrosis might result in even higher success rates than if conservative treatment is performed. Evaluating the results of this review and taking

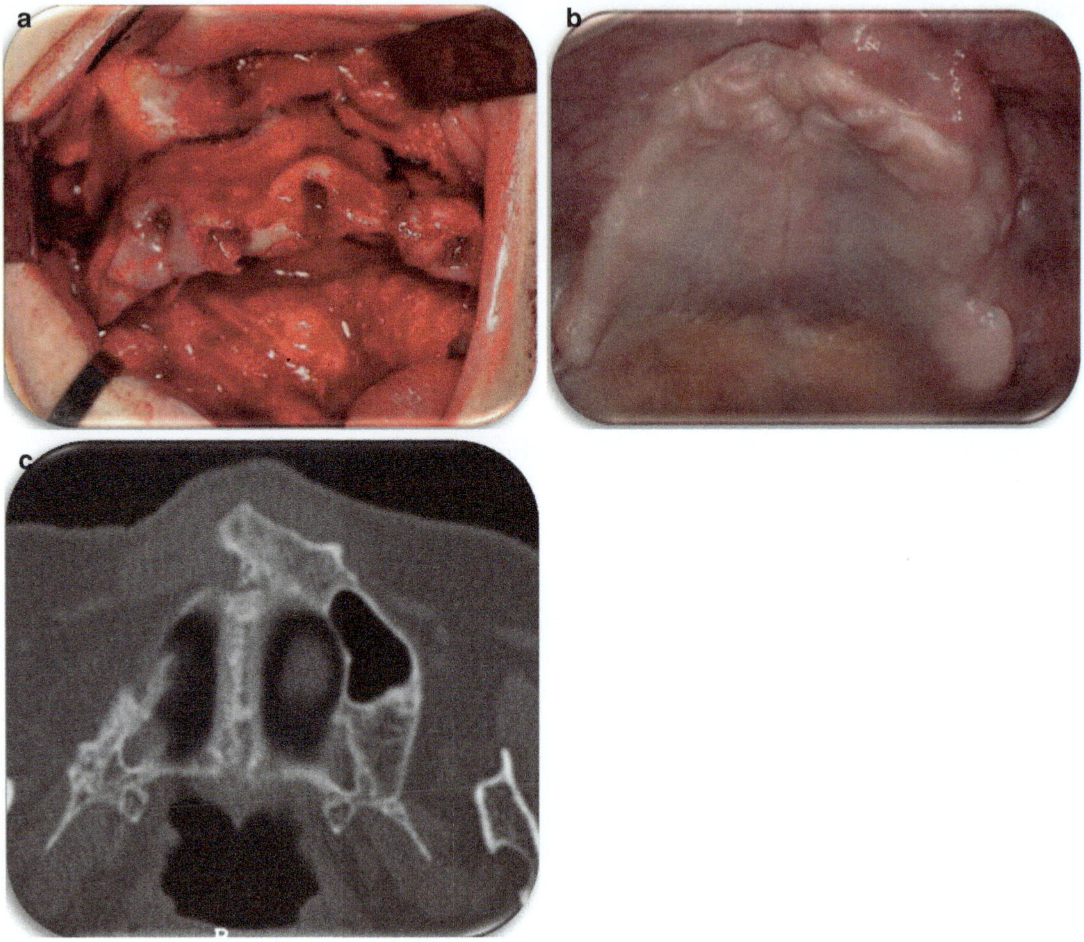

Fig. 14.2 (a) Lower right maxillectomy, followed by an accurate soft tissues suturing for a primary healing. (b) Intraoral view 6 months after the surgical treatment, with a good healing and relevant diminishing in pain. (c) Multislice CT performed at 6 months

our own experiences into account, we recommend conservative treatment as initial treatment for pain control and chronification of acute inflammatory signs before surgical treatment in any stage of ARONJ. Surgery, however, seems to be inevitable in most of the cases where complete and successful healing is the aim. Surgery may be avoided if complete healing appears during the initial phase of pain control, local disinfection (by mouth rinse or topical application of disinfectant paste), and administration of antibiotics. This, however, seems to be confined to a rather rare number of cases [63].

The histological analysis of bone margins is important to evaluate the appropriateness of bone resection as they were determined preoperatively only on the basis of CT and MR. Importantly the presence of osteomyelitis at one margin of resection was a predictor of ARONJ recurrence. It seems clear that clinical and radiological healing depend on the presence of healthy bone at the margins of resection. In fact, in the case series reported by Bedogni, all patients that relapsed during the follow-up had osteomyelitic involvement of the margins of resection. A resection margin was considered normal when its bone architecture was preserved and there were no signs of necrosis or inflammation. Presence of osteomyelitis in the resection margins is considered a predictor of ARONJ recurrence. CT signs of recurrent disease are apparent within 6 months after surgery and precede clinical manifestations of ARONJ [66].

The benefit of using ND:YAG laser stimulation or pulse application has not yet been proved. As yet there are no studies which have evaluated the level of evidence for trials published before 2010. The results of the present study show that the overall level of evidence concerning the incidence and treatment strategies for ARONJ is rather low [63].

It has been proposed that the serum C-terminal telopeptide (sCTX) levels, which reflect osteoclastic bone resorption, can be used as a useful biomarker for predicting the risk of ARONJ. CTX is a peptide fragment generated during collagen degradation by osteoclasts. Although type I collagen is found not only in mineralized matrix, sCTX levels are sensitive to bone resorption and, therefore, monitoring the sCTX level issued in some patients for assessing the efficacy of antiresorptive therapy. However, as individual wide variation exists in the levels of sCTX, it is difficult to assess the individual bone turnover state with a one-time point measurement. Without knowing sCTX levels at baseline (before antiresorptive therapy is commenced), it would be hard to infer the depth of osteoclast suppression from the sCTX levels of patients who are already on antiresorptive therapy. For these reasons, the use of sCTX as a risk predictor for ARONJ is not substantiated [52].

Follow-Up of Patients with BRONJ/ARONJ

Follow-up every 2–3 weeks is warranted by the American Association of Oral and Maxillofacial Surgeons [17].

In the publication by Bedogni, after surgical treatment is useful, the patients were followed up weekly for the first month, at 3-month intervals up to 1 year, and at 6-month intervals up to 2 years. At each visit, a visual analog score by Huskisson scale [67] for oral pain was obtained, and the oral mucosa inspected for early signs of ARONJ. At all visits a panoramic radiographs and CT scans were performed at 3, 6, 12, 18, and 24 months. CT and magnetic resonance (MR) imaging were used preoperatively to assess the degree of jawbone involvement and to define the margins of resection. CT signs of recurrent disease are apparent within 6 months after surgery and precede clinical manifestations of ARONJ [66].

Conclusions

In conclusion, despite the low frequency of this complication in patients receiving BP, ONJ can require a long time to recover and heal, sometimes interfering with the treatment of the oncological disease. For these reasons, dentists and maxillofacial surgeons need to work in close contact with oncohematologists, primary care physicians, and other specialists for the prevention and the treatment on BRONJ/ARONJ. Very few clear indications are available in the endodontic literature. Prevention is the cardinal point. Since endodontic surgery is an invasive procedure, and invasive procedures are considered a major risk factors for the development of this complication, it should be avoided, when possible, preferring other techniques. Once BRONJ/ARONJ manifests, we suggest to follow the major guidelines for conservative treatment, first, and eventually surgical procedures in the more advanced stages, with very close follow-up of the patients. A multidisciplinary approach of patients receiving antiresorptive agents is mandatory.

In conclusion, while nonsurgical retreatment is preferable, endodontic surgery might be a better and safer choice than extraction due to more frequent first-intention healing, less traumatic procedures, and possibly lower risk of infection, but no evidence-based data are currently available and future in vivo studies are necessary to support this hypothesis.

References

1. Brotons A, Penarrocha M. Orofacial neurogenic pain and maxillofacial ischemic osteonecrosis. A review. Med Oral. 2003;8(3):157–65.

2. Marx RE. Osteoradionecrosis: a new concept of its pathophysiology. J Oral Maxillofac Surg. 1983;41(5): 283–8.
3. Marx RE. Pamidronate (Aredia) and zoledronate (Zometa) induced avascular necrosis of the jaws: a growing epidemic. J Oral Maxillofac Surg. 2003; 61(9):1115–7.
4. Ruggiero SL, et al. Osteonecrosis of the jaws associated with the use of bisphosphonates: a review of 63 cases. J Oral Maxillofac Surg. 2004;62(5):527–34.
5. Migliorati CA, et al. Bisphosphonate-associated osteonecrosis of mandibular and maxillary bone: an emerging oral complication of supportive cancer therapy. Cancer. 2005;104(1):83–93.
6. Shlomi B, et al. Avascular necrosis of the jaw bone after bisphosphonate therapy. Harefuah. 2005;144(8): 536–9, 600, 599.
7. Vannucchi AM, et al. Osteonecrosis of the jaw associated with zoledronate therapy in a patient with multiple myeloma. Br J Haematol. 2005;128(6):738.
8. Purcell PM, Boyd IW. Bisphosphonates and osteonecrosis of the jaw. Med J Aust. 2005;182(8):417–8.
9. Bagan JV, et al. Jaw osteonecrosis associated with bisphosphonates: multiple exposed areas and its relationship to teeth extractions. Study of 20 cases. Oral Oncol. 2006;42(3):327–9.
10. Raje N, et al. Clinical, radiographic, and biochemical characterization of multiple myeloma patients with osteonecrosis of the jaw. Clin Cancer Res. 2008;14(8):2387–95.
11. Lazarovici TS, et al. Bisphosphonate-related osteonecrosis of the jaws: a single-center study of 101 patients. J Oral Maxillofac Surg. 2009;67(4):850–5.
12. Ruggiero SL. Guidelines for the diagnosis of bisphosphonate-related osteonecrosis of the jaw (BRONJ). Clin Cases Miner Bone Metab. 2007;4(1):37–42.
13. Drake MT, Clarke BL, Khosla S. Bisphosphonates: mechanism of action and role in clinical practice. Mayo Clin Proc. 2008;83(9):1032–45.
14. Rogers MJ, et al. Biochemical and molecular mechanisms of action of bisphosphonates. Bone. 2011;49(1): 34–41.
15. Pozzi S, Raje N. The role of bisphosphonates in multiple myeloma: mechanisms, side effects, and the future. Oncologist. 2011;16(5):651–62.
16. Ruggiero SL, et al. American Association of Oral and Maxillofacial Surgeons position paper on bisphosphonate-related osteonecrosis of the jaw – 2009 update. Aust Endod J. 2009;35(3):119–30.
17. Advisory Task Force on Bisphosphonate-Related Osteonecrosis of the Jaws, A.A.o.O. and S. Maxillofacial. American Association of Oral and Maxillofacial Surgeons position paper on bisphosphonate-related osteonecrosis of the jaws. J Oral Maxillofac Surg. 2007;65(3):369–76.
18. Colella G, Campisi G, Fusco V. American Association of Oral and Maxillofacial Surgeons position paper: Bisphosphonate-Related Osteonecrosis of the Jaws-2009 update: the need to refine the BRONJ definition. J Oral Maxillofac Surg. 2009;67(12):2698–9.
19. Bedogni A, et al. Learning from experience. Proposal of a refined definition and staging system for bisphosphonate-related osteonecrosis of the jaw (BRONJ). Oral Dis. 2012;18(6):621–3.
20. Troeltzsch M, et al. Physiology and pharmacology of nonbisphosphonate drugs implicated in osteonecrosis of the jaw. J Can Dent Assoc. 2012;78:c85.
21. Sivolella S, et al. Denosumab and anti-angiogenetic drug-related osteonecrosis of the jaw: an uncommon but potentially severe disease. Anticancer Res. 2013;33(5):1793–7.
22. Durie BG, Katz M, Crowley J. Osteonecrosis of the jaw and bisphosphonates. N Engl J Med. 2005;353(1):99–102; discussion 99–102.
23. Bamias A, et al. Osteonecrosis of the jaw in cancer after treatment with bisphosphonates: incidence and risk factors. J Clin Oncol. 2005;23(34):8580–7.
24. Dimopoulos MA, et al. Osteonecrosis of the jaw in patients with multiple myeloma treated with bisphosphonates: evidence of increased risk after treatment with zoledronic acid. Haematologica. 2006;91(7):968–71.
25. Pozzi S, et al. Bisphosphonate-associated osteonecrosis of the jaw: a review of 35 cases and an evaluation of its frequency in multiple myeloma patients. Leuk Lymphoma. 2007;48(1):56–64.
26. Zavras AI, Zhu S. Bisphosphonates are associated with increased risk for jaw surgery in medical claims data: is it osteonecrosis? J Oral Maxillofac Surg. 2006;64(6):917–23.
27. Wang EP, et al. Incidence of osteonecrosis of the jaw in patients with multiple myeloma and breast or prostate cancer on intravenous bisphosphonate therapy. J Oral Maxillofac Surg. 2007;65(7):1328–31.
28. Cafro AM, et al. Osteonecrosis of the jaw in patients with multiple myeloma treated with bisphosphonates: definition and management of the risk related to zoledronic acid. Clin Lymphoma Myeloma. 2008;8(2):111–6.
29. Hoff AO, et al. Frequency and risk factors associated with osteonecrosis of the jaw in cancer patients treated with intravenous bisphosphonates. J Bone Miner Res. 2008;23(6):826–36.
30. Borromeo GL, et al. A review of the clinical implications of bisphosphonates in dentistry. Aust Dent J. 2011;56(1):2–9.
31. Mavrokokki T, et al. Nature and frequency of bisphosphonate-associated osteonecrosis of the jaws in Australia. J Oral Maxillofac Surg. 2007;65(3):415–23.
32. McLeod NM, et al. Bisphosphonate osteonecrosis of the jaw: a literature review of UK policies versus international policies on the management of bisphosphonate osteonecrosis of the jaw. Br J Oral Maxillofac Surg. 2011;49(5):335–42.
33. Hsiao A, Glickman G, He J. A retrospective clinical and radiographic study on healing of periradicular lesions in patients taking oral bisphosphonates. J Endod. 2009;35(11):1525–8.
34. Gallego L, et al. Rubber dam clamp trauma during endodontic treatment: a risk factor of bisphosphonate-related osteonecrosis of the jaw? J Oral Maxillofac Surg. 2011;69(6):e93–5.

35. Goodell G. Bisphosphonate-associated osteonecrosis of the jaws and endodontic treatment: two case reports. J Mass Dent Soc. 2006;55(1):44–8.
36. Sarathy AP, Bourgeois Jr SL, Goodell GG. Bisphosphonate-associated osteonecrosis of the jaws and endodontic treatment: two case reports. J Endod. 2005;31(10):759–63.
37. Katz H. Endodontic implications of bisphosphonate-associated osteonecrosis of the jaws: a report of three cases. J Endod. 2005;31(11):831–4.
38. Campisi G, et al. BRONJ expert panel recommendation of the Italian Societies for Maxillofacial Surgery (SICMF) and Oral Pathology and Medicine (SIPMO) on Bisphosphonate-Related Osteonecrosis of the Jaws: risk assessment, preventive strategies and dental management. It J Maxillofac Surg. 2011;22(2):103–24.
39. Sedghizadeh PP, et al. Population pharmacokinetic and pharmacodynamic modeling for assessing risk of bisphosphonate-related osteonecrosis of the jaw. Oral Surg Oral Med Oral Pathol Oral Radiol. 2013;115(2):224–32.
40. Terpos E, et al. The use of bisphosphonates in multiple myeloma: recommendations of an expert panel on behalf of the European myeloma network. Ann Oncol. 2009;20(8):1303–17.
41. Van Poznak CH, Von Roenn JH, Temin S. American society of clinical oncology clinical practice guideline update: recommendations on the role of bone-modifying agents in metastatic breast cancer. J Oncol Pract. 2011;7(2):117–21.
42. National Osteoporosis Foundation. http://www.nof.org/files/nof/public/content/resource/913/files/580.pdf.
43. Marx RE, et al. Bisphosphonate-induced exposed bone (osteonecrosis/osteopetrosis) of the jaws: risk factors, recognition, prevention, and treatment. J Oral Maxillofac Surg. 2005;63(11):1567–75.
44. Statement, A.A.o.E.P. Endodontic implications of bisphosphonate-associated Osteonecrosis of the jaws. 2010;1–4.
45. Siqueira Jr JF. Aetiology of root canal treatment failure: why well-treated teeth can fail. Int Endod J. 2001;34(1):1–10.
46. Nair PN, et al. Intraradicular bacteria and fungi in root-filled, asymptomatic human teeth with therapy-resistant periapical lesions: a long-term light and electron microscopic follow-up study. J Endod. 1990;16(12):580–8.
47. Friedman S, Abitbol S, Lawrence HP. Treatment outcome in endodontics: the Toronto Study. Phase 1: initial treatment. J Endod. 2003;29(12):787–93.
48. Gutmann JL, Harrison JW. Posterior endodontic surgery: anatomical considerations and clinical techniques. Int Endod J. 1985;18(1):8–34.
49. Song M, Shin SJ, Kim E. Outcomes of endodontic micro-resurgery: a prospective clinical study. J Endod. 2011;37(3):316–20.
50. Tsesis I, et al. Outcomes of surgical endodontic treatment performed by a modern technique: an updated meta-analysis of the literature. J Endod. 2013;39(3):332–9.
51. Moinzadeh AT, et al. Bisphosphonates and their clinical implications in endodontic therapy. Int Endod J. 2013;46(5):391–8.
52. Yamashita J, McCauley LK. Antiresorptives and osteonecrosis of the jaw. J Evid Based Dent Pract. 2012;12(3 Suppl):233–47.
53. Kalra S, Jain V. Dental complications and management of patients on bisphosphonate therapy: a review article. J Oral Biol Craniofac Res. 2013;3(1):25–30.
54. Hellstein JW, et al. Managing the care of patients receiving antiresorptive therapy for prevention and treatment of osteoporosis: executive summary of recommendations from the American Dental Association Council on Scientific Affairs. J Am Dent Assoc. 2011;142(11):1243–51.
55. Fantasia JE. Bisphosphonates – what the dentist needs to know: practical considerations. J Oral Maxillofac Surg. 2009;67(5 Suppl):53–60.
56. Bedogni A, et al. Bisphosphonate-associated jawbone osteonecrosis: a correlation between imaging techniques and histopathology. Oral Surg Oral Med Oral Pathol Oral Radiol Endod. 2008;105(3):358–64.
57. Hutchinson M, et al. Radiographic findings in bisphosphonate-treated patients with stage 0 disease in the absence of bone exposure. J Oral Maxillofac Surg. 2010;68(9):2232–40.
58. O'Ryan FS, et al. Intravenous bisphosphonate-related osteonecrosis of the jaw: bone scintigraphy as an early indicator. J Oral Maxillofac Surg. 2009;67(7):1363–72.
59. Wilde F, et al. Prevalence of cone beam computed tomography imaging findings according to the clinical stage of bisphosphonate-related osteonecrosis of the jaw. Oral Surg Oral Med Oral Pathol Oral Radiol. 2012;114(6):804–11.
60. Khosla S, et al. Bisphosphonate-associated osteonecrosis of the jaw: report of a task force of the American Society for Bone and Mineral Research. J Bone Miner Res. 2007;22(10):1479–91.
61. American Dental Association Council on Scientific, A. Dental management of patients receiving oral bisphosphonate therapy: expert panel recommendations. J Am Dent Assoc. 2006;137(8):1144–50.
62. Migliorati CA, et al. Managing the care of patients with bisphosphonate-associated osteonecrosis: an American Academy of Oral Medicine position paper. J Am Dent Assoc. 2005;136(12):1658–68.
63. Kuhl S, et al. Bisphosphonate-related osteonecrosis of the jaws–a review. Oral Oncol. 2012;48(10):938–47.
64. Van den Wyngaert T, et al. Initial experience with conservative treatment in cancer patients with osteonecrosis of the jaw (ONJ) and predictors of outcome. Ann Oncol. 2009;20(2):331–6.
65. Thumbigere-Math V, et al. Bisphosphonate-related osteonecrosis of the jaw: clinical features, risk factors, management, and treatment outcomes of 26 patients. J Oral Maxillofac Surg. 2009;67(9):1904–13.
66. Bedogni A, et al. Long-term outcomes of surgical resection of the jaws in cancer patients with bisphosphonate-related osteonecrosis. Oral Oncol. 2011;47(5):420–4.
67. Huskisson EC. Measurement of pain. J Rheumatol. 1982;9(5):768–9.

Medicolegal Consideration in Endodontics: General and Surgical Aspects

15

Lars Bjørndal, Henrik Nielsen, and Vibe Rud

Abstract

Patient injuries in relation to medical treatment and in particular conventional or surgical endodontics might under certain circumstances trigger a wish for economical compensation. In many parts of the world, the patient would have to take the practitioner into a civil court to get compensation. However, in a number of countries, there is a legislation which deals with injuries in relation to medical treatment and compensation. Medicolegal considerations in relation to endodontic treatment are in a few countries particularly detailed. Endodontic complaints and insurance cases are relatively frequently occurring. A subcategorization of endodontic complaints shows that the suboptimal root filling represents a potential risk for complaints. Endodontic surgery as an area of claim per se seems lesser involved than conventional endodontics. Statistics about endodontic claims may indicate where risk management and educational efforts can be most effectively directed to improve the standard of care. "Lessons to learn" are presented only in cases where the "complained tooth" has been treated with the use of endodontic surgery.

L. Bjørndal, DDS, PhD, Dr Odont (✉)
Section of Cariology & Endodontics and Pediatric & Clinical Genetics, Department of Odontology, University of Copenhagen, Nørre Allé 20, Copenhagen N DK-2200, Denmark
e-mail: labj@sund.ku.dk

H. Nielsen, DDS, PhD
Department of Oral and Maxillofacial Surgery, Centre of Head and Orthopaedics, Rigshospitalet, Blegdamsvej 3, Østerbro DK-2100, Denmark
e-mail: henrik.paul.nielsen@rh.regionh.dk

V. Rud, DDS
Private Practice in Surgery and Endodontics, Puggaardsgade 17 st.th, Copenhagen DK-1573, Denmark
e-mail: rud@endokir.dk

Malpractice in a General Dental Practitioner Environment

From a historical perspective [1], it is a relatively new concept to be able to question the standard of care as carried out by a physician. In this chapter, we will describe the general complaint profile as well as the specific handling of endodontic claims and actual malpractice cases as experienced in some countries. Several recent reports (Table 15.1) have been published based on databases. This has brought more insight to how liability claims between the patient and the dentist have been managed. Although a detailed

I. Tsesis (ed.), *Complications in Endodontic Surgery*,
DOI 10.1007/978-3-642-54218-3_15,

Table 15.1 Medicolegal data from countries disclosing malpractice data, the different origin of the source, the study period, the total numbers of dental malpractice/complaint, and the proportion of the endodontic-related complaints

Reference	Country	Source of data	Study period	Total no. of dental malpractice/ complaints	Endodontic-related malpractice/ complaints no. (%)
René and Öwall [2]	Sweden	NHI[a] and Swedish DA[b]	1947–1983	1,599	206 (12.9)
Milgrom et al. [3]	USA	Self-reported questionnaire	1988–1992	215	39 (18.1)
Ozdemir et al. [4]	Turkey	Ministry of Health	1991–2000	11	2 (18.2)
Hapcook [5]	USA	Private insurance	2006	–	– (17.0)
Bjørndal and Reit [6]	Denmark	NHI and Danish DA[b]	1995–2004	5,407	742 (13.8)
Kiani and Sheikhazadi [7]	Iran	Expert committee	2002–2006	277	46 (16.6)
Givol et al. [8]	Israel	Insurance company	1992–2008	5,217	720 (13.8)
Pinchi et al. [9]	Italy	Insurance and ANDI[c]	2006–2010	1,230	237 (19.3)

[a]National Health Insurance
[b]Dental Association
[c]National Association of Italian Dentists

comparison is difficult, the proportion of the endodontic area is comparable in between the countries.

Furthermore, some lessons to be learned will be suggested in this chapter. What are the major reasons for claims within general endodontics as well as endodontic surgery per se? What is the typical fate of the "complained tooth," and how is it treated in the aspect of endodontic surgery?

The Medicolegal System Worldwide

The tradition of having a general dental practitioner (GDP)-related insurance, in case of treatment injuries, has in a few countries been an obligation. In other countries, the GDPs are mainly encouraged to be involved with an insurance company. Medicolegal activities may again in other countries only be dealt with in a civil court.

As evidenced from Israel and Italy [8, 9], most of the dental practitioners are obligated to report any incidence or suspicion of a legal action against them, as part of their professional liability insurance terms. In the USA, the GDPs are encouraged to handle dental office incidents and claims properly by early discussion with the insurance company [5]. Based on data from Turkey and Iran, it is apparent that only very few cases are enrolled in the published reports, being civil court cases, and these few cases do not reflect the actual number of complaint cases [4, 7]. In the Nordic countries, there is a complaint and an insurance system described below as "the Nordic model."

The Nordic Model

A brief description of complaint management with respect to medicolegal and insurance legislation in Denmark and Sweden follows. The Nordic model has been chosen, because the international tradition in covering complaints and insurance cases within a broader platform of legislation appears limited.

The Complaint System

In Denmark and Sweden, the medicolegal system handling complaints is closely related to health legislation. In both countries, complaints are managed by local committees or regional dental complaint boards (DCB) consisting of members from the Dental Association and officials. The committee makes administrative decisions based on best clinical practice and legislation [2, 6, 10]. Following a complaint from the patient and based on the patient file, the DCB gives a written statement, which includes a decision of malpractice or no malpractice. If the decision of the boards is consistent with malpractice, the dentist has to return the fee for the treatment to the patient. In other cases, the DCB may propose a settlement, where the dentist in question accepts to cover the patients' expenses for re-treatment provided by another practitioner. The dentist or the patient may appeal the decision to a national dental complaint board (NDCB). Besides dentists and laypeople, the NDCB also includes a civil court judge. The NDCB might temper, affirm, intensify, or reject the regional DCB's decision. If one of the parties still is dissatisfied, the decision can be brought to a civil court.

The Insurance System

In Denmark, patient insurance has been a part of health care legislation since 1992. With modification, the law now covers all kinds of treatment independently if the treatment is given in a private or public context. The financial resource for legislation and insurance is primarily founded by the government. However, the dentists pay a premium depending on their revenues.

The insurance in Denmark is a no-fault insurance. This means that it is not a matter of establishing if the practitioner has made a mistake. The important thing is to establish if the treatment per se leaves the patient in a situation where the status of the dentition has deteriorated. Additionally, a re-treatment is not possible to reestablish the patient's tooth/dentition. Finally, it is important to distinguish between well-known complications to a particular treatment and injuries. To do so, four principles are used:

1. Would another specialist have done it differently?
2. Could another method have been used?
3. Is the injury caused by apparatus fail?
4. Must the patient tolerate more discomfort than the average patient?

To describe the content of the four principles, the following should be observed:

Ad 1. Is it is possible to think of a hypothetical GDP who would have chosen another treatment based on best evidence and by that avoided the injury?

Ad 2. Is it be possible to treat the patient with another method and achieve the same result but without the risk of injury?

Ad 3. For example, if the injury is caused by a separated instrument or device.

Ad 4. It is a well-known fact that treatment often implies discomfort. However, a nerve injury in relation to conventional endodontics would be anticipated as more discomfort than the average patient would experience.

In Sweden, a similar no-fault compensation system has been introduced. The purpose has been to provide the patient who suffered a treatment injury with the right to be compensated, regardless of whether the injury had been established by negligence or not [11]. Concomitantly, the system can chase those dentists providing dental care where they were responsible for negligence under tort law.

In cases where the patient cannot accept the decision made in the insurance system, the Danish system has an appeal board. If it is still not acceptable to the patient, the patient can bring the decision to a civil court [12].

Hypotheses on Frequency and Areas of Malpractice Claims

Should we expect complaints within endodontics, some suggested hypotheses (H) are presented:

(*H1*) The frequency of root canal treatment has increased over the last decades [13]; therefore, the number of endodontically related malpractice claims should be rising.

(*H2*) Internationally, root fillings are often of substandard technical quality in a GDP environment [14–16] rarely performed with the use of rubber dam [17, 18], and a high frequency of persistent periapical inflammatory lesions is noted.

(*H3*) Molars predominate the treatment panorama, and if only a few endodontic specialists are available to refer complicated cases to (as in countries without endodontic specialist training), malpractice claims are expected to reflect this situation and to a substantial part be associated with the results of

Table 15.2 The top three most frequent areas of malpractice cases/complaint cases as described in actual references

René and Öwall [2]	Prosthodontics 36.8 %	Formalities 13.6 %	Endodontics 12.4 %
Milgrom et al. [3]	Oral surgery (21.9 %)	Prosthodontics (19.5 %)	Endodontics (18.1 %)
Ozdemir et al. [4]	Oral surgery (45.6 %)	Prosthodontics (36.4 %)	Endodontics (18.2 %)
Hapcook [5]	Prosthodontics (28 %)	Endodontics (17 %)	Restorative (16 %)
Bjørndal and Reit [6]	Prosthodontics (30.78 %)	Endodontics (13.8 %)	Diagnostics (12.3 %)
Kiani and Sheikhazadi [7]	Prosthodontics (27.8 %)	Oral surgery (23.5 %)	Endodontics (16.6 %)
Givol et al. [8]	Prosthodontics (28.0 %)	Oral surgery (16.0 %)	Endodontics (13.8 %)
Pinchi et al. [9]	Implant (25 %)	Prosthodontics (24 %)	Endodontics (19.3 %)

Notably, prosthodontics and endodontics have been present in all reports

defective root fillings and technical treatment complications.

(*H4*) Malpractice claims in endodontic surgery are seldom, because it is often introduced to save the "complained tooth" from extraction.

Frequency of Dental Malpractice Claims

In a study of Swedish malpractice cases, less than 1 malpractice case per 1,000 dentists was detected in the period from 1977 to 1983 [2]. In the USA, the number of general malpractice cases per 1,000 dentists increased from 11 to 27 malpractice cases in the period from 1988 to 1992 [3], and more recent statistics from 2007 shows that dentist with at least 1 filed claim increased from 27 per 1,000 dentist to 40 per 1,000 dentist [19].

In Denmark, from 1995 to 2004, the number of malpractice cases increased from 4 to 5 per 1,000 dentists [6]. Dental malpractice claims per 100,000 patients have been relatively constant covering a 10-year period from 1995 to 2004 in Denmark. However, in urban areas the frequency of claims was over the mean of the country (24.7 versus 13.1, respectively) [6]. A similar difference between urban and rural areas was reported in Sweden [2].

In short, medicolegal reports on endodontics are frequently received by the complaint boards and/or insurance systems/companies. As when it comes to the variation in claim frequency, the medicolegal systems vary between countries, and direct comparisons are difficult to make, but in general complaints from patients about dental treatments are internationally rising [7].

Areas of Malpractice Claims

Endodontic treatment and prosthodontics have been among the three most frequently listed complaint areas during the past decades (Table 15.2). Notably, oral surgery seems to be lesser involved within recent years, whereas implant placements are a new growing area of malpractice complaints. The latest report has implant as the number one most frequent claim area [9].

General Endodontics

A subcategorization of endodontic complaints has shown that a major problem is the inadequate root filling quality [6]. In particular, the short root filling appears to be dominating (Fig. 15.1). Perforations represent another high-risk area followed by intra-canal separated instruments. Also the inappropriate use of outdated medicaments produces malpractice claims. Paraformaldehyde application led in all reported cases in Denmark to a decision of malpractice [6].

Altered nerve sensation following root canal treatment is occurring in the mandibular. A typical profile for a complaint of an altered nerve sensation [20] is a female having problems in relation to a second mandibular molar associated with overfilling. Of particular interest, none of these claims were reported by the practitioner, and all cases were obtained as a result of the patient's demand for economical compensation, either by confronting the dentist or by legal actions [20].

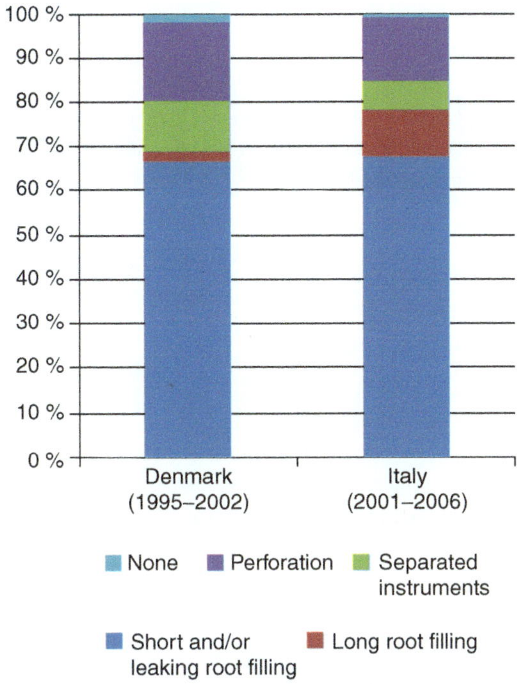

Fig. 15.1 Relative distribution of technical complications in endodontics (malpractice cases) based on data from Denmark and Italy

Vertical root fracture in root-filled teeth is another challenging complication clinically as well as medicolegally. In-depth analysis of vertical root fracture in endodontically treated teeth has shown that premolar and mandibular molar teeth are more prone to medicolegal claims. Moreover, a suboptimal root filling complicates the diagnosis of vertical root fracture, thus extending the required time for obtaining an accurate diagnosis and hereby increasing the medicolegal risk [21]. Data from the dental insurance appeals board in Denmark from 2008 to 2012 has been published [12] listing the number and the reasons of all the appeals. The frequency of the endodontic-related appeals comprises 20.2 % ($n=163$) of all the cases ($n=806$). These cases were further subcategorized into nerve damage, separated root canal instruments, root perforation, and fractured roots in root-filled teeth. Several additional endodontic-related appeals are listed as *causa sequela*. The primary pathology had progressed, and the actual problem is established by negligence.

Endodontic Surgery

Endodontic surgery is not one of the major reported claim areas, but injuries could be an improper flap design leading to gingival retraction or the presence of visible scar tissue. Also, altered nerve sensation may occur after endodontic surgery. Notably, complaints about altered nerve sensation happen most often in conventional endodontics as opposed to surgery, whereas surgery in relation to implant placement represents the most frequent complaints with respect to altered nerve sensation [20]. Other claim reasons for endodontic surgery could be a persistent pathology due to an insufficient retrograde root filling, or a treatment carried out on a wrong tooth.

The Fate of the "Complained Tooth"

From a medicolegal consideration, it appears that the gender of the clinician and the complainant as well as their communication in between plays an important role. In some reports an overrepresentation of male dentists is seen, but also an overrepresentation of female complainants has been observed [6, 20]. These data support the importance of the patient-doctor communication in these potential malpractice cases and indicate that the professional communication has a gender aspect [22–25]. Qualitative interview data confirms that a more patient-centered communication is found among female doctors [23] that might decrease the risk of being involved in liability claims. The so-called frustrating patient visit [26] may continue when a treatment decision of the "complained tooth" has to be carried out. In case of a critical relationship between the dentist and the patient, irrational treatment solutions may be chosen.

A common solution seems to be to extract the "complained tooth." Data indicate that close to 50 % of the teeth were extracted in case of a short root filling; almost 90 % were extracted if the actual tooth was perforated. Finally, all teeth were extracted, if a separated file was diagnosed [9]. Therefore, it is important to recall the reasonable prognosis for both surgical and nonsurgical endodontic re-treatment [27–29], including the

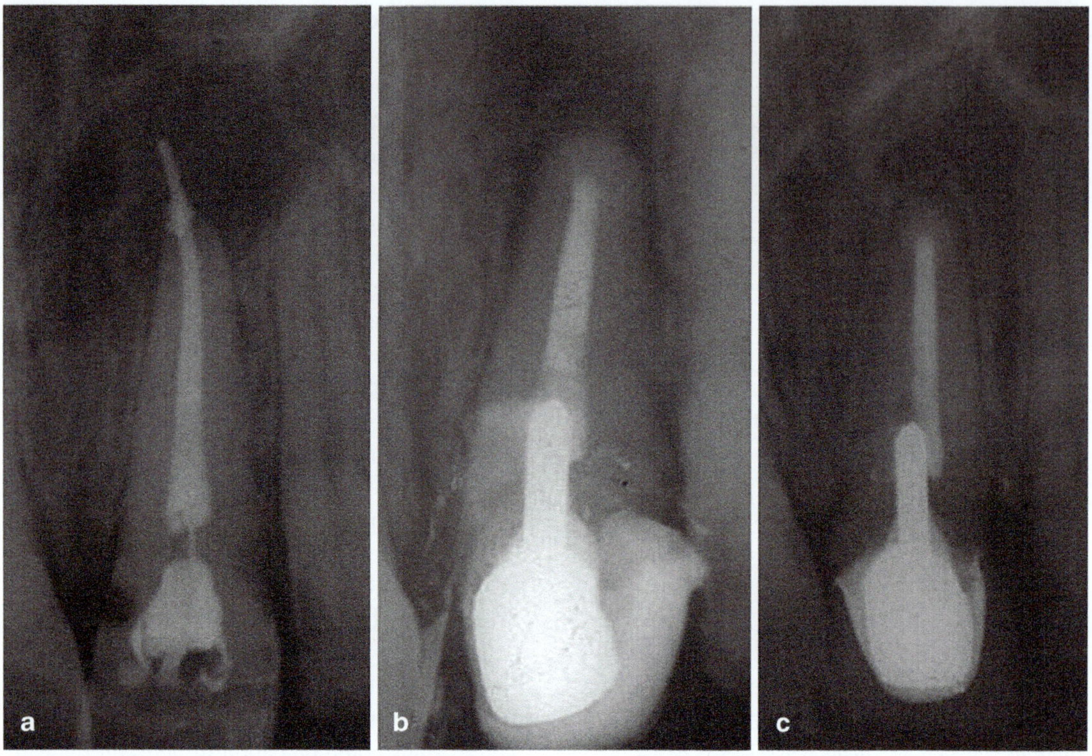

Fig. 15.2 Preoperative x-ray of first maxillary incisor with overfilling (**a**). Postoperative x-ray (**b**) showing the application of a retrograde root filling (composite with a dentin-bonding agent). A 9-year follow-up disclosing complete healing (**c**)

removal of intra-canal separated instruments [30]. Also, the sealing of perforations in the tooth may be performed with a good prognosis [31].

Taking the critical situation into account in between the complainant and the GDP, several teeth might be saved if conventional or surgical re-treatment is suggested, in contrast to extraction. To illustrate this dilemma, four cases are presented to show the use of endodontic surgery, as an alternative to extraction, including lessons to be learned.

Endodontic Surgery Case I

Subject: A sustained apical pathology is observed in relation to a first maxillary incisor. The primary dentist did not report about the overfilling. *Gender*: Male. *Age*: 17. *Year*: 1984.

Facts of the Case: The patient has made a complaint about a sustained infection in relation to a treated maxilla incisor (Fig. 15.2a).

Decision from GDP Insurance: The patient gets financial compensation for the treatment needed, as the patient was not informed about the suboptimal overfilling.

The Treatment of the Injured Teeth: The tooth was treated by apical surgery using a dentin-bonding agent and a composite resin. A 9- and 20-year follow-up are shown (Fig. 15.2b, c).

Lessons to Be Learned: Factors reducing the overfill include optimal measures on working length, such as an apex locator (combined with an x-ray confirmation), including an x-ray control of the master cone before obturation.

Endodontic Surgery Case II

Subject: A furcal radiolucency is noted after a crown and post restoration of a mandibular molar. The dentist was not aware of the complication. *Gender*: Female. *Age*: 45. *Year*: 1998.

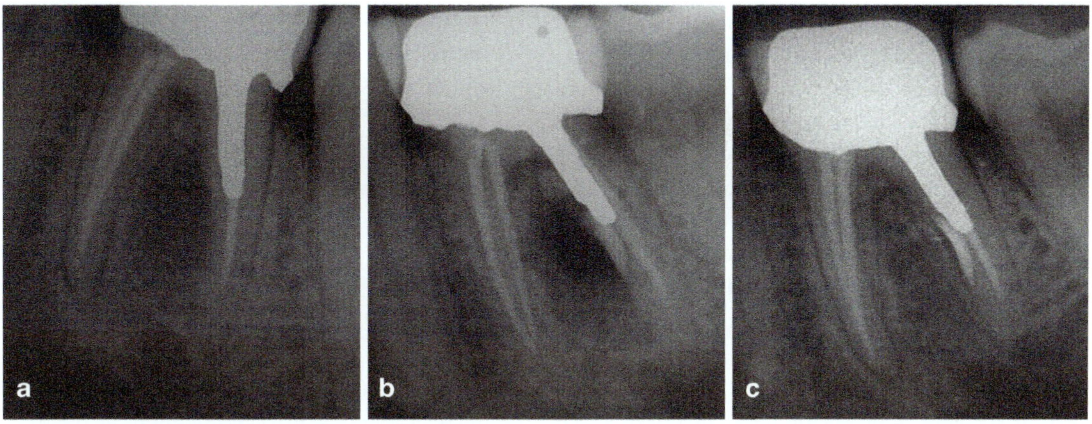

Fig. 15.3 Preoperative x-ray of first mandibular molar with a root perforation following a post preparation. Furcal radiolucency is noted at the distal root (**a**). Postoperative x-ray after endodontic surgery using composite with a dentin-bonding agent (**b**). A 1-year follow-up shows complete healing (**c**)

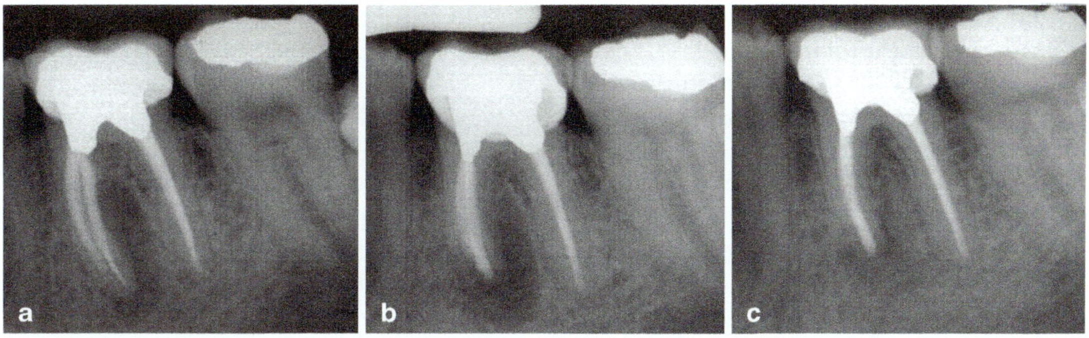

Fig. 15.4 Radiographical follow-up of first mandibular molar with a separated file in the mesial root. The patient has acute infection following the completed root canal treatment (**a**). Postoperative x-ray after endodontic surgery using MTA (**b**). A 1-year follow-up shows developing healing (**c**)

Facts of the Case: A new dentist discovers a radiolucency in between the roots following a radiographical control of the region (Fig. 15.3a). On this basis the patient makes a complaint about the tooth, and the new dentist suggests an implant placement.

Decision from GDP Insurance: It is decided that endodontic surgery is indicated. The patient gets financial support for the treatment needed.

The Treatment of the Injured Teeth: Based on a well-documented treatment protocol [30], the tooth was treated by apical surgery using a dentin-bonded composite resin (Fig. 15.3b, c).

Lessons to Be Learned: Knowledge about root morphology is essential during post preparation. In particular, the distal root of the mandibular molar may present different outlines of the root canals, and often they may have two orifices. Therefore, a central post preparation is critical and should be avoided. In fact, post should only be placed when essential for additional core support to avoid medicolegal risk [21].

Endodontic Surgery Case III

Subject: A file has separated in the mesial root component in a mandibular molar, and acute apical periodontitis has developed (Fig. 15.4a).

Facts of the Case: The patient has made a complaint about a sudden acute apical pathology in a previous root-filled tooth. A radiographical status discloses a separated instrument in the mesial root.

Decision from GDP Insurance: The patient gets financial support for the treatment needed.

The Treatment of the Injured Teeth: The mesial root was surgically treated using MTA. A 1-year follow-up compared to postoperative x-ray shows developing healing (Fig. 15.4b, c).

Lessons to Be Learned: When overfill or extrusion of the root filling material occurs, the risk of an additive altered sensation in the mandibular is present. Even though overfilling appears to be the least occurring root filling complication (Fig. 15.1), the following profile was identified in a retrospective analysis of patients [20]: A primary root canal treatment has been performed in the second mandibular molar, and in the vast majority of the cases, an overfill and altered sensation are present. None of the cases were reported by the GDP causing the problem. As the pain debut often is noted within the first 48 h after the treatment, it is very important to inform the patient about such a complication. Thus, in case of an overfilled root canal with the described details, the GDP should consider early action, which may include referral to endodontic surgery.

Conclusion

The specific medicolegal consideration is a changing entity due to new advances within the understanding of the specific disease causing the problem, and with this follows the adoption of new treatment technology. The medicolegal consideration should always be fully integrated with the perception of "standard of care," as well as an awareness of the patients' and dentists' rights.

Malpractice claim statistics may indicate where risk management and educational efforts can be most effectively directed to improve the standard of care.

Endodontic surgery is seemingly not the main cause of a malpractice case. However, endodontic surgery is typically involved to solve a complaint that has occurred in relation to a tooth. It is suggested that many teeth may be saved with a good prognosis if endodontic surgery is considered as opposed to extraction.

Taken together, the high prevalence of root fillings with substandard technical quality, in populations in general, represents the main reason for a medicolegal consideration in endodontics.

An Endodontic Surgery Protocol Where an Apical Box Preparation Is Impossible

As endodontic surgery may be the last option (otherwise the tooth will be extracted), a protocol follows that may save numerous teeth from extraction.

The protocol comprises the use of a composite and a dentin-bonding agent as retrograde root filling material (Case I and II). The protocol may be recommended for any case of apical surgery [31], but it is particularly applicable in cases where a traditional cavity preparation may be difficult, as following a root perforation (Fig. 15.3).

Preparation of the Root Surfaces: The resected surface is made slightly concave by the use of a large round bur. This approach facilitates the precise application of the composite retrograde filling material to the entire resected root surface. For preparation in conjunction with a post perforation, a well-defined zone of dentin is needed surrounding the perforation area (Case II, Fig. 15.3)

Hemostasis: Local anesthesia containing adrenaline is used. After osteotomy the bone cavity is cleaned with curettes and excavators and followed by meticulously removal of all granulation tissue. A hemostatic sponge moisture with maximum two to four drops of adrenaline (1 %) is placed for 2 min. in the bone cavity. Additional control of hemorrhage is applied using needle suction.

Application of EDTA and a Dentin-Bonding Agent: When hemostasis is established, EDTA is scrubbed on the resected root surface using a miniature brush soaked in 0.5 M EDTA (pH 7.4) for 20 s. After copious flow of saline and drying with compressed air, a dentin-bonding agent Gluma (Gluma Desensitizer, Heraeus Kulzer G.m.b.H, Wehrheim, Germany) is applied with a miniature brush to the resected surface/root perforation area for 20 s and thoroughly dried with compressed air.

Application of Composite: The resected root surface/root perforation area is covered with a thin layer of chemically curing composite resin (Retroplast™, Retroplast Trading, Rørvig, Denmark) by the use of a small excavator. After 2 min. curing, the unpolymerized surface layer is washed with 96 % ethanol and then rinsed with saline. The procedure with ethanol is repeated twice.

References

1. Medical malpractice, from world of health [Internet]. 2007 [Cited 2013 Mar 30]. Available from: http://www.bookrags.com/research/medical-malpractice.woh/.
2. René N, Öwall B. Dental malpractice in Sweden. J Law Ethics Dent. 1991;4:16–31.
3. Milgrom P, Fiset L, Whitney C, Conrad D, Cullen T, O'Hara D. Malpractice claims during 1988–1992: a national survey of dentists. J Am Dent Assoc. 1994;125:462–9.
4. Ozdemir MH, Saracoglu A, Ozdemir AU, Ergonen AT. Dental malpractice in Turkey during 1991–2000. J Clin Forensic Med. 2005;12:137–42.
5. Hapcook Sr CP. Dental malpractice claims. Percentages and procedures. J Am Dent Assoc. 2006;137:1444–5.
6. Bjørndal L, Reit C. Endodontic malpractice claims in Denmark 1995–2004. Int Endod J. 2008;41:1059–65.
7. Kiani M, Sheikhazadi A. A five-year survey for dental malpractice claims in Teheran, Iran. J Forensic Leg Med. 2009;16:76–82.
8. Givol N, Rosen E, Taicher S, Tsesis I. Risk management in endodontics. J Endod. 2010;36:982–4.
9. Pinchi V, PRadelle F, Gasparetto L, Norelli G-A. Trends in endodontic claims in Italy. Int Dent J. 2013;63:43–8.
10. Schwarz E. Patient complaints of dental malpractice in Denmark 1983–86. Community Dent Oral Epidemiol. 1988;16:143–7.
11. Cronström R, René N, Öwall B, Blomqvist A. The Swedish patient insurance scheme and guarantee insurance for prosthodontic treatment. Int Dent J. 1992;42:113–7.
12. Insurance appeals board on treatment injuries (Tandskadeankenævnet). Copenhagen Available from: http://www.tandskadeankenaevnet.dk/.
13. Bjørndal L, Reit C. The annual frequency of root fillings, tooth extractions and pulp-related procedures in Danish adults during 1977–2003. Int Endod J. 2004;37:782–8.
14. Kirkevang L-L, Hörsted-Bindslev P, Ørstavik D, Wenzel A. Periapical status and quality of root fillings and coronal restorations in a Danish population. Int Endod J. 2000;33:509–15.
15. Segura-Egea JJ, Jiménez-Pinzón A, Poyato-Ferrera M, Velasco-Ortega E, Ríos-Santos JV. Periapical status and quality of root fillings and coronal restorations in an adult Spanish population. Int Endod J. 2004;37:525–30.
16. Loftus JJ, Keating AP, McCartan BE. Periapical status and quality of endodontic treatment in an adult Irish population. Int Endod J. 2005;38:81–6.
17. Bjørndal L, Reit C. The adoption of new endodontic technology amongst Danish general dental practitioners. Int Endod J. 2005;38:52–8.
18. Lin H-C, Pai S-F, Hsu Y-Y, Chen C-S, Kuo M-L, Yang S-F. Use of rubber dams during root canal treatment in Taiwan. J Formos Med Assoc. 2011;110:397–400.
19. The statistics on dental malpractice claims. Am Dent Assoc. 2007. http://www.ada.org/prof/resources/topics/survey.pdf.
20. Givol N, Rosen E, Bjørndal L, Taschieri S, Ofec R, Tsesis I. Medico-legal aspects of altered sensation following endodontic treatment; a retrospective case series. Oral Surg Oral Med Oral Pathol Oral Radiol Endod. 2011;112:126–31.
21. Rosen E, Tsesis I, Tamse A, Bjørndal L, Taschieri S, Givol N. Medico-legal aspect of vertical root fractures in root filled teeth. Int Endod J. 2012;45:7–11.
22. Hall JA, Irish JT, Roter DL, Ehrlich CM, Miller LH. Satisfaction, gender, and communication in medical visits. Med Care. 1994;32:1216–31.
23. Levinson W, Roter DL, Mullooly JP, Dull VT, Frankel RM. Physician-patient communication. The relationship with malpractice claims among primary care physicians and surgeons. JAMA. 1997;277:553–9.
24. Hall JA, Horgan TG, Stein TS, Roter DL. Liking in the physician-patient relationship. Patient Educ Couns. 2002;48:69–77.
25. Roter DL, Hall JA, Aoki Y. Physician gender effects in medical communication a meta-analytic review. JAMA. 2002;288:756–64.
26. Milgrom P, Cullen T, Whitney C, Fiset L, Conrad D, Getz T. Frustrating patient visits. J Public Health Dent. 1996;56:6–11.
27. Kvist T, Reit C. Results of endodontic retreatment: a randomized clinical study comparing surgical and nonsurgical procedures. J Endod. 1999;25:814–7.
28. Del Fabbro M, Taschieri S, Testori T, Francette L, Weinstein RL. Surgical versus non-surgical endodontic re-treatment for periradicular lesions. Cochrane Database Syst Rev. 2007;(18):CD005511.
29. Torabinejad M, Corr R, Handysides R, Shabahang S. Outcomes of nonsurgical retreatment and endodontic surgery: a systematic review. J Endod. 2009;35:930–7.
30. Madarati AA, Hunter MJ, Dummer PM. Management of intracanal separated instruments. J Endod. 2013;39:569–81.
31. Rud J, Rud V, Munksgaard EC. Retrograde sealing of accidental root perforation with dentin-bonded composite resin. J Endod. 1998;24:671–7.

Guided Tissue Regeneration in Endodontic Surgery: Principle, Efficacy, and Complications

16

Louis M. Lin, Domenico Ricucci, and Thomas von Arx

Abstract

The concept of guided tissue regeneration (GTR) in endodontic surgery is derived from periodontal regenerative therapy for periodontal disease. Periapical tissue regeneration will occur predictably after endodontic surgery if intra- and extraradicular infections are controlled by adequate root-end resection and complete retrograde seal of the root canal. Indications for GTR technique in endodontic surgery are limited and should be clearly recognized to prevent misuse. They include: combined endodontic-periodontic lesions, through-and-through bone lesions, and large periapical lesions almost involving the alveolar crest bone. The materials, such as barrier membranes and bone grafts used in GTR technique should be biocompatible and approved by the FDA. Possible pre-surgical, intra-surgical, and post-surgical complications of GTR technique in endodontic surgery must be prevented to avoid failures. GTR technique in endodontic surgery could improve periapical wound healing in through-and through bone lesions and possibly in cases with large periapical lesions.

Introduction

Guided tissue regeneration (GTR) is a technique for enhancing and directing cell growth to repopulate specific parts of the periodontium that have been damaged by periodontal disease or trauma [51]. The concept of GTR technique in endodontic surgery is derived from that in periodontal regenerative therapy and has been shown to promote the rate of periapical wound healing in short-term observations [5, 55, 57, 72–74].

Application of GTR technique in endodontic surgery is more limited than that in periodontal

L.M. Lin, BDS, DMD, PhD (✉)
Department of Endodontics New York University College of Dentistry, 345 East 24th Street, New York, NY 10010, USA
e-mail: lml7@nyu.edu

D. Ricucci, MD, DDS
Private Practice, Piazza Calvario, 7, Cetraro, CS 87022, Italy
e-mail: dricucci@libero.it

T. von Arx, Prof. Dr. Med. Dent.
Department of Oral Surgery and Stomatology, School of Dental Medicine, University of Bern, Freiburgstrasse 7, Bern, Bern, Switzerland
e-mail: thomas.vonarx@zmk.unibe.ch

I. Tsesis (ed.), *Complications in Endodontic Surgery*,
DOI 10.1007/978-3-642-54218-3_16,

regenerative therapy [47, 77, 83, 86]. Although the composition of periodontal tissues, except gingival, is similar to that of periapical tissues and contains the alveolar bone, periodontal ligament (PDL), and cementum, the wound healing of periodontal lesions after using GTR technique in periodontal regenerative therapy is more complex than that of periapical lesions after application of GTR technique in endodontic surgery. Periodontal regenerative therapy is constantly challenged by direct bacterial threat from the oral cavity. In addition, open-flap debridement of periodontal lesions alone without using GTR technique is not able to achieve satisfactorily periodontal regeneration [48, 49]. In contrast, periapical tissue regeneration occurs predictively after endodontic surgery of periapical lesions alone without using GTR technique if intra- and extraradicular infections are controlled by adequate root-end resection and complete retrograde seal of the root canal [78]. Therefore, unlike periodontal disease, GTR in endodontic surgery is limited.

Barrier membranes, bone grafts, or local application of exogenous growth factors/cytokines has been used to help promote host's wound healing potential in GTR technique in periodontal and endodontic therapy [7]. To prevent and manage complications of GTR technique in endodontic surgery, it is necessary to fully understand the biology of periapical wound healing after endodontic surgery because evidence-based information using GTR technique in endodontic surgery is scarce and has no consensus agreement [77, 86]. In addition, reproducible results, long-term observations, and well-designed clinical studies of GTR technique in endodontic surgery are lacking [83, 86]. Therefore, application of GTR technique in endodontic surgery should be carefully evaluated biologically prior to discussion of prevention and management of complications to avoid misuse and unnecessary complications of GTR technique. It is important to emphasize that the size of the bony defect is not always necessarily an indication of GTR technique in endodontic surgery.

Size of Defect and Bone Wound Healing

It has been shown that through-and-through jawbone lesions involving both buccal and lingual bone plates after surgery were often associated with incomplete healing or scar tissue formation in short-term animal experiments [16, 17, 31, 62]. In studying the influence of various factors upon healing after endodontic surgery, it was found that the size of the jawbone lesions had only a minor importance in relation to the development of scar tissue [62].

Huh et al. [33] studied the critical size of bone defects in the canine and showed when the periosteum was removed, mandibular defects greater than 15 mm failed to heal across the entire defect. However, when the periosteum was preserved, mandibular defects needed to be greater than 50 mm to fail to heal. In testing the critical size of calvarial bone defects in mice and rats, it was suggested that the critical size of bone defects in animal experiments had only a limited clinical applicability and only served to standardize the research methodology. Therefore, the use of the term "critical-size defect" should be discontinued [15]. The definition of critical-size defect basically implies the smallest size of an intraosseous wound in a particular bone and species of animal that will not heal spontaneously during the lifetime of the animal. Regardless of the size of bone defect, blood clot and granulation tissue are able to completely fill the defects as a wound healing process. Vascularity and availability of osteoprogenitor cells are important in wound healing of large bone defects [12].

Scar tissue formation is a sequel of wound healing process, which is not fully understood. It has been demonstrated that scar tissue formation could be caused by persistent inflammation, overproduction of extracellular matrix [89], dysregulation of apoptosis of myofibroblasts [18, 36], upregulation of TGF-β [37, 39, 89], upregulation of VEGF [35, 88], or downregulation of matrix metalloproteinase [46, 80, 89]. Fibroblasts stimulated by TGF-ß and cellular fibronectin are capable of differentiating into myofibroblasts [64, 66]. In addition, myofibroblasts can also be differentiated from resident mesenchymal cells, bone marrow mesenchymal stem cells, and epithelial-mesenchymal transition [64]. When myofibroblasts complete their task and are no longer needed at the remodeling stage of wound healing, they are eliminated by apoptosis or programmed cell death. In normal wound healing, collagen production by myofibroblasts and collagen degradation by matrix metalloproteinase are in balance; therefore, there is no net collagen gain. Functional impairments of fibroblasts/myofibroblasts might play an important role in pathological scarring in bone repair [64].

It has been shown that large or through-and-through bone lesions or defects in the jawbone would not always result in scar tissue formation if barrier membrane were not used after apical surgery [72]. The size of the jawbone lesions might be a factor [84, 85] but is not a mechanism of scar tissue formation in bone wound healing. For example, regardless of size of myocardial infarct, the myocardium is always repaired with scar tissue [71]. After partial hepatectomy, the liver is able to regenerate [14]. Therefore, it is not the size of the lesion but the microenvironment (e.g., neighboring cells, extracellular matrix, soluble and insoluble bioactive molecules) and availability of the stem/progenitor cells in the injured tissue that play a crucial role in tissue regeneration or scar formation during wound healing.

Barrier Membranes in Endodontic Surgery

Many types of absorbable and bioabsorbable membranes have been used in dentistry [7]. Barrier membranes used in endodontic surgery are assumed to prevent epithelial cells or fibroblasts in the mucoperiosteal flap from proliferating into the surgical bony crypt, thus interfering with new bone formation (Fig. 16.1).

Can barrier membranes prevent epithelial cells in the mucoperiosteal flap from migrating into the surgical bony crypt? Indeed it can, but is it necessary? The basal cells of epithelium attach to a layer of connective tissue called basement membrane (BM) by hemidesmosome. BM consists of basal lamina (laminin, type IV collagen) and reticular lamina (type III collagen). BM is very resistant to penetration by proliferating basal cells caused by inflammatory or benign hyperplasia. Only malignant epithelial cells, such in carcinoma, are capable of degrading basement membrane by producing proteolytic enzymes (matrix metalloproteinases, collagenase) and invade the underlying connective tissue [32]. Therefore, epithelial cells in the mucoperiosteal flap are not able to penetrate into the surgical bony crypt even without using barrier membranes after endodontic surgery.

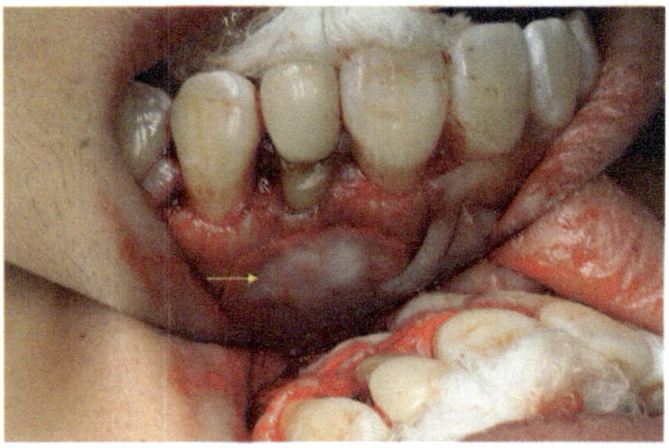

Fig. 16.1 Surgical bone crypt covered by a barrier membrane

It is generally believed that fibroblasts move faster than osteoblasts to occupy the bony crypt after apical surgery. Consequently, a scar tissue is formed in large bone defects after periapical wound healing [17, 56]. Barrier membranes are presumably utilized in apical surgery to prevent proliferation of fibroblasts from the surrounding tissue into the bony crypt [16, 17, 56]. Cell movement is a complex biologic process and does not simply depend on cell mobility. Cell surface integrins, extracellular matrix molecules, and gradient of chemokines as well as growth factors regulate cell movement ([38]). Fibroblast is one of the slow-moving cells. It has been demonstrated that fibroblasts move slower than keratinocytes and leukocytes because they apply force to bind to the extracellular matrix much larger than the force required for their movement [38]. In addition, the speed of cell migration depends on substratum ligand level, cell integrin expression level, and integrin-ligand binding affinity [53]. For example, if very few extracellular matrix ligands expressing RGD-sequence-containing peptide are available, cell surface integrins cannot get a strong enough grip to ligands and enable them to move. If there are too many extracellular matrix ligands, cell surface integrins bind firmly to ligands and get stuck in place [53]. Importantly, during periapical bone wound healing after apical surgery, the newly differentiated osteoblasts are derived from bone marrow mesenchymal stem cells and osteoprogenitor cells lining the endosteum, which are in the bony crypt [31]. These osteoblasts do not have to compete with fibroblasts from surrounding tissue to occupy the surgical bony crypt.

There are studies showing significantly more new bone formation after apical surgery when barrier membrane was used as compared to controls in short-term clinical follow-up or animal experiment [5]. On the contrary, other studies have demonstrated no beneficial effect by utilizing barrier membrane to improve new bone formation after apical surgery [10, 24, 43, 72]. When both buccal and lingual bone plates of the jawbone were perforated at the time of endodontic surgery, it was demonstrated that the defects were significantly related to later development of scar tissue in a human study [62]. Similar findings were also observed in clinical case studies [56, 73]. Histologically, it has been shown that fibrous connective tissue from the surrounding mucoperiosteum could proliferate into the through-and-through bone defects artificially created in the jawbone and formed a scar tissue if barrier membrane was not used in short-term animal experiments [6, 16, 17, 31]. However, osseous regeneration with ingrowth of fibrous connective tissue was also observed in three of eight cases with barrier membrane at 9 weeks of animal experiments [16]. The studies of Grung et al. [27], Halse et al. [29], and Molven et al. [45] showed that there was a difference in incomplete healing of bone lesions in periapical surgery after comparing 1- and 4-year outcomes. The incomplete healing group had a tendency to reduce in size if follow-up time was extended. Most studies of GTR technique in endodontic surgery are to compare the rate of new bone formation during the course of wound healing and not to evaluate the efficacy of bone remodeling between experimental and control groups. Large periapical lesions take a longer time to heal after surgical endodontic therapy if root canal infection is under control [62]. Therefore, a longer period of clinical follow-up or experimental observation is needed to assess the outcome of periapical bone wound healing when a barrier membrane is used in endodontic surgery.

An important question is: Can barrier membranes in endodontic surgery completely exclude fibroblasts from proliferating into the bone crypt? Apical surgery involves not only cortical bone but also trabecular bone. Blood clot and granulation (fibrovascular) tissue formation in the bony crypt after apical surgery are essential components of the process of bone wound healing [20] and precede bone matrix production by osteoblasts. Fibroblasts in the granulation tissue in the bony crypt are from several sources, such as the periosteum, bone marrow stromal compartment, and PDL. In addition, bone marrow mesenchymal stem cells are capable of differentiating into fibroblasts [22, 30]. Therefore, barrier membranes might be able to prevent fibroblasts in the surrounding tissue from proliferating into the bony crypt but cannot exclude fibroblasts originating from the bone marrow and PDL, which are already present in the bony crypt.

Application of barrier membranes in through-and-through bony crypts after endodontic surgery might create a microenvironment, which is conducive for osteogenesis in a short-term experimental observation or clinical follow-up as compared to without barrier membranes. However, the cellular and molecular biology of wound healing of through-and-through bone lesions after endodontic surgery and scar formation is not fully understood.

Based on limited information in the literature, through-and-through bone defects could benefit from application of GTR technique using bioabsorbable barrier membranes after endodontic surgery to improve the rate of new bone formation in short-term observation [77, 83, 86]. Barrier membranes should be approved according to the Food and Drug Administration (FDA). The use of barrier membranes must follow manufacturer's instructions. The barrier membrane should cover the bone defect at least 3 mm beyond the margins of the defect and be stable to avoid collapse into the bone defect. Foreign materials such as barrier membranes can easily invite infection [23, 50]; therefore, contamination should be avoided during surgical placement of the barrier membrane.

Bone Grafts in Endodontic Surgery

Bone grafts are used as a matrix or scaffold to fill the bone defect (Fig. 16.2) and to improve new bone formation in orthopedic surgery, craniofacial surgery, periodontal surgery, and apical surgery [54]. Extracellular matrixes, such as bone grafts, are capable of regulating tissue-specific stem cell differentiation [13]. Autologous bone, the gold standard of bone grafting, provides optimal osteoconductive, osteoinductive, and osteogenic properties [25]. It has the capability to regenerate bone from bone-forming cells (bone marrow mesenchymal stem cells) [19, 25]. However, autologous bone grafts have several disadvantages, such as donor site morbidity [82, 84, 85], limited availability, and cosmetic problems [25, 54]. Accordingly, bone graft substitutes have become a popular and alternative choice. Bone graft substitutes can be divided according to their properties of osteoinduction and osteoconduction (7, 19, 54]). Osteoinductive bone grafts, for example, demineralized bone, are capable of supporting the mitogenesis of adult mesenchymal stem cells, leading to the formation of osteoprogenitor cells with the capacity to form new bone [1, 19]. Osteoconductive bone grafts, such as calcium sulfate, are able to support the attachment of osteoprogenitor cells for subsequent bone formation [1, 19].

Fibrin clot and granulation tissue are important components of bone wound healing process

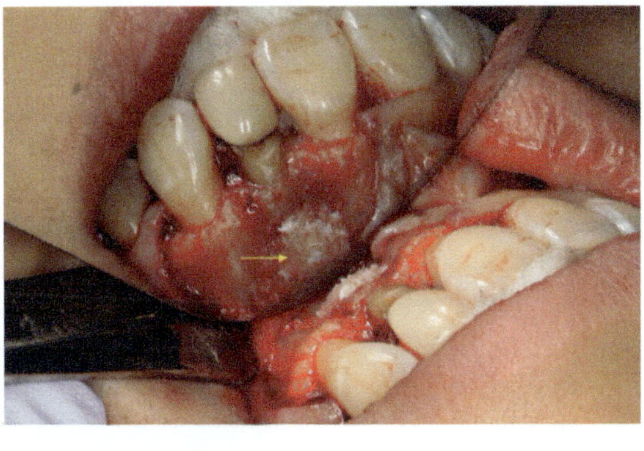

Fig. 16.2 Surgical bony crypt filled with bone graft

[20]. Bone graft substitutes must be able to keep fibrin clot and granulation tissue at the wound site; otherwise, osteoprogenitor cells might not be able to migrate to and survive at the wound site because of lack of growth factors, chemokines, collagen matrix, and angiogenesis. The cell surface integrins of osteoprogenitor cells cannot attach to the synthetic bone graft substitutes (e.g., calcium sulfate, hydroxyapatite, bioactive glass) because these graft substitutes do not express RGD-sequence-containing protein, such as collagen, fibronectin, laminin, or osteopontin [13, 69]. Therefore, synthetic bone graft substitutes have to absorb fibrin clot and allow ingrowth of granulation tissue to become osteoconductive [3, 44]. Bone graft substitutes might enhance the rate of new bone formation in bone wound healing. Radiographically, the problem of using bone graft substitutes in endodontic surgery is the difficulty of differentiating incomplete healing (scar tissue) from uncertain healing (no healing) because bone graft substitutes are radiopaque [73]. Bone graft substitutes alone without blood clot and granulation tissue formation in the bony crypt after endodontic surgery would not induce new bone formation. This is best exemplified, for example, with dry socket after tooth extraction because of absence of blood clot and granulation tissue formation.

Most studies using bone graft substitutes in endodontic surgery are case reports or animal studies. Some studies demonstrated favorable new bone formation using bone graft substitutes as compared to controls in short-term observation [55, 57, 58, 63, 90]. In contrast, other studies showed no difference [4, 8, 70, 72]. Only a few controlled clinical trials using bone graft substitutes in apical surgery are available [55, 57, 72–74]. These clinical studies have a small sample and no standard radiographic evaluation, and their follow-up observation is only 1 year [86]. A trend of better outcome was found when GTR technique was used compared to control cases, but the results were not statistically significant. Additional large-scale prospective clinical studies are needed to further evaluate possible benefits of GTR techniques in endodontic surgery [77]. Similar to GTR technique with barrier membranes in endodontic surgery, the studies evaluate the rate of new bone formation during periapical bone wound healing and not the efficacy of bone remodeling. Like in orthopedic surgery, prospective, randomized controlled studies are needed to provide reliable information regarding the use of bone graft substitutes in endodontic surgery [12, 19, 34].

The bone grafts may be used to support barrier membranes from collapsing into through-and-through or large periapical bone defects after endodontic surgery. The bone grafts must be approved according to the FDA. Preparation of bone grafts should follow manufacturer's instruction. The ideal bone grafts should be biocompatible, biodegradable, osteoconductive, osteoinductive, and structurally similar to bone [25, 34]. They should be disease-free and contain minimal antigenic factors. In addition, the bone graft substitutes should be porous, and the pore size is ideally 300–500 *u*m with interconnection to allow ingrowth of granulation tissue and osteoprogenitor cells into the three-dimensional bone scaffold [19, 25]. The rate of degradation of bone grafts should be closely corresponding to the rate of new bone formation by newly differentiated osteoblasts. Importantly, the bone grafts should be able to mimic normal process of bone formation during bone wound healing.

Growth/Differentiation Factors in Endodontic Surgery

Growth/differentiation factors play an important role in tissue wound healing [28, 87]. They are capable of signaling adult mesenchymal stem cells to differentiate into tissue-committed cells [79]. Growth factors are multifunctional and often have more than one target cell [87]. Most growth factors affect more than a single cellular activity, and most cellular activities are often a response to the summation of several growth factors [28, 87]. The biologic functions of growth factors might be synergistic or antagonistic and depend on the presence or absence of other factors [28, 87]. Many growth factors are involved at the same or different stages of wound healing. The temporal and spatial expression of growth/differentiation factors and their exact target cells during tissue wound healing is complex.

The bone growth factors or bone morphogenetic proteins have level 1 evidence of osteoinductive properties in orthopedic surgery [19]. However, there are conflicting results using bone growth/differentiation factors in apical surgery [9, 61]. Bone growth/differentiation factors might improve new bone formation in a short-term animal experiment or clinical observation after endodontic surgery. Nevertheless, long-term experiments are required before clinical application can be recommended. Biologically, exogenous growth factors are similar to natural growth factors and have a promising prospect in endodontic surgery. However, it is not easy to control the release of exogenous growth factor/factors incorporated in the carriers, such as barrier membranes or bone grafts, with regard to time and space as well as concentration during periapical wound healing in endodontic surgery.

Other Clinical Conditions Recommended for Using GTR Technique in Endodontic Surgery

There are other clinical conditions, in which barrier membranes and/or bone graft substitutes are recommended in endodontic surgery [83]. Barrier membranes are used to improve periodontal tissue regeneration and avoid periodontal involvement during endodontic surgery in combined endodontic-periodontic lesions [11, 26, 52, 75] and large periapical lesions extending almost to the alveolar crest bone (<3 mm crest bone remaining) [60]. Barrier membranes and/or bone graft substitutes could be used in cases of buccal bone dehiscence to regenerate bone attachment in endodontic surgery [21, 59, 65, 68]. In cases of large periapical lesions penetrating through both buccal and palatal cortical bone plates, GTR technique has been shown to improve outcome of bone regeneration following surgical endodontic treatment in a systematic review [77].

Prevention and Management of Complications of GTR Technique in Endodontic Surgery

Limited information is available in this area in the literature. Complications of GTR technique in endodontic surgery are rare and usually associated with complications of endodontic surgery, which include maxillary sinus exposure, accidental injury to neurovascular bundles emerging from the mental foramen or the greater palatal foramen resulting in paresthesia [40, 41], or postoperative infection.

The following are possible complications of GTR technique in endodontic surgery:

Presurgical complications – inappropriate patient and case selection, uncontrolled root canal infection and marginal periodontitis, bleeding disorders, radiation therapy of the head and neck [81], or long-term intravenous bisphosphonate therapy [2]

Intra-surgical complications – vertical root fracture

Postsurgical complications – untreated extra canal/canals, membrane exposure, and bone graft contamination

Management of complications of GTR in endodontic surgery is basically similar to that of endodontic surgery without using GTR technique. Handling of barrier membrane and/or bone grafts should be careful to avoid contamination. Prior to GTR in endodontic surgery, root canal infection and marginal periodontitis should be eliminated; otherwise, periapical wound healing would be compromised even using GTR technique. Excessive bleeding, due to surgical trauma and not hemophilia, can be controlled by using various hemostatic agents, for example, cotton pellets soaked with 2 % lidocaine containing 1:50,000 epinephrine, before placement of bone graft and/or barrier membrane. However, it must be emphasized that blood clot formation is a necessary process of wound healing after endodontic surgery [20, 42]. Without blood clot formation, wound healing can be compromised. Postoperative infection, pain, or swelling can be managed with antibiotics or anti-inflammatory analgesics.

Conclusion

GTR technique in periodontal therapy can produce a significant improvement over conventional open-flap debridement in regeneration of the attachment apparatus because the outcome of open-flap debridement alone is poor due to direct challenge by oral microorganisms and apical migration of junctional epithelium [48]. GTR technique in implant dentistry is able to improve the rate of new bone formation so that the dental implant can be placed as soon as possible. GTR in endodontic surgery is to help the host create a favorable environment to improve the rate of periapical wound healing. If intraradicular infection is controlled by adequate orthograde and retrograde fillings, the periapical wound should heal satisfactorily after endodontic surgery even without using GTR technique [67, 76]. However, in cases of through-and-through periapical lesions, GTR may have a beneficial effect on the outcome of periapical bone healing [77]. Scar tissue sometimes may be formed in the periapical area after endodontic surgery of large periapical lesions but is not considered a treatment failure.

Based on limited information in the literature, through-and-through bone lesions or defects of the jawbone [77] and combined endodontic-periodontic lesions appear to be able to benefit from GTR technique to promote the rate of periapical wound healing after endodontic surgery. However, if root-end management is inadequately performed during endodontic surgery, GTR technique, for example, bone graft placement may obscure the destructive pathological process. This would lead to delayed diagnosis of the treatment failure and further compromise the long-term outcome as well as jeopardize the success of future retreatment (Fig. 16.3, 16.4 and 16.5).

GTR technique does not necessarily enhance the successful outcome (absence of signs and symptoms and resolution of apical periodontitis) of endodontic surgery, which requires elimination of intra- and/or extraradicular infection [62]. Nevertheless, GTR technique in endodontic surgery appears to be able

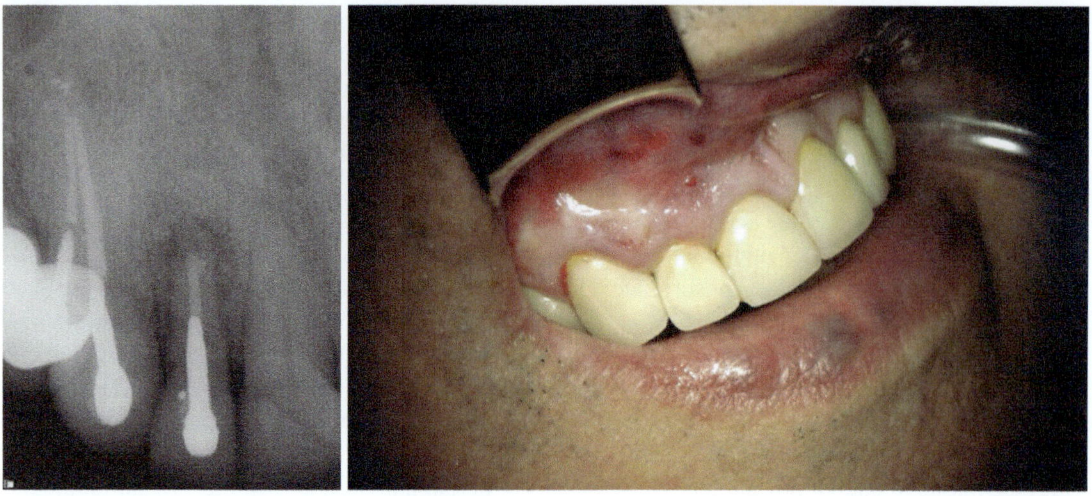

Fig. 16.3 Complication of endodontic surgery performed in a traditional technique using GTR. Preoperative examination: Maxillary right lateral incisor 6 months following endodontic surgery performed using the traditional technique; the patient presented with signs and symptoms of symptomatic apical periodontitis. The periapical bony lesion is masked by the radiopaque appearance of the bone substitute grafting material

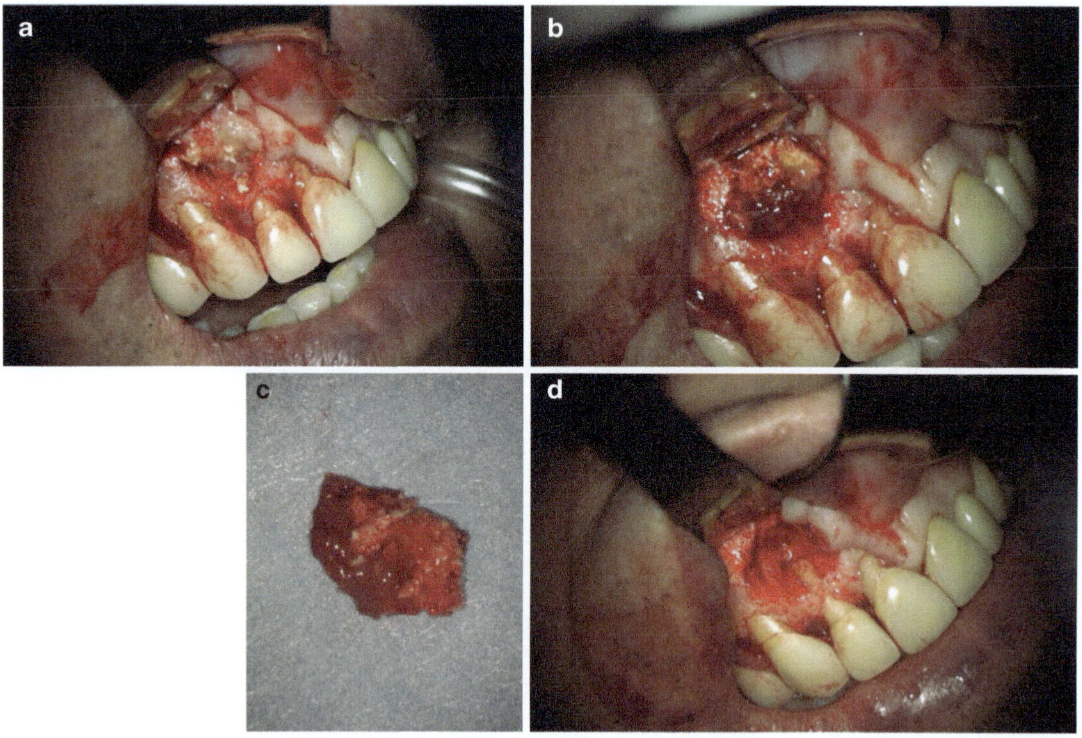

Fig. 16.4 Complication of endodontic surgery performed in a traditional technique using GTR. Intraoperative: Surgical retreatment: following flap elevation pathological fenestration of cortical plate (**a**), a large bony defect filled with granulation tissue and remnants of the grafting material (**b**). The granulation tissue and the grafting material were removed (**c**); the root end was surgically retreated using a modern technique (**d**)

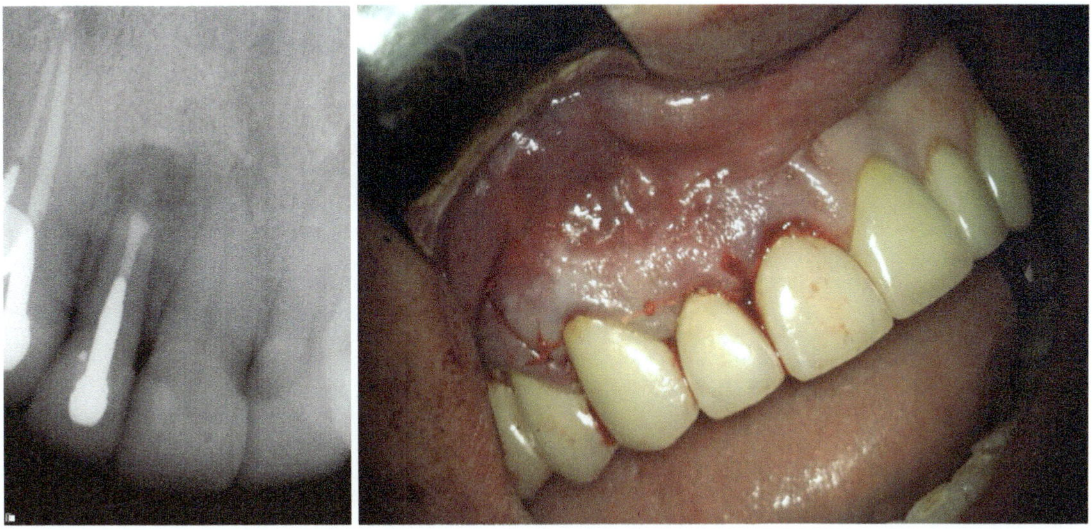

Fig. 16.5 Complication of endodontic surgery performed in a traditional technique using GTR. Postoperative: Sutures were placed, and a routine postoperative management protocol was applied

to promote the rate of periapical bone healing in large periapical lesions eroding both buccal and palatal cortical bone plates. Long-term prospective, controlled clinical trials are needed to carefully evaluate the successful outcome, safety, efficacy, and cost-effectiveness of GTR technique in endodontic surgery.

References

1. Albrektsson T, Johansson C. Osteoinduction, osteoconduction and osseointegration. Eur Spine J. 2001; 10:S96–101.
2. American Association of Oral and Maxillofacial Surgeons. Position paper on bisphosphonate-related osteonecrosis of the jaw – 2009 update. 2009. Available at: www.aaoms.org/docs/position-papers/bronj-update.
3. Anselme K. Osteoblast adhesion on biomaterials. Biomaterials. 2000;21:667–81.
4. Apaydin ES, Torabinejad M. The effect of calcium sulfate on hard tissue healing after periapical surgery. J Endod. 2004;30:17–20.
5. Artzi Z, Wasersprung N, Weinreb M, et al. Effect of guided tissue regeneration on newly formed bone and cementum in periapical tissue healing after endodontic surgery: an *in vivo* study in the cat. J Endod. 2012; 38:163–9.
6. Baek S-H, Kim S. Bone repair of experimentally induced through-and-through defects by Gore-Tex, Guidor, and Vicryl in ferrets: a pilot study. Oral Surg Oral Med Oral Pathol Oral Radiol Endod. 2001;91: 710–4.
7. Bashutski JD, Wang H-L. Periodontal and endodontic regeneration. J Endod. 2009;35:321–8.
8. Beck-Coon RJ, Newton CW, Kafrawy AH. An in vivo study of the use of nonresorbable ceramic hydroxyapatite as an alloplastic graft material in periapical surgery. Oral Surg Oral Med Oral Pathol. 1991;71:483–8.
9. Bergenholtz G, Wikesjö UME, Sorensen RG, et al. Observation on healing following endodontic surgery in nonhuman primates (Macaca fascicularis): effect of rhBMP-2. Oral Surg Oral Med Oral Pathol Oral Radiol Endod. 2006;101:116–25.
10. Bernabé PF, Gomes-Filho JE, Cintra LT, et al. Histologic evaluation of the use of membrane, bone graft, and MTA in apical surgery. Oral Surg Oral Med Oral Pathol Oral Radiol Endod. 2010;109:309–14.
11. Britian SK, von Arx T, Schenk RK, et al. The use of guided tissue regeneration principles in endodontic surgery for induced chronic periodontic-endodontic lesions: a clinical, radiographic and histological evaluation. J Periodontol. 2005;76:450–60.
12. Calori GM, Mazza E, Colombo M, et al. The use of bone-graft substitutes in large bone defects: Any specific need? Injury. 2011;42:S56–63.
13. Chastain SR, Kundu AK, Dhar S, et al. Adhesion of mesenchymal stem cells to polymer scaffolds occurs via distinct ECM ligands and controls their osteogenic differentiation. J Biomed Mater Res A. 2006;78: 73–85.
14. Chen M-F, Hwang T-L, Hung C-F. Human liver regeneration after major hepatectomy. Ann Surg. 1991;3:227–9.

15. Cooper GM, Mooney MP, Gosain AK, et al. Testing the critical size in calvarial bone defects: revisiting the concept of a critical-size defect. Plast Reconstr Surg. 2010;125:1685–92.
16. Dahlin C, Linde A, Gottlow J, Nyman S. Healing of bone defects by guided tissue regeneration. Plast Reconstr Surg. 1988;81:672–6.
17. Dahlin C, Gottlow J, Linde A, Nyman S. Healing of maxillary and mandibular bone defects using a membrane technique: an experimental study in monkeys. Scand J Plast Reconstr Surg Hand Surg. 1990;24:13–9.
18. Douglass A, Wallace K, Parr R, et al. Antibody-targeted myofibroblast apoptosis reduces fibrosis during sustained liver injury. J Hepatol. 2008;49:88–98.
19. De Long Jr WG, Einhorn TA, Koval K, et al. Bone grafts and bone graft substitutes in orthopaedic trauma surgery. J Bone Joint Surg Am. 2007;89:649–58.
20. Dimitrious R, Tsiridis E, Giannoudis PV. Current concepts of molecular aspects of bone healing. Injury. 2005;36:1392–404.
21. Douthitt JC, Gutmann JL, Witherspoon DE. Histologic assessment of healing after the use of a bioresorbable membrane in the management of buccal bone loss concomitant with periapical surgery. J Endod. 2001;27:404–10.
22. Ebihara Y, Masuya M, Larue AC, et al. Hematopoietic origin of fibroblasts: II – in vitro studies of fibroblasts, CFU-F, and fibrocytes. Exp Hematol. 2006;34:219–29.
23. Elek SD, Conen PE. The virulence of Staphylococcus pyogenes for man. A study of the problems of wound infection. Br J Exp Pathol. 1957;38:573–88.
24. Garrett K, Kerr M, Hartwell G, et al. The effect of bioresorbable matrix barrier in endodontic surgery on the rate of periapical healing: an in vivo study. J Endod. 2002;28:503–6.
25. Giannoudis PV, Dinopoulos H, Tsiridis E. Bone substitutes: an update. Injury. 2005;365:S20–7.
26. Goyal B, Tewari S, Duhan J, et al. Comparative evaluation of platelet-rich plasma and guided tissue regeneration membrane in the healing of apicomarginal defects: a clinical study. J Endod. 2011;37:773–80.
27. Grung B, Molven O, Halse A. Periapical surgery in a Norwegian county hospital: follow-up findings of 477 teeth. J Endod. 1990;16:411–7.
28. Gurtner GC, Werner S, Barrandon Y, et al. Wound repair and regeneration. Nature. 2008;453:314–21.
29. Halse A, Molven O, Grung B. Follow-up after periapical surgery: the value of the one-year control. Dent Traumatol. 1991;7:246–50.
30. Haniffa MA, Collin MP, Buckley CD, Dazzi F. Mesenchymal stem cells: the fibroblasts's new clothes? Haematologica. 2009;94:258–63.
31. Hjorting-Hansen E, Andreasen JO. Incomplete bone healing of experimental cavities in dog mandibles. Br J Oral Surg. 1971;9:33–40.
32. Hotary K, Lin X-Y, Allen E, et al. A cancer cell metalloproteinase regulates the basement membrane transmigration program. Genes Dev. 2006;20:2673–86.
33. Huh JY, Choi BH, Kim BY, et al. Critical size defect in the canine mandible. Oral Surg Oral Med Oral Pathol Oral Radiol Endod. 2005;100:296–301.
34. Janicki P, Schmidmaier G. What should be the characteristics of the ideal bone graft substitute? Combining scaffold with growth factors and/or stem cells. Injury. 2011;42:S77–81.
35. Kalluri R, Sukhatme VP. Fibrosis and angiogenesis. Curr Opin Nephrol Hypertens. 2000;9:413–8.
36. Kissin E, Korn JH. Apoptosis and myofibroblasts in the pathogenesis of systemic sclerosis. Curr Rheumatol Rep. 2002;4:129–35.
37. Krummel TM, Michna BA, Thomas BL, et al. Transforming growth factor beta (TGF-β) induces fibrosis in a fetal wound healing. J Pediatr Surg. 1988;23:647–52.
38. Lauffenburger DA, Horwitz AF. Cell migration: a physically integrated molecular process. Cell. 1996;84:359–69.
39. Leask A, Abraham DT. TGF-ß signaling and fibrotic response. FASEB J. 2004;18:816–27.
40. Lin L, Skribner J, Shovlin F, Langeland K. Periapical surgery of mandibular posterior teeth: anatomical and surgical considerations. J Endod. 1983;9:496–501.
41. Lin L, Chance K, Shovlin F, et al. Oroantral communication in periapical surgery of maxillary posterior teeth. J Endod. 1985;11:40–4.
42. Lin L, Chen MY-H, Ricucci D, et al. Guided tissue regeneration in periapical surgery. J Endod. 2010;36:618–25.
43. Maguire H, Torabinejad M, McMillan P, et al. Effects of resorbable membrane placement and human osteogenic protein-1 on hard tissue healing after periapical surgery in cats. J Endod. 1998;24:720–5.
44. Matsura T, Hosokawa R, Okamoto K, et al. Diverse mechanisms of osteoblast spreading on hydroxyapatite and titanium. Biomaterials. 2000;21:1121–7.
45. Molven O, Halse A, Grung B. Incomplete healing (scar tissue) after periapical surgery – radiographic findings 8 to 12 years after treatment. J Endod. 1996;22:264–8.
46. Mutsaers SE, Bishop JE, McGrouther G, et al. Mechanisms of tissue repair: from wound healing to fibrosis. Int J Biochem Cell Biol. 1997;29:5–17.
47. Naylor J, Mines P, Anderson A, Kwon D. The use of guided tissue regeneration techniques among endodontists: a web-based survey. J Endod. 2011;37:1495–8.
48. Needleman IG, Giedrys-Leeper E, Tucker RJ, Worthington NV. Results of guided tissue regeneration are highly variable. Evid Based Dent. 2002;3:12–23.
49. Needleman IG, Worthington HV, Giedrys-Leeper E, Tucker RJ. Guided tissue regeneration for periodontal infra-bony defects. Cochrane Database Syst Rev. 2006;(2);CD001724.
50. Noble WC. The production of subcutaneous staphylococcal skin lesions in mice. Br J Exp Pathol. 1965;46:254–62.

51. Nyman S, Gottlow J, Lindhe J, et al. New attachment formation by guided tissue regeneration. J Periodontal Res. 1987;22:252–4.
52. Oh S-L, Fouad AF, Park S-H. Treatment strategy for guided tissue regeneration in combined endodontic-periodontic lesions: case report and literature review. J Endod. 2009;35:1331–6.
53. Palecek SP, Loftus JC, Ginsberg MH, et al. Integrin-ligand binding properties govern cell migration speed through cell-substratum adhesiveness. Nature. 1997; 385:537–40.
54. Parikh SN. Bone graft substitutes: past, present, future. J Postgrad Med. 2002;48:142–8.
55. Pecora G, Kim S, Celletti R, Davarpanah M. The guided tissue regeneration principle in endodontic surgery: one-year postoperative results of large periapical lesions. Int Endod J. 1995;28:41–6.
56. Pecora G, Baek S-H, Rethnam S, Kim S. Barrier membrane techniques in endodontic surgery. Dent Clin N Am. 1997;41:585–602.
57. Pecora G, de Leonardis D, Ibrahim N, et al. The use of calcium sulfate in the surgical treatment of a "through and through" periapical lesion. Int Endod J. 2001; 34:189–97.
58. Pinto VS, Zuolo ML, Mellonig JT. Guided bone regeneration in the treatment of a large periapical lesion: a case report. Pract Periodontics Aesthet Dent. 1995;7:76–81.
59. Pompa DG. Guided tissue repair of complete buccal dehiscence associated with periapical defects: a clinical prospective study. J Am Dent Assoc. 1997;128: 989–97.
60. Rankow HJ, Krasner PR. Endodontic applications of guided tissue regeneration in endodontic surgery. J Endod. 1996;22:34–43.
61. Regan JD, Gutmann JL, Lacopino AM, et al. Response of periradicular tissue to growth factors introduced into the surgical site in the root-end filling material. Int Endod J. 1999;32:171–82.
62. Rud J, Andreasen JO, Moller-Jensen JE. A multivariate analysis of the influence of various factors upon healing after endodontic surgery. Int J Oral Surg. 1972;1:258–71.
63. Saad AY, Abdellatief EM. Healing assessment of osseous defects of periapical lesions associated with failed endodontically treated teeth with use of freeze-dried bone allograft. Oral Surg Oral Med Oral Pathol. 1991;71:612–7.
64. Sarrazy V, Billet F, Micallef L, et al. Mechanisms of pathological scarring: role of myofibroblasts and current development. Wound Repair Regen. 2011; 19:S10–5.
65. Schwartz F, Herten M, Ferrari D, et al. Guided tissue regeneration at dehiscence-type defects using biphasic hydroxyapatite + beta tricalcium phosphate (Bone Ceramic) or a collagen-coated natural bone mineral (BioOss Collagen): an immunohistochemical study in dogs. Int J Oral Maxillofac Surg. 2007;36:1198–206.
66. Serini G, Bochaton-Piallat M-L, Ropraz P, et al. The fibronectin domain ED-A is crucial for myofibroblastic phenotype induction by transforming growth factor-ß1. J Cell Biol. 1998;142:873–81.
67. Setzer FC, Shah SB, Kohli MR, et al. Outcome of endodontic surgery: a meta-analysis of the literature – part 1: comparison of traditional root-end surgery and endodontic microsurgery. J Endod. 2010;36:1757–65.
68. Shi H, Ma J, Zhao N, et al. Periodontal regeneration in experimentally-induced alveolar bone dehiscence by an improved porous biphasic calcium phosphate ceramic in beagle dogs. J Mater Sci Mater Med. 2008;19:3515–24.
69. Siebers MC, ter Brugge PJ, Walboomers XF, et al. Integrins as linker proteins between osteoblasts and bone replacement materials. A critical review. Biomaterials. 2005;26:137–46.
70. Stassen LFA, Hislop WS, Still DM, et al. Use of anorganic bone in periapical defects following apical surgery: a prospective trial. Br J Oral Maxillofac Surg. 1994;32:83–5.
71. Sun Y, Weber KT. Infarct scar: a dynamic tissue. Cardiovasc Res. 2000;46:250–6.
72. Taschieri S, del Fabbro M, Testori T, et al. Efficacy of xenogenic bone grafting with guided tissue regeneration in the management of bone defects after surgical endodontics. J Oral Maxillofac Surg. 2007;65:1121–7.
73. Taschieri S, del Fabbro M, Testori T, et al. Efficacy of guided tissue regeneration in the management of through-and-through lesions following surgical endodontics: a preliminary study. Int J Periodontics Restorative Dent. 2008;28:265–71.
74. Tobon SL, Arismendi JA, Marin ML, et al. Comparison between a conventional technique and two bone regeneration techniques in periradicular surgery. Int Endod J. 2002;35:635–41.
75. Tseng CC, Harn WM, Chen YH, et al. A new approach to the treatment of true combined endodontic-periodontic lesions by the guided tissue regeneration technique. J Endod. 1996;22:693–6.
76. Tsesis I, Faivishevsky V, Kfir A, Rosen E. Outcomes of surgical endodontic treatment performed by a modern technique: a meta-analysis of the literature. J Endod. 2009;35:1505–11.
77. Tsesis I, Rosen E, Tamse A, et al. Effect of guided tissue regeneration on the outcome of surgical endodontic treatment: a systematic review and meta-analysis. J Endod. 2011;37:1039–45.
78. Tsesis I, Rosen E, Taschieri S, et al. Outcomes of surgical endodontic treatment performed by a modern technique: an updated meta-analysis of the literature. J Endod. 2013;39:332–9.
79. Urist MR, DeLange RJ, Finerman GA. Bone cell differentiation and growth factors. Science. 1983;220: 680–6.
80. Van der Veer WM, Bloemen MC, Ulrich MM, et al. Potential cellular and molecular causes of hypertrophic scar formation. Burns. 2009;35:15–29.
81. Vissink A, Burlage FR, Spijkervert FKL, et al. Prevention and treatment of the consequences of head and neck radiotherapy. Crit Rev Oral Biol Med. 2003;14:213–25.

82. von Arx T, Häfliger J, Chappuis V. Neurosensory disturbances following bone harvesting in the symphysis. A prospective clinical study. Clin Oral Implants Res. 2005;16:432–9.
83. von Arx T, Cochran DL. Rationale for the application of the GTR principle using a barrier membrane in endodontic surgery: a proposal of classification and literature review. Int J Periodontics Restorative Dent. 2001;21:127–39.
84. von Arx T, Chappuis V, Winzap-Kälin C, Bornstein MM. Laser Doppler flowmetry for assessment of anterior mandibular teeth in conjunction with bone harvesting in the symphysis: a clinical pilot study. Int J Oral Maxillofac Implants. 2007;22:383–9.
85. von Arx T, Hänni S, Jensen SS. Correlation of bone defect dimensions with healing outcome one year after apical surgery. J Endod. 2007;33:1044–8.
86. von Arx T, AlSaeed M. The use of regenerative techniques in apical surgery: a literature review. Saudi Dent J. 2011;23:113–27.
87. Werner S, Grose R. Regulation of wound healing by growth factors and cytokines. Physiol Rev. 2003;83:835–70.
88. Wilgus TA, Ferreira AM, Oberyszyn TM, et al. Regulation of scar formation by vascular endothelial growth factor. Lab Invest. 2008;88: 579–90.
89. Wynn T. Cellular and molecular mechanisms of fibrosis. J Pathol. 2008;214:199–210.
90. Yoshikawa G, Murashima Y, Wadachi R, et al. Guided bone regeneration (GBR) using membrane and calcium sulfate after apicectomy: a comparative histomorphometrical study. Int Endod J. 1991; 26:255–63.

Index

I. Tsesis (ed.), *Complications in Endodontic Surgery*,
DOI 10.1007/978-3-642-54218-3, © Springer-Verlag Berlin Heidelberg 2014

GPSR Compliance

The European Union's (EU) General Product Safety Regulation (GPSR) is a set of rules that requires consumer products to be safe and our obligations to ensure this.

If you have any concerns about our products, you can contact us on ProductSafety@springernature.com

In case Publisher is established outside the EU, the EU authorized representative is:

Springer Nature Customer Service Center GmbH
Europaplatz 3
69115 Heidelberg, Germany

Batch number: 10607946

Printed by Printforce, the Netherlands